Male Infertility

Stefan S. du Plessis • Ashok Agarwal
Edmund S. Sabanegh Jr.
Editors

Male Infertility

A Complete Guide to Lifestyle and Environmental Factors

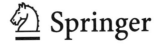

Editors
Stefan S. du Plessis, BSc (Hons), MSc,
  MBA, PhD (Stell)
Division of Medical Physiology
Department of Biomedical Sciences
Faculty of Medicine and Health Sciences
Stellenbosch University
Tygerberg, South Africa

Ashok Agarwal, PhD, HCLD, (ABB),
  ELD (ACE)
Center for Reproductive Medicine
Andrology Center
Glickman Urological and Kidney Institute
Cleveland Clinic
Cleveland, OH, USA

Edmund S. Sabanegh Jr., MD
Glickman Urological and Kidney
  Institute
Cleveland Clinic
Cleveland, OH, USA

ISBN 978-1-4939-1039-7   ISBN 978-1-4939-1040-3 (eBook)
DOI 10.1007/978-1-4939-1040-3
Springer New York Heidelberg Dordrecht London

Library of Congress Control Number: 2014944131

© Springer Science+Business Media New York 2014
This work is subject to copyright. All rights are reserved by the Publisher, whether the whole or
part of the material is concerned, specifically the rights of translation, reprinting, reuse of
illustrations, recitation, broadcasting, reproduction on microfilms or in any other physical way,
and transmission or information storage and retrieval, electronic adaptation, computer software,
or by similar or dissimilar methodology now known or hereafter developed. Exempted from this
legal reservation are brief excerpts in connection with reviews or scholarly analysis or material
supplied specifically for the purpose of being entered and executed on a computer system, for
exclusive use by the purchaser of the work. Duplication of this publication or parts thereof is
permitted only under the provisions of the Copyright Law of the Publisher's location, in its
current version, and permission for use must always be obtained from Springer. Permissions for
use may be obtained through RightsLink at the Copyright Clearance Center. Violations are liable
to prosecution under the respective Copyright Law.
The use of general descriptive names, registered names, trademarks, service marks, etc. in this
publication does not imply, even in the absence of a specific statement, that such names are
exempt from the relevant protective laws and regulations and therefore free for general use.
While the advice and information in this book are believed to be true and accurate at the date of
publication, neither the authors nor the editors nor the publisher can accept any legal responsibility
for any errors or omissions that may be made. The publisher makes no warranty, express or
implied, with respect to the material contained herein.

Printed on acid-free paper

Springer is part of Springer Science+Business Media (www.springer.com)

Foreword

Male infertility is on the rise. Most providers are familiar with the well-known causes of infertility, such as varicoceles. Lifestyle and environment, although postulated in having a role in the etiology of male infertility, has not been well studied. This book seeks to bring to light the various factors that can impact male fertility and sperm function. The editors, Drs. Du Plessis, Agarwal, and Sabanegh, have assembled a wide range of experts to contribute to this unique text. Topics include epidemiology, the impact of smoking and alcohol, obesity, exercise, vitamins and supplements, illegal drugs, heat, STIs, psychological stress, electronic devices, pesticides, endocrine disruptors, radiation, iatrogenic treatment, and age. These are all areas that have been implicated at some time with male infertility for which convincing evidence is lacking or conflicting. The editors have done a fine job of bringing together all of these varied topics and presenting balanced views of the literature regarding their potential impact on male fertility. Each of the editors is well known for their contributions to the field of andrology and infertility, and their expertise, along with that of their chosen authors, makes this book unique. This book should add to the armamentarium of all providers who see patients of reproductive age.

Milwaukee, WI, USA

Jay I. Sandlow, MD
Professor and Vice-Chairman
Department of Urology
Medical College of Wisconsin

Preface

Male infertility is on the upsurge worldwide, thereby contributing progressively more to couple infertility. There is growing evidence supporting causal links between the environment, lifestyle choices, general male health, systemic disease, and male reproductive health. Due to increased environmental pressures and unhealthy modern lifestyle choices, this combined set of factors can accumulate over time and contribute significantly to adverse impact on male reproductive issues.

With the advent of ICSI these concerns may be circumvented and marginalized. However, ART procedures do not address the root of the problem and it is important to focus on environmental and lifestyle issues such as pesticides, dietary habits, sexually transmitted infections, cell phone radiation, alcohol, tobacco, and recreational drug use to name but a few.

With this first of a kind textbook we aim to provide a comprehensive yet concise review of various environmental and lifestyle factors which impact male infertility with specific emphasis on the mechanisms contributing to decreased sperm production and impaired function. The book consists of 16 different yet applicably themed topics. Each chapter was written by internationally recognized scientists and clinicians in an easy to follow, informal yet scientific style thereby making the text ideal for those seeking to increase their general knowledge of the field. We hope that this book will have a broad and global appeal as it would be used not only as a reference for basic scientists, andrologists, and embryologists, but may also act as a clinical guideline for physicians and infertility experts.

We would like to thank all of the contributing authors for their inputs and are especially grateful to Michael D. Sova (developmental editor) for his tireless efforts in reviewing and preparing each of the manuscripts for production. We would also like to acknowledge the Division of Medical Physiology at Stellenbosch University and the Glickman Urological Institute at the Cleveland Clinic for their institutional support towards this endeavor. Finally we would like to express our gratitude towards our families for their support and patience in allowing us to complete this book. We trust that this book will become an important resource for reproductive professionals around the world.

Tygerberg, South Africa	Stefan S. du Plessis
Cleveland, OH	Ashok Agarwal
Cleveland, OH	Edmund S. Sabanegh Jr.

Contents

1 Epidemiology and Evidence of Declining Male Fertility 1
Marcello Cocuzza and Sandro C. Esteves

Part I Lifestyle/Personal Factors

2 The Effect of Smoking on Male Infertility 19
Omar Haque, Joseph A. Vitale, Ashok Agarwal,
and Stefan S. du Plessis

3 BMI and Obesity 31
Karishma Khullar, Ashok Agarwal, and Stefan S. du Plessis

4 The Impact of Physical Exercise on Male Fertility 47
Diana Maria Vaamonde Martin, Marzo Edir Da Silva-Grigoletto,
Asghar Abbasi, and Juan Manuel García Manso

**5 The Importance of Diet, Vitamins, Malnutrition,
and Nutrient Deficiencies in Male Fertility** 61
Landon W. Trost, Ahmet Gudeloglu, Edmund Y. Ko,
and Sijo J. Parekattil

6 The Effect of Alcohol Consumption on Male Infertility 83
Edson Borges Jr. and Fábio Firmbach Pasqualotto

**7 Drugs: Recreational and Performance Enhancing
Substance Abuse** 93
Fanuel Lampiao, Taryn Lockey, Collins E. Jana,
David Moon Lee, and Stefan S. du Plessis

8 Testicular Heat Stress and Sperm Quality 105
Damayanthi Durairajanayagam, Rakesh K. Sharma,
Stefan S. du Plessis, and Ashok Agarwal

**9 Sexual Issues: Role of Sexually Transmitted
Infections on Male Factor Fertility** 127
William B. Smith II, Landon W. Trost, Yihan Chen,
Amanda Rosencrans, and Wayne J.G. Hellstrom

10 Psychological Stress and Male Infertility 141
S.C. Basu

Part II Occupational Exposure

11 The Impact of Cell Phone, Laptop Computer, and Microwave Oven Usage on Male Fertility 161
John J. McGill and Ashok Agarwal

Part II Occupational Exposure

12 Pesticides and Heavy Metal Toxicity 181
Lidia Mínguez-Alarcón, Jaime Mendiola, and Alberto M. Torres-Cantero

13 Endocrine Disruptors and Male Infertility 193
Riana Bornman and Natalie Aneck-Hahn

14 Ionizing Radiation 211
Pieter Johann Maartens, Margot Flint, and Stefan S. du Plessis

Part III Other Factors Affecting Male Fertility

15 Risks from Medical and Therapeutic Treatments 227
Yagil Barazani and Edmund S. Sabanegh Jr.

16 The Aging Male: Longevity and Subsequent Implications 247
Sonja Grunewald and Uwe Paasch

Index 257

Contributors

Asghar Abbasi Division of Exercise Immunology and Genetics, Institute of Clinical and Experimental Transfusion Medicine (IKET)/University Hospital Tübingen, Tuebingen, Germany

Ashok Agarwal, PhD Center for Reproductive Medicine, Cleveland Clinic Foundation/Glickman Urological and Kidney Institute, Cleveland, OH, USA

Natalie Aneck-Hahn, DTech Department of Urology, University of Pretoria, Pretoria, South Africa

Yagil Barazani, MD Department of Urology, Cleveland Clinic, Cleveland, OH, USA

S.C. Basu, MBBS, FRCS (Edinburgh), FRCS (England), FICS, FACS Surgery and Urology, Consultant Urologist and Male Infertility Specialist, Fortis C-DOC Healthcare Ltd, New Delhi, India

Edson Borges Jr., MD, PhD Clinical Department, Fertility—Centro de Fertilização Assistida, São Paulo, São Paulo, Brazil

Riana Bornman, MBChB, PhD Department of Urology, University of Pretoria, Pretoria, South Africa

Yihan Chen, BA Department of Urology, Tulane University School of Medicine, New Orleans, LA, USA

Marcello Cocuzza, MD, PhD Human Reproduction Center and Department of Andrology, University of São Paulo, São Paulo, São Paulo, Brazil

Marzo Edir Da Silva-Grigoletto, PhD Department of Physical Education, Federal University of Sergipe, Aracaju, Sergipe, Brazil

Damayanthi Durairajanayagam, PhD Center for Reproductive Medicine, Cleveland Clinic, Cleveland, OH, USA

Stefan S. du Plessis, BSc (Hons), MSc, MBA, PhD (Stell) Division of Medical Physiology, Department of Biomedical Sciences, Faculty of Medicine and Health Sciences, Stellenbosch University, Tygerberg, Western Cape, South Africa

Sandro C. Esteves, MD, PhD ANDROFERT, Andrology and Human Reproduction Clinic, Referral Center for Male Reproduction, Campinas, São Paulo, Brazil

Margot Flint, BSc, BSc (Hons), MSc Division of Medical Physiology, Faculty of Medicine and Health Sciences, Stellenbosch University Tygerberg, Western Cape, South Africa

Sonja Grunewald, MD Department of Dermatology, University of Leipzig, European Training Centre of Andrology, Leipzig, Saxony, Germany

Ahmet Gudeloglu, MD Department of Urology, University of Florida & Winter Haven Hospital, Winter Haven, FL, USA

Omar Haque, BS Center for Reproductive Medicine, Cleveland Clinic, Foundation/Glickman Urological and Kidney Institute, Cleveland, OH, USA

Wayne J.G. Hellstrom, MD, FACS Department of Urology, Tulane University School of Medicine, New Orleans, LA, USA

Collins E. Jana, MSc Department of Basic Medical Sciences, College of Medicine, University of Malawi, Blantyre, Malawi

Karishma Khullar, BA Center for Reproductive Medicine, Cleveland Clinic Foundation/Glickman Urological and Kidney Institute, Cleveland, OH, USA

Edmund Y. Ko, MD Department of Urology, Loma Linda University, Loma Linda, CA, USA

Fanuel Lampiao, PhD Department of Basic Medical Sciences, College of Medicine, University of Malawi, Blantyre, Malawi

Juan Manuel García Manso, BS, MS, PhD Department of Physical Education, Universidad de Las Palmas de GranCanaria, Las Palmas de Gran Canaria, Islas Canarias (Gran Canaria), Spain

David Moon Lee, BA Center for Reproductive Medicine, Cleveland Clinic Foundation, Winter Haven, FL, USA

Taryn Lockey, BSc, BSc (Hons) Division of Medical Physiology, Department of Biomedical Sciences, Faculty of Medicine and Health Sciences, Stellenbosch University, Tygerberg, Western Cape, South Africa

Pieter Johann Maartens, BSc, BSc (Hons), MSc Division of Medical Physiology, Department of Biomedical Sciences, Stellenbosch University, Tygerberg, Western Cape, South Africa

Diana Maria Vaamonde Martin, BS, MS, PhD Department of Morphological Sciences, University of Cordoba, Cordoba, Spain

John J. McGill, MD Urology Institute, University Hospitals—Case Medical Center, Cleveland, OH, USA

Jaime Mendiola, PhD Department of Preventive Medicine and Public Health, University of Murcia, Espinardo, Murcia, Spain

Lidia Mínguez-Alarcón, PhD Department of Preventive Medicine and Public Health, University of Murcia, Espinardo, Murcia, Spain

Uwe Paasch, MD, PhD Department of Dermatology, University of Leipzig, European Training Centre of Andrology, Leipzig, Saxony, Germany

Sijo J. Parekattil, MD Department of Urology, University of Florida & Winter Haven Hospital, Winter Haven, FL, USA

Fábio Firmbach Pasqualotto, MD, PhD Departamento de Urologia, Universidade de Caxias do Sul e Conception - Centro de Reprodução Assistida, Caxias do Sul, Rio Grande do Sul, Brazil

Amanda Rosencrans, MS, BA Department of Urology, Tulane University School of Medicine, New Orleans, LA, USA

Edmund S. Sabanegh Jr., MD Glickman Urological and Kidney Institute, Cleveland Clinic, Cleveland Clinic Main Campus, Cleveland, OH, USA

Rakesh K. Sharma, PhD Center for Reproductive Medicine, Cleveland Clinic, Cleveland, OH, USA

William B. Smith II, MBA, BA Department of Urology, Tulane University School of Medicine, New Orleans, LA, USA

Alberto M. Torres-Cantero, MD, DrPH Department of Preventive Medicine and Public Health, University of Murcia, Espinardo, Murcia, Spain

Landon W. Trost, MD Department of Urology, Mayo Clinic, Rochester, MN, USA

Joseph A. Vitale Center for Reproductive Medicine, Cleveland Clinic Foundation, Cleveland, OH, USA

About the Editors

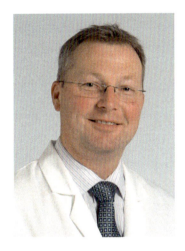

Professor Stefan S. du Plessis is Head of the Division of Medical Physiology in the Faculty of Medicine and Health Sciences at Stellenbosch University (South Africa), where he is actively involved in undergraduate teaching and postgraduate training. He also heads up the Stellenbosch University Reproductive Research Group (SURRG), and his research interests include male gamete function and factors that can influence it (oxidative stress, antioxidants, obesity, diabetes, nicotine and STIs). To date, he has published more than 50 peer-reviewed scientific articles and numerous book chapters. He serves on the editorial board of two leading international journals and regularly acts as an ad hoc reviewer for various scientific journals and funding agencies as well as moderator and examiner to several national and international universities. Prof. du Plessis is an NRF-rated researcher and Fulbright Research Scholar awardee.

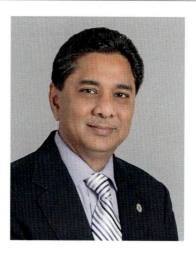

Ashok Agarwal is a Professor at Lerner College of Medicine, Case Western Reserve University and the head of the Andrology Center. He is the Director of Research at the Center for Reproductive Medicine, Cleveland Clinic, USA. He has researched extensively on oxidative stress and its implications on human fertility and his group has published over 500 research articles. Dr. Agarwal serves on the editorial boards of several key journals in human reproduction. His current research interests are the study of molecular markers of oxidative stress, DNA fragmentation and apoptosis using proteomics and bioinformatics tools, as well as fertility preservation in patients with cancer, and the efficacy of certain antioxidants in improving male fertility.

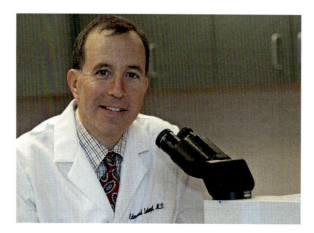

Edmund S. Sabanegh Jr., MD is Chairman of the Department of Urology, leading one of the top-ranked Urology Departments in the United States. He is also Director of the Center of Male Fertility for the Glickman Urological and Kidney Institute at the Cleveland Clinic. His surgical interests include microsurgical reconstruction of the male reproductive tract and advanced sperm harvest techniques. His research interests include complex reconstructions for obstruction of the reproductive tract, fertility preservation in cancer patients, varicoceles and environmental influences on fertility. Dr. Sabanegh has published more than 140 scientific articles and chapters in peer-reviewed journals and textbooks and has authored two books. He is a Professor of Urology at the Lerner College of Medicine of Case Western Reserve University. He is the Assistant Editor for *UROLOGY* and has served as a reviewer for the *Journal of Andrology*, *Urology*, *British Journal of Urology* and *Fertility and Sterility*.

Abbreviations

AA	Arachidonic acid
ABP	Androgen-binding protein
ADMA	Asymmetric dimethylarginine
AGD	Anogenital distance
ALA	Alpha-lipoic acid
APEs	Alkylphenolethoxylates
ART	Assistive reproductive technology
BBB	Blood–brain barrier
BBP	Butyl benzyl phthalate
BMI	Body mass index
BPA	Bisphenol-A
BTB	Blood-testis barrier
BzBP	Benzylbutyl phthalate
CIS	Carcinoma in situ
CoQ10	Co-enzyme Q10
DBP	Dibutyl phthalate
DCHP	Dicyclohexylphthalate
DDE	Dichlorodiphenyldichloroethane
DDT	Dichlorodiphenyltrichloroethane
DEHP	Di-2-ethylhexyl phthalate
DEP	Diethyl phthalate
DES	Diethylstilbestrol
DHA	Docosahexaenoic acid
DHT	Dihydrotestosterone
DIGE	Difference gel electrophoresis
DiNP	Di-isononyl phthalate
DMP	Dimethyl phthalate
DOP	Di-*n*-octyl phthalate
DRE	Digital rectal examination
EDCs	Endocrine disrupting chemicals
EMWs	Electromagnetic waves
EPC	Eppin protein complex
FSH	Follicle-stimulating hormone
GHz	Gigahertz

GnRH	Gonadotropin-releasing hormone
Gy	Gray
HPG axis	The hypothalamic–pituitary–gonadal (HPG) axis
hsp	Heat shock protein
ICSI	Intracytoplasmic sperm injection
IL-6	Interleukin-6
IR	Ionizing radiation
IVF	In vitro fertilization
kV/m	Kilovolts/meter
LAC	L-Acetyl carnitine
LC	L-Carnitine
LH	Luteinizing hormone
MBP	Mono-n-butyl phthalate
MBzP	Mono-benzyl phthalate
MEHP	Mono-ethylhexyl phthalate
MEP	Mono-ethyl phthalate
MHz	Megahertz
MIS	Müllerian-inhibiting substance
MMP	Mitochondrial membrane potential
MRH	Male reproductive health
mSv	Millisievert
NAC	N-Acetyl cysteine
NMDRCs	Nonmonotonic dose response curves
NO	Nitric oxide
NOS	Nitric oxide synthase
NP	Nonylphenol
NPEs	Nonylphenolethoxylates
NTP	National toxicology program
OAT	Oligoasthenoteratospermia
8-OH-2G	8-Hydroxy-2deoxyguanasine
OP	Octylphenol
OPEs	Octylphenolethoxylates
OS	Oxidative stress
PBDEs	Polybrominateddiphenyl ethers
PCBs	Polychlorinated biphenyls
PDE	Phosphodiesterase
PKC	Protein kinase C
POPs	Persistent organic pollutants
PPAR	Peroxisome proliferators
PSA	Prostate-specific antigen
PUFA	Polyunsaturated fatty acid
RCT	Randomized controlled trials
RF	Radiofrequency
ROS	Reactive oxygen species
SA	Semen analysis
SAR	Specific absorption rate
SHBG	Sex-hormone-binding globulin

(SOCS-3) pathway	Suppressor of cytokine signaling 3 pathway
SRY	Sex-determining region Y
StAR	Steroid acute regulatory protein
STP	Sewage treatment plant
TAC	Total antioxidant capacity
TDS	Testicular dysgenesis syndrome
TGCTs	Testicular germ cell tumors
TGF-β	Transforming growth factor-β
TNF-α	Tumor necrosis factor-alpha
UDT	Undescended testes
UMI	Unexplained male infertility
W/kg	Watts/kg
WBC	White blood cells
WHO	World Health Organization
WHR	Waist-to-hip ratio
WMD	Weighted mean difference

Epidemiology and Evidence of Declining Male Fertility

1

Marcello Cocuzza and Sandro C. Esteves

Introduction

Significance

A paper by Carlsen and coworkers showed evidence of a decline in semen quality and thus raised controversy over the topic. The aforementioned study opened the debate and several other studies have been added [1, 2]. In fact, more than 100 articles have been published in the peer-reviewed literature in the past 50 years on this topic. Although many studies have reported a decline in sperm quality over time, others could not detect any changes [2]. The issue is still controversial since some previous studies were criticized for methodological errors, including bias in the recruitment of the population and in the methods applied for the seminal analysis [3]. As male fertility is to some extent correlated to sperm count, it is therefore important to assess whether these findings are indeed reflecting an overall reduction in male fertility [4].

Among fertile men, there are reports suggesting that the decline in human seminal parameters over the last decades is independent of aging. Also, these changes in semen quality seemed to have not been geographically homogeneously distributed, and these variations support the idea that specific factors, presented in some areas but not in others, may be related to a decline in the seminal parameters [5]. The significant deterioration in male genitourinary function is more likely to occur due to environmental rather than genetic factors. Such geographical differences might be related to pollution, occupational exposure to industrial agents or heavy metals, and lifestyle risk factors including smoking, caffeine intake, or alcohol.

There are many other factors that could be involved in decreasing semen quality. It seems that malfunction of the male reproductive system could represent a high-quality sensitive marker of different hazards. The biological significance of these changes over time is emphasized by a concomitant increase in the incidence of genitourinary abnormalities such as testicular cancer and possibly also cryptorchidism and hypospadias, thus suggesting a growing impact of unknown factors with serious effects on male gonadal function [6].

The human spermatozoa is the end result of a sophisticated biological process that is hormonally regulated and produced by a highly specialized cell line, initiated at puberty and continued throughout the man's entire life span in cycles.

M. Cocuzza, MD, PhD (✉)
Human Reproduction Center and Department of Andrology, University of São Paulo, Alameda Casa Branca, 456 apto 41, São Paulo 01408 000, São Paulo, Brazil
e-mail: mcocuzza@uol.com.br

S.C. Esteves, MD, PhD
ANDROFERT, Andrology and Human Reproduction Clinic, Referral Center for Male Reproduction, Av. Dr. Heitor Penteado, 1464, Campinas, São Paulo 13075-460, Brazil
e-mail: s.esteves@androfert.com.br

S.S. du Plessis et al. (eds.), *Male Infertility: A Complete Guide to Lifestyle and Environmental Factors*, DOI 10.1007/978-1-4939-1040-3_1, © Springer Science+Business Media New York 2014

As a result, semen is a sensitive indicator of environmental, occupational, and lifestyle exposures that can exert direct toxic effects and hormonal disruption. Although, damage may occur at any stage of life, early fetal life is a mainly critical time period, when the endocrine system is established and organs are developing [7]. Nonetheless, many questions remain, and we still know little about the effect of many other factors on male fertility.

Objective of Chapter

This chapter explores in detail the issue of a supposed decline in semen quality over time that can directly impact the society in some ways. First, we examine a possible impact of a real decline in semen quality, and thus human fertility, to human well-being. Second, we critically analyze the basis of the "anti-endocrine disruptor theory" as a cause of semen quality decline. Last, we discuss the uncertainty and misinformation concerning semen quality that still prevails in lay and professional circles.

Epidemiological Trends

In Favor of a Decline in the Seminal Parameters

As early as the 1980s, many scientists/clinicians reported an emerging concern about deteriorating semen quality [8–11]. To better elucidate the problem, a meta-analysis of 61 articles including 14,947 men with no previous history of infertility was published by Carlsen and coworkers, in 1992. The authors concluded that the mean sperm count of healthy men had declined by 1 % per year between 1938 and 1990 [1]. Furthermore, they reported a statistically significant decrease of a nearly 50 % reduction in the mean sperm count from 113×10^6 mL^{-1} in 1940 to 66×10^6 mL^{-1} in 1990 and in the seminal volume from 3.40 to 2.75 mL, using linear regression of data weighted by the number of men in each study. These results indicated an even more pronounced decrease in sperm production than expressed by the decline in sperm density.

From 1995 and onwards, many were skeptical about these findings, and this prompted several researchers to study trends in their own countries, mostly based on data from semen banks or semen donor registries. The resulting papers reported heterogeneous findings, with some confirming a decreasing trend in semen quality, and others not [12, 13].

In 1997, Swan and coworkers published a reanalysis of global trend data [14]. The authors found significant declines in sperm density in the United States and Europe/Australia after controlling for abstinence time, age, percent of men with proven fertility, and specimen collection method. The decline in the sperm density in the United States (approximately 1.5 % per year) and Europe/Australia (approximately 3 % per year) was somewhat greater than the average decline reported by Carlsen and coworkers (approximately 1 % per year) [1]. However, Swan and coworkers found no decline in sperm densities in non-Western countries, for which data were very limited. In 2000, an updated comprehensive meta-analysis was undertaken by the same aforesaid authors who confirmed the downward trend [15]. The authors used similar methods to analyze an expanded set of studies, including 47 English language studies published from 1934 to 1996, in addition to those that they had reported in their previous study. They showed that an average decline in sperm count was virtually unchanged from that reported previously by Carlsen and coworkers, and data were similar to their previous findings. The authors suggested that the reported trends were not dependent on the particular studies included by Carlsen and coworkers and that the observed trends previously reported in the 1938–1990 were also seen in the 1934–1996 one [1, 14, 15]. During the same period, there was a strong evidence for a worldwide increase in the incidence of testicular germ-cell cancer, a disease linked to a decreased semen quality [6, 16, 17].

In Finland, a disappointing temporal decrease in semen quality in men from the general population has been observed in the period 1998–2006.

Table 1.1 Summary of studies finding an unambiguous decline in sperm count published from 1995

Date	Author	Location	Study period	Sample size
1995	Auger [23]	France	1973–1992	1,351
1996	Irvine [24]	Scotland	1984–1995	577
1996	Van Waeleghem [25]	Belgium	1977–1995	416
1996	de Mouzon [26]	France	1989–1994	7,714
1996	Menchini-Fabris [27]	Italy	1970–1990	4,518
1996	Adamopoulos [28]	Greece	1977–1993	2,385
1999	Ulstein [29]	Norway	1975–1994	4,072
1998	Bonde [30]	Denmark	1986–1995	1,196
1999	Bilotta [31]	Italy	1981–1995	1,068
1999	Zhang [32]	China	1983–1996	9,292
2003	Almagor [33]	Israel	1990–2000	2,638
2003	Vicari [34]	Italy	1982–1999	716
2005	Lackner [35]	Austria	1986–2003	7,780
2007	Sripada [36]	Scotland	1994–2005	4,832
2008	Liang [37]	China	1980–2005	5,834
2009	Feki [38]	Tunisia	1996–2007	2,940
2010	Molina [39]	Argentina	1995–2004	9,168
2012	Geoffroy-Siraudin [40]	France	1988–2007	10,932
2012	Haimov-Kochman [41]	Israel	1995–2009	2,182
2013	Mendiola [42]	Spain	2001–2011	273

Men born more recently had decreased seminal parameters compared with the cohort that was only a few years older [18]. Furthermore, in 2012, Jorgensen and coworkers published a study, initiated in 1996, which assessed the reproductive health of men from the general population to monitor changes in semen quality over time [19]. In this large, prospective and well-controlled study of semen quality of annual cohorts of young men from the general Danish population, a total of 4,867 individuals have been included. Statistically significant increases in the sperm concentration and total sperm counts over the past 15 years were detected. However, it was noted that men from the general population had significantly lower sperm concentrations, and also total sperm counts, than recently examined fertile men and men of a historical cohort of male partners of infertile couples. Still, only one in four men had optimal semen quality. Thus, the aforementioned authors concluded that there is reason for concern about the future fertility of young Danish men. Less impact cross-sectional studies involving men of the general popular comparable high incidence of low sperm counts in other European countries [18, 20, 21].

Therefore, reduced semen quality seems to be a widespread observable fact. This understanding is in line with the elevated and the growing need of fertility treatment in Denmark [22]. Table 1.1 summarized the major studies finding an unambiguous decline in sperm count trends published from 1995. The extent of the reported declines in terms of total count as well as sperm concentration varied from a 16 % decline to a 31.5 % decline in the study period.

Contrary Opinion

Before 1992, many regional studies of men seeking infertility suggested a decline in sperm counts or other semen parameters in primarily European countries [6–15]. In the same period, Macleod and Wang published a large study in the United States showing no consistent trend in seminal parameters detected over time [43]. The discrepancy in the results of these studies remained a topic of debate during these decades, albeit not achieving notable importance. However, the publication of the aforementioned paper of Carlsen and coworkers from the University of Copenhagen changed this scenario [1]. Their meta-analysis of 61 previous studies gained worldwide media attention due to the surprising enormity of the findings that showed a nearly 50 % drop in sperm count from 1940 to 1990. In addition, the authors suggested that the causes for the decline were the compounds with estrogen-like activity and other environmental pollutants. Although the medical community reacted with skepticism about such results and criticized the methodology, the conclusions have had a huge negative impact on the popular imagination. Although the study has been analyzed by many scientists, a summary of the main criticisms is presented in the next paragraph.

First, a potential selection bias may have occurred with the 61 assembled studies, in such a way that they are not representative of their underlying populations. In fact, the authors failed to include studies that showed no declines in the sperm counts, despite being available at the time of the meta-analysis. Surprisingly, the total population of subjects with no decline in semen parameters was ten times larger than that in which a decline was found. Second, the authors failed to account for geographic variation among the studies. Before 1970, all studies were from the United States, and 80 % of these were from New York, where sperm counts were the highest. After 1970, only three studies were from the United States, and many were from third world countries, where sperm counts were the lowest. A reanalysis of the meta-analysis accounting for this geographic variation showed no decline in sperm counts [44]. Third, the application of an inappropriate statistical analysis may have contributed to the findings. A comprehensive statistical reanalysis of the Carlsen and coworkers study showed that the linear regression model used was inappropriate. A variety of other mathematical models could perform statistically better than the linear model at describing the data and thus offer substantial different hypotheses [45]. In truth, the data were robust for the last 20 years of the studied period only, in which all the models, except the linear model, suggested a constant or slightly increased sperm count [44]. Some argue that given the number of methodological flaws

encountered, the study by Carlsen and coworkers should be excluded from any review of data supporting a decline in sperm counts or other semen parameters. Its importance is limited to promoting a real incentive for additional careful researchers to explore the complex issue of semen quality [3].

Although we cannot change the data quality collected in the past, we can better plan studies to come. Toward this end, the Danish data, collected annually over a 15-year period, provide the best longitudinal semen data yet available [19]. Such a prospectively collected data from a well-defined population, and examined according to a uniform protocol, offer a much better basis for the evaluation of secular trends than retrospective data. The Danish study provided no indication that semen quality has changed during the past 15 years. However, it is of concern that men from the general population had significantly lower seminal parameters, in the new millennium, than recently examined fertile men as well as men of a historical cohort of male partners of infertile couples. Unfortunately, historical data on the semen quality of men from the general population do not exist, and the only Danish semen data available for comparison was obtained by the pioneer of modern Danish andrology, Dr. Richard Hammen, who studied semen quality of men 70 years ago [19]. Although the methods used for counting sperm concentration in historical cohorts were very similar to that used in present investigations and are in accordance with the current recommendations by the WHO, early semen specimens were obtained from male partners of infertile couples [46].

Table 1.2 summarized the major studies finding no decline or an increase in sperm count trends published from 1995. As can be seen from Table 1.1, 20 studies with a combined number of 79,884 subjects reported an unambiguous decline in sperm count, whereas, as can be seen from Table 1.2, 24 studies with a combined number of 107,701 subjects reported no decline or an increase in sperm count. In comparison, the studies reporting no decline or an increase in sperm count comprise approximately 30 % more subjects than studies reporting no decline in sperm count published from 1995. All the studies

1 Epidemiology and Evidence of Declining Male Fertility

Table 1.2 Summary of studies finding no decline or an increase in sperm count, published from 1995

Date	Author	Location	Study period	Sample size	Sperm count[a]
1996	Bujan [47]	France	1977–1992	302	NC
1996	Vierula [48]	Finland	1967–1994	5,719	NC
1996	Paulsen [49]	United States	1972–1993	510	NC
1996	Fisch [50]	United States	1970–1994	1,283	↑
1997	Berling [51]	Sweden	1985–1995	718	↑
1997	Benshushan [52]	Israel	1980–1995	188	NC
1997	Handelsman [53]	Australia	1980–1995	689	NC
1997	Rasmussen [54]	Denmark	1950–1970	1,055	NC
1997	Zheng [55]	Denmark	1968–1992	8,608	NC
1998	Emanuel [56]	United States	1971–1994	374	NC
1998	Younglai [57]	Canada	1984–1996	48,968	NC
1999	Andolz [58]	Spain	1960–1996	20,411	NC
1999	Gyllenborg [59]	Denmark	1977–1995	1,927	↑
1999	Ulstein [29]	Norway	1975–1994	1,108	NC
1999	Zorn [60]	Slovenia	1983–1996	2,343	NC
2000	Acacio [61]	United States	1951–1997	1,347	NC
2001	Itoh [62]	Japan	1975–1998	711	NC
2002	Costello [63]	Australia	1983–2001	448	NC
2003	Marimuthu [64]	India	1990–2000	1,176	NC
2003	Chen [65]	United States	1989–2000	551	↑
2005	Carlsen [66]	Denmark	1996–2001	158	NC
2010	Mukhopadhyay [67]	India	1980–2000	3,729	NC
2011	Axelsson [21]	Sweden	2000–2010	511	NC
2012	Jorgensen [19]	Denmark	1996–2010	4,867	↑

[a]*Note*: ↑ significant increase, *NC* no significant change

included in the table attempted as best as they could to control for some of the confounding variables discussed below.

Confounders Which May Influence Human Sperm Production

Studies of semen quality have been hampered by three fundamental sources of possible error. First, semen quality is highly variable. Attributes such as sperm concentration, seminal volume, and sperm morphology vary widely not only between individuals but also within individuals [46, 68]. Second, it is difficult to recruit men to volunteer for reproductive studies that involve semen analysis, and the selection biases involved are well recognized. Studied populations have been selected from men who have provided semen samples for reasons such as donation to sperm

banks, general population, evaluation for male factor infertility, and pre-vasectomy evaluation [46]. None of these populations represent a random sample of the population at large, and each presents a selection bias, although some of these study populations are more likely to be biased than others [46, 69]. Third, the literature on human semen quality hardly indicates that seminal parameters have varied significantly by geographic region [50, 70, 71]. The inability to include a truly random population due to the wide and unpredictable geographic variations in semen quality represents an important source of potential methodological error [44]. At present, no data exist to elucidate the observed geographic variations in semen parameters.

The authors of the best-published studies concerning semen quality trends are aware of some or all of these potential sources of error [12, 13]. Several studies have attempted to control for variables such as abstinence time, semen analysis methods, or protocols used for sperm collection and measurement. Longer abstinence periods result in seminal parameter modifications, including higher sperm counts, higher semen volumes, and a higher percentage of sperm displaying abnormal morphology [23, 72, 73]. Also important, intra- and inter-technician and laboratory variation exists [74]. Similarly, intraindividual variation also exists, and therefore, at least two semen analysis should be included [74, 75]. Since sperm concentration is not normally distributed, proper transformations using logarithmic or cubic root should be applied to increase the power of the statistical analyses [75]. When confounding factors such as age, number of participants enrolled, and season of the year are available, they might be taken into account to better compare data from different centers [12]. Few studies of semen quality have shown seasonal fluctuations mainly in sperm concentrations, with averages highest in springtime and lowest in the summer [59].

Another source of potential error is the inability to control for lifestyle factors, such as cigarette smoking or recreational drug use. An association between cigarette smoking and reduced seminal quality has been identified [76, 77]. Harmful substances including alkaloids, nitrosamines, nicotine, and hydroxycotinine are present in cigarettes and produce free radicals [78]. Men who smoke cigarettes present higher seminal oxidative stress than nonsmokers, possibly due to the significant increase in leukocyte concentration in their semen [79]. Significantly higher levels of DNA strand breaks have also been identified in smokers which may be resultant from the presence of carcinogens and mutagens in cigarette smoke [80]. Chronic use of marijuana has also been associated with a trend toward elevated seminal fluid leukocytes [79]. Both, experimental and human studies, have demonstrated deleterious effects of tetrahydrocannabinol on sperm parameters including sperm concentration [81]. Varying regional or temporal trends in the use of marijuana might be a confounding factor in numerous studies of semen quality.

Table 1.3 Confounding factors in semen quality studies

Characteristics of the study population	Method
Geographic variations in semen quality	Semen analysis methods
Intra- and interindividual variability	Intra- and inter-technician variability
Medication and diseases	Season at sample delivery
Lifestyle factors	Statistical methods
Study population inclusion criteria	Abstinence period
Age	Number of semen analysis

The aforementioned shortcomings would serve to cast the results of a scientific study in doubt when taken alone; however, taken together, they justify a deep skepticism regarding some of the studies of semen quality in the past 50 years. Many studies have not taken these potential sources of error into account, and thus, the results lack credibility. Some of the possible confounders which may influence semen values, including the characteristics of a study population and methodology, are listed in Table 1.3.

Changes of Clinical Reference Values over Time

Although semen analysis is one of the most important predictors in determining the fertility potential of a man, the true litmus test for male fertility remains the ability to cause pregnancy in vivo [82]. Proper laboratory semen testing is important in the evaluation of men presenting with infertility. However, seminal parameters do not allow for the definitive classification of patients into fertile or infertile [83].

It is important to understand that although the statistical chance of conception decreases as the semen quality decline, it does not reach zero. Also, clinical research has shown that normal semen analysis may not reflect defects in sperm function, and men with poor sperm parameters are still able to generate spontaneous pregnancies [84]. Routine semen parameters such as sperm count, percentage motility, and morphology have limited value mainly because they merely represent the distribution of a given patient population, as determined by the WHO in the last decades [46, 85, 86].

The definition of normal semen quality has varied over time. The most recent WHO guidelines have adhered to the common laboratory standards, in the sense that the "normal" reference range was defined as the one that covers 95 % of a population [46]. The most recent WHO guidelines have reduced the reference limits for sperm concentration from 20 to 15 million/mL. Reference limits based on 95 % of the population may be relevant in relation to certain clinical tests including levels of sodium or potassium in serum but are unsuitable for public health issues in which secular changes may affect the whole population.

Seminal parameters provided from donors with known fertility status reveal a significant overlap in the sperm characteristics between fertile and subfertile men [83, 87]. The current normal values fail to satisfy clinical and statistical standards and pose the risk of misclassifying a subject's true fertility status [87]. Moreover, the introduction of these new values to the clinical practice is likely to result in a reclassification of many infertile couples [84]. Specifically, those couples previously classified as having male factor infertility with sperm parameters greater than the new reference limits, but less than the previous values, will now be diagnosed as having unexplained or female factor infertility. In fact, using the WHO current cutoff values most likely result in some patients previously categorized as having an abnormal semen analysis to be considered "normal," with referral for evaluation postponed or not undertaken [69, 84]. In conclusion, the current WHO guidelines for normal semen quality should be used with caution, because many men with sperm count above the lower limit of the normal range defined by WHO may in fact be subfertile.

It is tempting to suggest that the lower reference limits of semen parameters, as proposed by the 2010 WHO manual, are part of gradual declines in sperm count extensively reported over the past two decades [88]. However, there are two other possible explanations that may explain the difference in the reference values between the current and previous WHO manuals. The first is the adherence by many laboratories to higher-quality control standards, especially when assessing sperm morphology. The second reason is that previous WHO reference values were obtained mainly based on the clinical experience of investigators who have studied populations of healthy fertile men of unknown time to pregnancy rather than controlled populations of fertile men as in the current WHO edition [46, 85]. For these reasons, one must exercise caution when concluding that the newly proposed lowered WHO reference values can be justified by the suggested decline in global sperm quality. It is more probable that such differences are instead related to a methodological bias created by different ways of generating reference values [84].

We must keep in mind that the interpretation of the new reference ranges for seminal parameters, as proposed by the WHO in 2010, requires an understanding that seminal parameters within the 95 % reference interval do not guarantee fertility nor do the values outside those limits necessarily indicate male infertility [46]. This may illustrate an urgent need for new tools in the assessment of these men and also to evaluate the possible decline in semen quality over time.

The Impact of Environmental Factors and Occupational Exposures on Male Reproduction System

The real impact of environmental and occupational exposure on spermatogenesis is extremely complicated to prove and measure. During the past decades, the rapid growth of the chemical industry in both the developed and developing worlds has resulted in the release of a plethora of xenobiotics into the environment [7]. Xenobiotics are any alien molecules that are foreign to biological systems. Such substances, including pesticides, herbicides, cosmetics, preservatives, cleaning materials, private waste, and pharmaceutical products, have worked their way into our lives in a variety of forms. Even though consciousness of the biological risks of chemical toxicity has increased considerably in recent years, the majority of these chemicals have long half-lives, and they have been detected in the environment decades after they were released.

Although the biological fallout from environmental pollution has usually centered on the risks of induction of some kinds of cancer, it is becoming progressively more evident that another major target of this chemical barrage is the reproductive system, particularly in the male. The male reproductive system can be affected by a multiplicity of mechanisms that have an effect on hormone balance and other metabolic systems.

The disruption of germ-cell differentiation and thus the sperm quality decrease seem to involve two fundamentally different routes of exposure.

First, xenobiotics and other environmental factors such as radiation can act straight on male germ cells within the mature testis. The extremely effective proofreading and repair of DNA in the stem cells that generate sperm mean that the male germ line has one of the lowest spontaneous mutation rates in the body [89]. However, as these cells go through meiosis, their capacity for DNA repair is condensed, and their ability to respond to such damage by undergoing programmed cell death is gradually lost. As a consequence, once spermatozoa are released from the germinal epithelium, they can no longer rely on the protection previously afforded by the Sertoli cells. The male germ-cell line is committed to spend a long journey of about 2–12 days in the epididymis and then up to 2 days of swimming around the female reproductive tract searching for the oocyte. During this period, sperms are mainly vulnerable to DNA damage by a variety of environmental factors [90]. Thus, there is no doubt that the spermatozoon is much more susceptible to damage than the oocyte, due to its prolonged lonely existence and relative lack of protection, repair, and self-destruct mechanisms.

The second route by which xenobiotics exert an influence on male reproduction is less direct, through the exposure of women during pregnancy and subsequent disruption of reproductive tract development in male embryos. Such action is thought to affect both the germ cells and the somatic tissues of the male tract, and the consequences comprise a complex array of pathological changes collectively known as the testicular dysgenesis syndrome in the offspring. The features of testicular dysgenesis syndrome include poor semen quality, hypospadia, testicular cancer, and cryptorchidism. Although this syndrome originates in the fetal life, the exact mechanisms involved are not known; however, its incidence seems to be increasing [91]. Experimental evidence of the xenobiotic induction of testicular dysgenesis comes from studies in which a testicular toxicant, as dibutyl phthalate, is administered to pregnant rats. This substance produces testicular dysgenesis-like tissue abnormalities in the testes of male offspring. Abnormal development of Sertoli cells, leading to abnormalities in other cell types, is hypothesized as the explanation for the abnormal changes in dibutyl phthalate-exposed animals [91]. The various features of the testicular dysgenesis syndrome, such as low birth weight and retained placenta, have common risk factors, thus supporting the idea that they share the same pathophysiologic mechanism involving the perturbation of normal fetal development [92]. At present, we know very little about the nature of the xenobiotic-metabolizing enzymes in the male germ line, and thus, the potential that different groups of compounds have for inducing genetic damage by oxidative stress mechanisms is uncertain [7]. However, if xenobiotics are involved in causing testicular dysgenesis, they must act relatively early in fetal development.

Many agents including heavy metals, organic solvents, and pesticides, such as dibromochloropropane, have been associated with gonadotoxicity [93, 94]. Also, industrial lead exposure exerts direct harmful effects on both seminiferous tubules and the hypothalamic pituitary axis, resulting in decreased sperm counts, motility, as well as morphology and ultimately leading to infertility [94–96]. Furthermore, an association between aromatic solvents and impaired semen parameters has been demonstrated, irrespective of the exposure assessment method used [95]. Environmental estrogen is currently one of the most intensively researched compounds.

These phenolic compounds are usually found in plants. However, they also can be found in man-made products and competitively interact with the body's receptors for the natural estrogen, a steroid hormone. The original "estrogen hypothesis" postulated that the apparent increase in human male reproductive developmental disorders includes low sperm counts, which might have occurred due to increased estrogen exposure during the neonatal period [97]. As a result, reduced sperm counts may be associated with the capacity of environmental estrogens to suppress the production of follicle-stimulating hormone (FSH) by the fetal pituitary gland. As FSH stimulates the growth of Sertoli cells in the developing testes, the number of these cells is consequently decreased [98]. Sertoli cells usually do not replicate, and each cell can only support the differentiation of a finite number of spermatozoa. Hence, a reduction in the size of this cell population can have an irreversible impact on male germ-cell development [97].

Environmental pollution is a major source of ROS production and has been implicated in the pathogenesis of poor sperm quality [99]. In a study conducted by De Rosa and coworkers, toll-gate workers with continuous environmental pollutant exposure had inversely correlated blood methemoglobin and lead levels to sperm parameters in comparison to local male inhabitants not exposed to comparable automobile pollution levels. These findings suggest that nitrogen oxide and lead, both present in the composition of automobile exhaust, adversely affect semen quality [100]. In addition, the increase of industrialization has resulted in an elevated deposition of highly toxic heavy metals into the atmosphere. Paternal exposure to heavy metals such as lead, arsenic, and mercury is associated with decreased fertility and pregnancy delay according to relatively recent studies [101, 102]. Oxidative stress is hypothesized to play an important role in the development and progression of adverse health effects due to such environmental exposure [96].

Environmental factors that appear to be involved in the increase in abnormal sperm morphology are not particularly related to geographical area. Future research will show whether this adverse trend continues, but if aspects of altered semen function were linked to a specific environmental influence, it would be susceptible to correction.

Why Has the Incidence of Genitourinary Abnormalities Changed During the Last Decades?

Systemic diseases in adulthood can affect fertility through a number of diverse mechanisms. Neoplasms in general can induce marked impairment of spermatogenesis due to numerous reasons, including endocrine disturbances, malnutrition, hypermetabolism with associated fever, and immunologic factors [103]. Moreover, specific malignancies such as Hodgkin disease and testicular germ-cell tumors produce significant direct gonadotoxic effects.

Several reports indicate that an increase in the incidence of testis cancer has occurred in the last 50 years, although there are considerable differences among countries, being particularly higher in industrialized ones [17, 18, 104, 105]. This increase, however, was most notable among some European-descended populations. East Asian populations, in contrast, continued to have low rates of testis cancer that remained stable or declined [6]. Of note, the incidence of female reproductive tract cancers such as ovarian and uterine cancer has remained constant while the incidence of cervical cancer has decreased during the same period of time [7]. Comparable trends have been seen in all developed countries where data are available [17]. As a consequence of the global tendency of an increased incidence of testicular cancer, we should be aware that the male reproductive system is under attack, in contrast to the female reproductive tract.

Although no solitary hypothesis can be put forward to account for an unexpected increase in the incidence of testicular cancer, one of the possible explanations is the widespread use of ultrasound as a screening method in all fields of medical practice, including scrotal ultrasonography in urology [105, 106]. Another possible explanation could be the fact that people are living longer. However, we feel that such justifications are of limited value because testicular cancer is a disease of young men and is easily detected by self-examination. Although testicular cancer is a rare disease, its rising incidence is certainly a cause for concern.

Suggestions of a potential link between low sperm counts and testicular cancer come from the discrepancies in the incidence of male reproductive pathologies between men from Denmark and those from Finland [18]. Danish men have the lowest sperm counts in Europe and also the highest incidence of testicular cancer and malformations of the genital tract such as hypospadias [107]. In contrast, the frequency of testicular cancer in Finnish men is practically three times lower. In addition, genital malformations are rare and the mean sperm counts are among the highest reported [108]. As such, male reproductive problems thus seem to coincide as men from countries with high frequencies of testicular cancer appear to have lower average semen quality compared with those from countries with a lower cancer incidence [107]. Currently, there is no convincing explanation why the reproductive fate of men in these two countries is so different [107]. Nevertheless, recent studies on smoking during pregnancy indicate strong geographical and temporal association between female smoking and testicular cancer in the offspring [109]. These increased trends could be alleviated by primary prevention, although a satisfactory valid assessment of the hypothesis is still lacking [109].

Of note, the increases in testicular cancer rates, especially over the last 40-year period, argue in favor of a negative impact of environmental risk factors. Even though the large variation in the incidence of testicular cancer among men of different racial and ethnic background suggests that genetic susceptibility might also be a significant determinant [6]. Such recent increases in testicular cancer in most industrialized countries should guide urologists and andrologists to give more awareness to testicular symptoms, such as a painless testicular mass, testicular pain, swelling, hardness, or orchitis, and also to be more prone to recommend a testicular self-examination, particularly in adolescents and young adults [17].

Conclusions

It has been suggested that the sperm production and sperm quality in humans are declining over the last decades. These changes might be responsible for a possible decline in fertility rates in the industrialized world. The inter- and intraindividual biological variability of sperm production, the heterogeneity of the studied population, the small sample-sized evaluation, the paucity of information on subject characteristics, and the uncertainty in the quality and standardization of methods used for semen analyses make the interpretation of secular trends in semen quality extremely difficult as most studies have not taken these potentials sources of error into account.

Despite of that, the reported decline in semen quality is a matter of great interest because it has been associated with an adverse trend for an increased incidence of other male disorders, including testis cancer and undescended testis. A critical appraisal of the available evidence indicates that it is unsound to assume that such trends may be linked to lifestyle and environmental exposures to endocrine disrupters.

Occupational exposure to several agents, including heavy metals, organic solvents, and pesticides such as dibromochloropropane, have been widely associated with reproductive dysfunction in males as well as in females. The possible mechanisms for explaining the negative effects of chemicals on the male reproductive health include both a direct effect on reproductive organs and an indirect effect resulting in a hormonal imbalance that is crucial for growth, sexual development, as well as many other essential physiological functions. Although environmental factors, whatever the route of exposure, can undoubtedly affect the development and function of the male reproductive tract, we must be aware of the wide range of behavioral, medical, and other factors that can potentially damage the male reproductive health. All these factors may contribute to a decrease in the fertility rates, and the necessary research to elucidate this phenomenon is complex and requires nontraditional collaboration between demographers, epidemiologists, clinicians, biologists, wildlife researchers, geneticists, and molecular biologists. This research effort can hardly be carried out without major support from governments and granting agencies, making it possible to fund collaborative projects within novel research networks of scientists.

Taking into account the weakness as well as the qualities of all the studies included in this chapter, there is sufficient power to provide reliable data. If there was a genuine decline in sperm counts in these study populations, these analyses would be able to identify it. Therefore, two conclusions can be drawn from this chapter. Firstly, there is not enough data to confirm a worldwide decline in sperm counts or other semen parameters. Secondly, to date, there is no truly scientific connection about a causative role for endocrine disruptors in the decline of sperm production over time. We strongly believe that a definite conclusion will not be achieved on how much the quality of sperm has changed during the late twentieth century. These uncertainties emphasize the need of continuing good quality research not only concerning the semen quality, reproductive hormones, and xenobiotics but also on defining better indicators of couple fecundity, such as time to pregnancy.

References

1. Carlsen E, Giwercman A, Keiding N, Skakkebaek NE. Evidence for decreasing quality of semen during past 50 years. BMJ. 1992;305(6854):609–13.
2. Skakkebaek NE, Andersson AM, Juul A, Jensen TK, Almstrup K, Toppari J, Jorgensen N. Sperm counts, data responsibility, and good scientific practice. Epidemiology. 2011;22(5):620–1.
3. Fisch H. Declining worldwide sperm counts: disproving a myth. Urol Clin North Am. 2008;35(2):137–46, vii.
4. Joffe M. Decreased fertility in Britain compared with Finland. Lancet. 1996;347(9014):1519–22.
5. Skakkebaek NE, Jorgensen N, Main KM, Rajpert-De Meyts E, Leffers H, Andersson AM, Juul A, Carlsen E, Mortensen GK, Jensen TK, Toppari J. Is human fecundity declining? Int J Androl. 2006;29(1):2–11.
6. Chia VM, Quraishi SM, Devesa SS, Purdue MP, Cook MB, McGlynn KA. International trends in the incidence of testicular cancer, 1973-2002. Cancer Epidemiol Biomarkers Prev. 2010;19(5):1151–9.
7. Aitken RJ, Koopman P, Lewis SE. Seeds of concern. Nature. 2004;432(7013):48–52.
8. Menkveld R, Van Zyl JA, Kotze TJ, Joubert G. Possible changes in male fertility over a 15-year period. Arch Androl. 1986;17(2):143–4.
9. Osser S, Liedholm P, Ranstam J. Depressed semen quality: a study over two decades. Arch Androl. 1984;12(1):113–6.
10. James WH. Secular trend in reported sperm counts. Andrologia. 1980;12(4):381–8.
11. Murature DA, Tang SY, Steinhardt G, Dougherty RC. Phthalate esters and semen quality parameters. Biomed Environ Mass Spectrom. 1987;14(8):473–7.
12. Jouannet P, Wang C, Eustache F, Kold-Jensen T, Auger J. Semen quality and male reproductive health: the controversy about human sperm concentration decline. APMIS. 2001;109(5):333–44.
13. Merzenich H, Zeeb H, Blettner M. Decreasing sperm quality: a global problem? BMC Public Health. 2010;10:24.
14. Swan SH, Elkin EP, Fenster L. Have sperm densities declined? A reanalysis of global trend data. Environ Health Perspect. 1997;105(11):1228–32.
15. Swan SH, Elkin EP, Fenster L. The question of declining sperm density revisited: an analysis of 101 studies published 1934-1996. Environ Health Perspect. 2000;108(10):961–6.
16. Schmiedel S, Schuz J, Skakkebaek NE, Johansen C. Testicular germ cell cancer incidence in an immigration perspective, Denmark, 1978 to 2003. J Urol. 2003;183(4):1378–82.
17. Huyghe E, Matsuda T, Thonneau P. Increasing incidence of testicular cancer worldwide: a review. J Urol. 2003;170(1):5–11.
18. Jorgensen N, Vierula M, Jacobsen R, Pukkala E, Perheentupa A, Virtanen HE, Skakkebaek NE, Toppari J. Recent adverse trends in semen quality and testis cancer incidence among Finnish men. Int J Androl. 2011;34(4 Pt 2):e37–48.
19. Jorgensen N, Joensen UN, Jensen TK, Jensen MB, Almstrup K, Olesen IA, Juul A, Andersson AM, Carlsen E, Petersen JH, Toppari J, Skakkebaek NE. Human semen quality in the new millennium: a prospective cross-sectional population-based study of 4867 men. BMJ Open. 2012;2(4):e000990.
20. Jorgensen N, Asklund C, Carlsen E, Skakkebaek NE. Coordinated European investigations of semen quality: results from studies of Scandinavian young men is a matter of concern. Int J Androl. 2006;29(1):54–61; discussion 105–8.
21. Axelsson J, Rylander L, Rignell-Hydbom A, Giwercman A. No secular trend over the last decade in sperm counts among Swedish men from the general population. Hum Reprod. 2011;26(5):1012–6.
22. Jensen TK, Sobotka T, Hansen MA, Pedersen AT, Lutz W, Skakkebaek NE. Declining trends in conception rates in recent birth cohorts of native Danish women: a possible role of deteriorating male reproductive health. Int J Androl. 2008;31(2):81–92.

23. Auger J, Kunstmann JM, Czyglik F, Jouannet P. Decline in semen quality among fertile men in Paris during the past 20 years. N Engl J Med. 1995;332(5):281–5.

24. Irvine S, Cawood E, Richardson D, MacDonald E, Aitken J. Evidence of deteriorating semen quality in the United Kingdom: birth cohort study in 577 men in Scotland over 11 years. BMJ. 1996;312(7029): 467–71.

25. Van Waeleghem K, De Clercq N, Vermeulen L, Schoonjans F, Comhaire F. Deterioration of sperm quality in young healthy Belgian men. Hum Reprod. 1996;11(2):325–9.

26. de Mouzon J, Thonneau P, Spira A, Multigner L. Declining sperm count. Semen quality has declined among men born in France since 1950. BMJ. 1996;313(7048):43; author reply 4–5.

27. Menchini-Fabris F, Rossi P, Palego P, Simi S, Turchi P. Declining sperm counts in Italy during the past 20 years. Andrologia. 1996;28(6):304.

28. Adamopoulos DA, Pappa A, Nicopoulou S, Andreou E, Karamertzanis M, Michopoulos J, Deligianni V, Simou M. Seminal volume and total sperm number trends in men attending subfertility clinics in the greater Athens area during the period 1977-1993. Hum Reprod. 1996;11(9):1936–41.

29. Ulstein M, Irgens A, Irgens LM. Secular trends in sperm variables for groups of men in fertile and infertile couples. Acta Obstet Gynecol Scand. 1999;78(4):332–5.

30. Bonde JP, Ramlau-Hansen CH, Olsen J. Trends in sperm counts: the saga continues. Epidemiology. 1998;22(5):617–9.

31. Bilotta P, Guglielmo R, Steffe M. [Analysis of decline in seminal fluid in the Italian population during the past 15 years]. Minerva Ginecol. 1999;51(6):223–31.

32. Zhang SC, Wang HY, Wang JD. Analysis of change in sperm quality of Chinese fertile men during 1981-1996. Reprod Contracept. 1999;10(1):33–9.

33. Almagor M, Ivnitzki I, Yaffe H, Baras M. Changes in semen quality in Jerusalem between 1990 and 2000: a cross-sectional and longitudinal study. Arch Androl. 2003;49(2):139–44.

34. Vicari E, Conticello A, Battiato C, La Vignera S. [Sperm characteristics in fertile men and healthy men of the south-east Sicily from year 1982 to 1999]. Arch Ital Urol Androl. 2003;75(1):28–34.

35. Lackner J, Schatzl G, Waldhor T, Resch K, Kratzik C, Marberger M. Constant decline in sperm concentration in infertile males in an urban population: experience over 18 years. Fertil Steril. 2005;84(6): 1657–61.

36. Sripada S, Fonseca S, Lee A, Harrild K, Giannaris D, Mathers E, Bhattacharya S. Trends in semen parameters in the northeast of Scotland. J Androl. 2007;28(2):313–9.

37. Liang XW, Lu WH, Chen ZW, Wang XH, Zhao H, Zhang GY, Gu YQ. [Changes of semen parameters in Chinese fertile men in the past 25 years]. Zhonghua Nan Ke Xue. 2008;14(9):775–8.

38. Feki NC, Abid N, Rebai A, Sellami A, Ayed BB, Guermazi M, Bahloul A, Rebai T, Ammar LK. Semen quality decline among men in infertile relationships: experience over 12 years in the South of Tunisia. J Androl. 2009;30(5):541–7.

39. Molina RI, Martini AC, Tissera A, Olmedo J, Senestrari D, de Cuneo MF, Ruiz RD. Semen quality and aging: analysis of 9.168 samples in Cordoba. Argentina. Arch Esp Urol. 2010;63(3):214–22.

40. Geoffroy-Siraudin C, Loundou AD, Romain F, Achard V, Courbiere B, Perrard MH, Durand P, Guichaoua MR. Decline of semen quality among 10 932 males consulting for couple infertility over a 20-year period in Marseille, France. Asian J Androl. 2012;14(4):584–90.

41. Haimov-Kochman R, Har-Nir R, Ein-Mor E, Ben-Shoshan V, Greenfield C, Eldar I, Bdolah Y, Hurwitz A. Is the quality of donated semen deteriorating? Findings from a 15 year longitudinal analysis of weekly sperm samples. Isr Med Assoc J 14(6):372–7.

42. Mendiola J, Jorgensen N, Minguez-Alarcon L, Sarabia-Cos L, Lopez-Espin JJ, Vivero-Salmeron G, Ruiz-Ruiz KJ, Fernandez MF, Olea N, Swan SH, Torres-Cantero AM. Sperm counts may have declined in young university students in Southern Spain. Andrology. 2013;1(3):408–13.

43. MacLeod J, Wang Y. Male fertility potential in terms of semen quality: a review of the past, a study of the present. Fertil Steril. 1979;31(2):103–16.

44. Olsen GW, Bodner KM, Ramlow JM, Ross CE, Lipshultz LI. Have sperm counts been reduced 50 percent in 50 years? A statistical model revisited. Fertil Steril. 1995;63(4):887–93.

45. Bahadur G, Ling KL, Katz M. Statistical modelling reveals demography and time are the main contributing factors in global sperm count changes between 1938 and 1996. Hum Reprod. 1996;11(12):2635–9.

46. World Health Organization (WHO). WHO laboratory manual for the examination and processing of human semen. 5th ed. Geneva, Switzerland: WHO Press; 2010.

47. Bujan L, Mansat A, Pontonnier F, Mieusset R. Time series analysis of sperm concentration in fertile men in Toulouse, France between 1977 and 1992. BMJ. 1996;312(7029):471–2.

48. Vierula M, Niemi M, Keiski A, Saaranen M, Saarikoski S, Suominen J. High and unchanged sperm counts of Finnish men. Int J Androl. 1996; 19(1):11–7.

49. Paulsen CA, Berman NG, Wang C. Data from men in greater Seattle area reveals no downward trend in semen quality: further evidence that deterioration of semen quality is not geographically uniform. Fertil Steril. 1996;65(5):1015–20.

50. Fisch H, Goluboff ET, Olson JH, Feldshuh J, Broder SJ, Barad DH. Semen analyses in 1,283 men from the United States over a 25-year period: no decline in quality. Fertil Steril. 1996;65(5):1009–14.

51. Berling S, Wolner-Hanssen P. No evidence of deteriorating semen quality among men in infertile

relationships during the last decade: a study of males from Southern Sweden. Hum Reprod. 1997; 12(5):1002–5.

52. Benshushan A, Shoshani O, Paltiel O, Schenker JG, Lewin A. Is there really a decrease in sperm parameters among healthy young men? A survey of sperm donations during 15 years. J Assist Reprod Genet. 1997;14(6):347–53.

53. Handelsman DJ. Sperm output of healthy men in Australia: magnitude of bias due to self-selected volunteers. Hum Reprod. 1997;12(12):2701–5.

54. Rasmussen PE, Erb K, Westergaard LG, Laursen SB. No evidence for decreasing semen quality in four birth cohorts of 1,055 Danish men born between 1950 and 1970. Fertil Steril. 1997;68(6): 1059–64.

55. Zheng Y, Bonde JP, Ernst E, Mortensen JT, Egense J. Is semen quality related to the year of birth among Danish infertility clients? Int J Epidemiol. 1997; 26(6):1289–97.

56. Emanuel ER, Goluboff ET, Fisch H. MacLeod revisited: sperm count distributions in 374 fertile men from 1971 to 1994. Urology. 1998;51(1):86–8.

57. Younglai EV, Collins JA, Foster WG. Canadian semen quality: an analysis of sperm density among eleven academic fertility centers. Fertil Steril. 1998;70(1):76–80.

58. Andolz P, Bielsa MA, Vila J. Evolution of semen quality in North-eastern Spain: a study in 22,759 infertile men over a 36 year period. Hum Reprod. 1999;14(3):731–5.

59. Gyllenborg J, Skakkebaek NE, Nielsen NC, Keiding N, Giwercman A. Secular and seasonal changes in semen quality among young Danish men: a statistical analysis of semen samples from 1927 donor candidates during 1977-1995. Int J Androl. 1999; 22(1):28–36.

60. Zorn B, Virant-Klun I, Verdenik I, Meden-Vrtovec H. Semen quality changes among 2343 healthy Slovenian men included in an IVF-ET programme from 1983 to 1996. Int J Androl. 1999;22(3):178–83.

61. Acacio BD, Gottfried T, Israel R, Sokol RZ. Evaluation of a large cohort of men presenting for a screening semen analysis. Fertil Steril. 2000;73(3): 595–7.

62. Itoh N, Kayama F, Tatsuki TJ, Tsukamoto T. Have sperm counts deteriorated over the past 20 years in healthy, young Japanese men? Results from the Sapporo area. J Androl. 2001;22(1):40–4.

63. Costello MF, Sjoblom P, Haddad Y, Steigrad SJ, Bosch EG. No decline in semen quality among potential sperm donors in Sydney, Australia, between 1983 and 2001. J Assist Reprod Genet. 2002; 19(6):284–90.

64. Marimuthu P, Kapilashrami MC, Misro MM, Singh G. Evaluation of trend in semen analysis for 11 years in subjects attending a fertility clinic in India. Asian J Androl. 2003;5(3):221–5.

65. Chen Z, Isaacson KB, Toth TL, Godfrey-Bailey L, Schiff I, Hauser R. Temporal trends in human semen parameters in New England in the United States, 1989-2000. Arch Androl. 2003;49(5):369–74.

66. Carlsen E, Swan SH, Petersen JH, Skakkebaek NE. Longitudinal changes in semen parameters in young Danish men from the Copenhagen area. Hum Reprod. 2005;20(4):942–9.

67. Mukhopadhyay D, Varghese AC, Pal M, Banerjee SK, Bhattacharyya AK, Sharma RK, Agarwal A. Semen quality and age-specific changes: a study between two decades on 3,729 male partners of couples with normal sperm count and attending an andrology laboratory for infertility-related problems in an Indian city. Fertil Steril. 2010;93(7):2247–54.

68. Ombelet W, Bosmans E, Janssen M, Cox A, Vlasselaer J, Gyselaers W, Vandeput H, Gielen J, Pollet H, Maes M, Steeno O, Kruger T. Semen parameters in a fertile versus subfertile population: a need for change in the interpretation of semen testing. Hum Reprod. 1997;12(5):987–93.

69. Andersen AG, Jensen TK, Carlsen E, Jorgensen N, Andersson AM, Krarup T, Keiding N, Skakkebaek NE. High frequency of sub-optimal semen quality in an unselected population of young men. Hum Reprod. 2000;15(2):366–72.

70. Jorgensen N, Andersen AG, Eustache F, Irvine DS, Suominen J, Petersen JH, Andersen AN, Auger J, Cawood EH, Horte A, Jensen TK, Jouannet P, Keiding N, Vierula M, Toppari J, Skakkebaek NE. Regional differences in semen quality in Europe. Hum Reprod. 2001;16(5):1012–9.

71. Jorgensen N, Carlsen E, Nermoen I, Punab M, Suominen J, Andersen AG, Andersson AM, Haugen TB, Horte A, Jensen TK, Magnus O, Petersen JH, Vierula M, Toppari J, Skakkebaek NE. East-West gradient in semen quality in the Nordic-Baltic area: a study of men from the general population in Denmark, Norway, Estonia and Finland. Hum Reprod. 2002;17(8):2199–208.

72. Blackwell JM, Zaneveld LJ. Effect of abstinence on sperm acrosin, hypoosmotic swelling, and other semen variables. Fertil Steril. 1992;58(4):798–802.

73. Agarwal A, Sidhu RK, Shekarriz M, Thomas Jr AJ. Optimum abstinence time for cryopreservation of semen in cancer patients. J Urol. 1995; 154(1):86–8.

74. Auger J, Eustache F, Ducot B, Blandin T, Daudin M, Diaz I, Matribi SE, Gony B, Keskes L, Kolbezen M, Lamarte A, Lornage J, Nomal N, Pitaval G, Simon O, Virant-Klun I, Spira A, Jouannet P. Intra- and inter-individual variability in human sperm concentration, motility and vitality assessment during a workshop involving ten laboratories. Hum Reprod. 2000;15(11):2360–8.

75. Berman NG, Wang C, Paulsen CA. Methodological issues in the analysis of human sperm concentration data. J Androl. 1996;17(1):68–73.

76. Kunzle R, Mueller MD, Hanggi W, Birkhauser MH, Drescher H, Bersinger NA. Semen quality of male smokers and nonsmokers in infertile couples. Fertil Steril. 2003;79(2):287–91.

77. Sadeu JC, Hughes CL, Agarwal S, Foster WG. Alcohol, drugs, caffeine, tobacco, and environmental contaminant exposure: reproductive health consequences and clinical implications. Crit Rev Toxicol. 2010;40(7):633–52.
78. Traber MG, van der Vliet A, Reznick AZ, Cross CE. Tobacco-related diseases. Is there a role for antioxidant micronutrient supplementation? Clin Chest Med. 2000;21(1):173–87, x.
79. Close CE, Roberts PL, Berger RE. Cigarettes, alcohol and marijuana are related to pyospermia in infertile men. J Urol. 1990;144(4):900–3.
80. Potts RJ, Newbury CJ, Smith G, Notarianni LJ, Jefferies TM. Sperm chromatin damage associated with male smoking. Mutat Res. 1999;423(1–2):103–11.
81. Nahas GG, Frick HC, Lattimer JK, Latour C, Harvey D. Pharmacokinetics of THC in brain and testis, male gametotoxicity and premature apoptosis of spermatozoa. Hum Psychopharmacol. 2002;17(2):103–13.
82. Aziz N, Fear S, Taylor C, Kingsland CR, Lewis-Jones DI. Human sperm head morphometric distribution and its influence on human fertility. Fertil Steril. 1998;70(5):883–91.
83. Guzick DS, Overstreet JW, Factor-Litvak P, Brazil CK, Nakajima ST, Coutifaris C, Carson SA, Cisneros P, Steinkampf MP, Hill JA, Xu D, Vogel DL. Sperm morphology, motility, and concentration in fertile and infertile men. N Engl J Med. 2001;345(19):1388–93.
84. Esteves SC, Zini A, Aziz N, Alvarez JG, Sabanegh Jr ES, Agarwal A. Critical appraisal of World Health Organization's new reference values for human semen characteristics and effect on diagnosis and treatment of subfertile men. Urology. 2012;79(1):16–22.
85. World Health Organization (WHO). WHO laboratory manual for the examination of human semen and sperm-cervical mucus interaction. New York, NY: Cambridge University Press; 1999.
86. World Health Organization (WHO). WHO laboratory manual for the examination of human semen and sperm-cervical mucus interaction. Cambridge, UK: Cambridge University Press; 1992.
87. Nallella KP, Sharma RK, Aziz N, Agarwal A. Significance of sperm characteristics in the evaluation of male infertility. Fertil Steril. 2006;85(3):629–34.
88. Bromwich P, Cohen J, Stewart I, Walker A. Decline in sperm counts: an artefact of changed reference range of "normal"? BMJ. 1994;309(6946):19–22.
89. Hill KA, Buettner VL, Halangoda A, Kunishige M, Moore SR, Longmate J, Scaringe WA, Sommer SS. Spontaneous mutation in Big Blue mice from fetus to old age: tissue-specific time courses of mutation frequency but similar mutation types. Environ Mol Mutagen. 2004;43(2):110–20.
90. Aitken RJ, Sawyer D. The human spermatozoon—not waving but drowning. Adv Exp Med Biol. 2003;518:85–98.

91. Fisher JS, Macpherson S, Marchetti N, Sharpe RM. Human 'testicular dysgenesis syndrome': a possible model using in-utero exposure of the rat to dibutyl phthalate. Hum Reprod. 2003;18(7):1383–94.
92. Skakkebaek NE. Testicular dysgenesis syndrome: new epidemiological evidence. Int J Androl. 2004;27(4):189–91.
93. Lipshultz LI, Ross CE, Whorton D, Milby T, Smith R, Joyner RE. Dibromochloropropane and its effect on testicular function in man. J Urol. 1980;124(4):464–8.
94. Kumar S. Occupational exposure associated with reproductive dysfunction. J Occup Health. 2004;46(1):1–19.
95. Tielemans E, Burdorf A, te Velde ER, Weber RF, van Kooij RJ, Veulemans H, Heederik DJ. Occupationally related exposures and reduced semen quality: a case-control study. Fertil Steril. 1999;71(4):690–6.
96. Fowler BA, Whittaker MH, Lipsky M, Wang G, Chen XQ. Oxidative stress induced by lead, cadmium and arsenic mixtures: 30-day, 90-day, and 180-day drinking water studies in rats: an overview. Biometals. 2004;17(5):567–8.
97. Sharpe RM. The 'oestrogen hypothesis'—where do we stand now? Int J Androl. 2003;26(1):2–15.
98. Sharpe RM, Rivas A, Walker M, McKinnell C, Fisher JS. Effect of neonatal treatment of rats with potent or weak (environmental) oestrogens, or with a GnRH antagonist, on Leydig cell development and function through puberty into adulthood. Int J Androl. 2003;26(1):26–36.
99. Gate L, Paul J, Ba GN, Tew KD, Tapiero H. Oxidative stress induced in pathologies: the role of antioxidants. Biomed Pharmacother. 1999;53(4):169–80.
100. De Rosa M, Zarrilli S, Paesano L, Carbone U, Boggia B, Petretta M, Maisto A, Cimmino F, Puca G, Colao A, Lombardi G. Traffic pollutants affect fertility in men. Hum Reprod. 2003;18(5):1055–61.
101. Sallmen M, Lindbohm ML, Anttila A, Taskinen H, Hemminki K. Time to pregnancy among the wives of men occupationally exposed to lead. Epidemiology. 2000;11(2):141–7.
102. Sallmen M, Lindbohm ML, Nurminen M. Paternal exposure to lead and infertility. Epidemiology. 2000;11(2):148–52.
103. Costabile RA, Spevak M. Cancer and male factor infertility. Oncology (Williston Park). 1998;12(4):557–62, 65; discussion 66–8, 70.
104. Coleman MP, Esteve J, Damiecki P, Arslan A, Renard H. Trends in cancer incidence and mortality. IARC Sci Publ. 1993;121:1–806.
105. Carmignani L, Gadda F, Mancini M, Gazzano G, Nerva F, Rocco F, Colpi GM. Detection of testicular ultrasonographic lesions in severe male infertility. J Urol. 2004;172(3):1045–7.
106. Horstman WG, Haluszka MM, Burkhard TK. Management of testicular masses incidentally discovered by ultrasound. J Urol. 1994;151(5):1263–5.

107. Nordkap L, Joensen UN, Blomberg Jensen M, Jorgensen N. Regional differences and temporal trends in male reproductive health disorders: semen quality may be a sensitive marker of environmental exposures. Mol Cell Endocrinol. 2012;355(2):221–30.

108. Slama R, Eustache F, Ducot B, Jensen TK, Jorgensen N, Horte A, Irvine S, Suominen J, Andersen AG, Auger J, Vierula M, Toppari J, Andersen AN, Keiding N, Skakkebaek NE, Spira A, Jouannet P. Time to pregnancy and semen parameters: a cross-sectional study among fertile couples from four European cities. Hum Reprod. 2002;17(2):503–15.

109. Pettersson A, Kaijser M, Richiardi L, Askling J, Ekbom A, Akre O. Women smoking and testicular cancer: one epidemic causing another? Int J Cancer. 2004;109(6):941–4.

Part I

Lifestyle/Personal Factors

The Effect of Smoking on Male Infertility

2

Omar Haque, Joseph A. Vitale, Ashok Agarwal, and Stefan S. du Plessis

Introduction

The detrimental effects of cigarette smoking on human longevity, respiratory and cardiovascular physiology, and general health are well documented. However, a less publicized aspect of smoking is its link to male infertility. In a society where one third of the world's population over the age of 15 smokes cigarettes daily and the highest prevalence is among young adult males in their reproductive years [1], it becomes critical to determine whether or not the compounds in cigarette smoke can lead to infertility issues for males. Although 30 % of men and 35 % of women of reproductive age in the United States smoke, current evidence cannot conclusively verify the causative relationship between smoking and male reproductive problems. However, there is a consensus in medical literature that cigarette smoke is an infertility risk factor [2]. A major reason why this debate has persisted is because the biological mechanisms through which chemicals and gases in cigarette smoke lead to male infertility are largely unknown.

Based on this current situation, the objective of this chapter is fourfold. First, the myriad of fertility factors that are adversely affected by cigarette smoke will be discussed. Next, the evidence that challenges the causative link between smoking and male infertility will be analyzed in the effort to provide explanations for the continued inconsistencies seen in medical literature. Afterwards, this chapter will summarize the possible mechanisms through which smoking can lead to male infertility. Finally, the chapter will conclude with a discussion regarding how this area of research should advance to meet the clinical needs of infertile smokers.

O. Haque, BS • J.A. Vitale • A. Agarwal, PhD
Center for Reproductive Medicine, Cleveland
Clinic Foundation/Glickman Urological and Kidney
Institute, 10681 Carnegie Avenue, Cleveland,
OH 44195, USA
e-mail: ohaque2@gmail.com; vitale.40@osu.edu;
agarwaa@ccf.org

S.S. du Plessis, BSc (Hons), MSc, MBA,
PhD (Stell) (✉)
Division of Medical Physiology, Department
of Biomedical Sciences, Faculty of Medicine and
Health Sciences, Stellenbosch University,
Tygerberg, Western Cape, South Africa
e-mail: ssdp@sun.ac.za

Content of Cigarette Smoke

The contents of cigarette smoke have shown substantial effects on male infertility worldwide. Around 4,000 compounds are released by a lit cigarette consisting of gases, vaporized liquids, and particles through the processes of hydrogenation, pyrolysis, oxidation, decarboxylation, and dehydration. Cigarette smoke consists of two phases: gaseous and particulate phases. Nicotine and tar are released in the particulate phase, while carbon monoxide emerges

S.S. du Plessis et al. (eds.), *Male Infertility: A Complete Guide to Lifestyle and Environmental Factors*,
DOI 10.1007/978-1-4939-1040-3_2, © Springer Science+Business Media New York 2014

in the gaseous phase [3]. Radioactive polonium, benzopyrene, dimethylbenzanthracene, naphthalene, methylnaphthalene, polycystic aromatic hydrocarbons, and cadmium (Cd) are common carcinogens and mutagens that are present in cigarettes [4, 5]. In fact, elevated seminal Cd levels have been seen in smokers who consumed more than 20 cigarettes per day [6, 7]. A known environmental hazard and a risk factor for early hypertension, Cd has been linked with male infertility, and seminal Cd levels in normozoospermics have been directly correlated with cigarette consumption per day [8].

Next, there are two types of smoke that are generated when a cigarette is lit: main stream and sidestream smoke. When smoke is drawn from the cigarette and filtered through the user's lungs, mainstream smoke emerges. Sidestream smoke is merely a byproduct of cigarette burning [9]. High levels of ROS such as hydroxyl anion, hydrogen peroxide, and hydroxyl radicals were found to be an active component in cigarette smoke [1]. In addition, carcinogens such as N-nitrosamine (TSNA), N'-nitrosonornicotine (NNN), and 4-(methylnitrosamino)-1-(3-pyridyl)-1-butanone (NNK) were identified in smokeless tobacco (including snuff and chewing tobacco) as well. Finally, 3-methylnitrosamino-propion-aldehyde (MNPA), also found in smokeless tobacco, negatively impacted DNA by breaking single strands. Many harmful compounds and active ingredients found in smoking tobacco (nicotine, Cd, and benzene) are present in chewing tobacco as well [10].

Effect of Smoking on Male Infertility

The consensus in medical literature indicates that smoking can negatively affect virtually every aspect of the male reproductive system. Due to a multitude of factors that will be presented in the following sections, the spermatozoa of chronic smokers have a decreased fertilization capability (see Fig. 2.1) and, when coupled to form an embryo, display lower successful implantation rates [11, 12].

Semen Parameters

The harmful effects of cigarette smoke shift virtually all semen parameters (count, motility, and morphology) away from normal physiological levels. Furthermore, some people have reported that there is no "safe" amount of cigarette smoke intake with regard to semen quality and that some semen parameters such as volume are inversely related to the amount of cigarette use [13]. Nicotine, an alkaloid compound found in nightshade plants, has a negative effect on both sperm morphology and count (since human spermatozoa have nicotine receptors) and is found in higher concentrations among smokers [14]. In rats, the compound has a negative dose-dependent effect on sperm parameters, reducing fertility; moreover, nicotine withdrawal helps lessen the effects, suggesting a causative relationship [15]. Numerous clinical studies on humans have also reported that smokers have lower sperm counts [16–19] and significantly lower sperm concentrations [6, 20–23]. These studies indicate that smokers suffer from oligospermia or even azoospermia, causing infertility problems due to lack of viable spermatozoa. Studies have also found that spermatozoa from smokers exhibit lower motility [16, 18, 19, 22, 24–28] and quality (in relation to semen parameters) [21] before and after swim-up [4] compared to the spermatozoa of nonsmokers. More specifically, the spermatozoa of smokers displayed reduced progressive motility [23], higher deviations in their straight-line motility [29], and after ejaculation, faster deterioration as well [13]. Lastly, the semen from smokers appeared to contain larger counts of morphologically abnormal spermatozoa [20, 22, 24, 29]. These alterations include more oval spermatozoa [16], head defects [6, 27], and cytoplasmic droplets [30] compared to normal semen samples. Thus, in addition to oligospermia and azoospermia, heavy smoking can also lead to teratozoospermia [13].

Spermatozoa Structure and Proteins

While semen parameters are a convenient way to assess the reproductive capability of spermato-

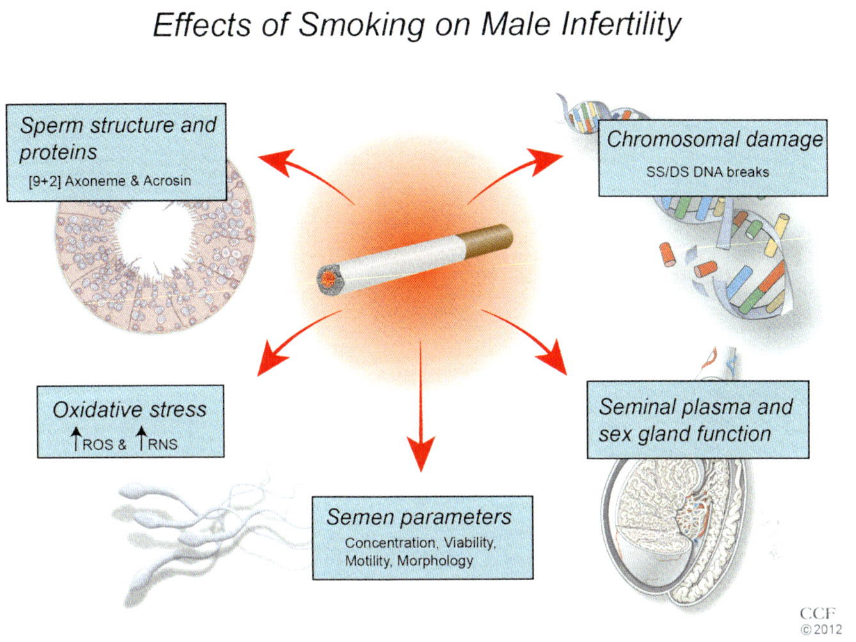

Effects of Smoking on Male Infertility

Fig. 2.1 A summary of the general categorical effects of smoking on male infertility. The contents of cigarette smoke have been shown to (*clockwise*) lead to DNA single-stranded and double-stranded breaks, reduced quality in seminal plasma, lower sex gland function, reduced semen parameters, higher levels of ROS and RNS, and abnormal morphology of sperm axonemes. (*ROS* reactive oxygen species, *RNS* reactive nitrogen species) [Reprinted with permission, Cleveland Clinic Center for Medical Art & Photography © 2012. All Rights Reserved]

zoa, they are often highly variable between different men. Thus, to further assess the effect of cigarette smoke on spermatozoa, a biological lens is required. To begin, studies have found fluctuations in both amount and positioning of axonemal microtubules in smokers [31]. The axoneme is the cytoskeleton comprised of microtubules in the classic $9 + 2$ arrangement (nine doublets encircling two central pairs) in motile cilia and flagella. Thus, the smoke-induced alterations to the normal axoneme structure (such as coiling of tail filaments) could impede flagellar beating, leading to the sperm motility pathologies seen in smokers [32].

Next, the catalytic role of acrosin in smokers seems to be affected [33]. Acrosin is a digestive enzyme encoded by the ACR gene that acts as a protease to degrade the zona pellucida of the oocyte. It is released during the acrosome reaction and aids the penetration of the spermatozoa into the ovum by degrading the oolemma. Smokers displayed lower acrosin activity in the

presence of normal semen parameters compared to nonsmokers [33]. The reduced level of acrosin activity in smokers relays a fundamental point when assessing male infertility—even with perfectly normal semen, men can be infertile due to the other biological factors such as a failure of proper enzymatic function.

Seminal Plasma and Sex Glands

Seminal plasma, the fluid component of the ejaculate, also plays a major role in male fertility. This complex fluid contains a huge variety of molecules, both organic and inorganic, providing the spermatozoa nutrition and protection during their travel through the female reproductive tract. Experiments indicate that when spermatozoa from nonsmokers come into contact with the seminal fluid of smokers, the spermatozoa display reduced motility and acrosome reaction. However, when spermatozoa from smokers come into contact with the seminal plasma of non-smokers, the results were insignificant [34]. From these experiments, it becomes clear that poor seminal plasma can contribute to male infertility, and spermatozoa quality is not the only factor to take into consideration when clinically advising infertile male smokers.

Accessory sex glands, responsible for producing seminal plasma, are an aggregate of cells that are specialized to secrete chemicals and compounds to meet the biological and metabolic needs of an organism. The male accessory sex glands include the seminal vesicles, prostate gland, and bulbourethral glands that together lubricate the ducts of the male reproductive system, provide nourishment to the spermatozoa, and act as a medium for sperm transport. The seminal vesicles produce a fructose-enriched fluid that gives spermatozoa energy and facilitates their motility. The prostate secretes an alkaline, milky fluid that comprises up to 30 % of semen volume, and the bulbourethral glands (also called the Cowper glands) secrete a clear fluid that nourishes the spermatozoa. Studies have analyzed the function of these three glands by examining the ejaculate contents with various glandular markers (total phosphate for the seminal vesicles, zinc acid phosphatase for the prostate gland, and alpha-1,4,glucosidase for the epididymis). Statistically significant findings showed reduced vesicular and prostatic parameters in smokers [35]. This result reiterates the point that smoking's effect on male reproduction stretches well past merely affecting sperm parameters and quality.

Reactive Oxygen Species, Reactive Nitrogen Species, and Oxidative Stress

Reactive oxygen species (ROS) are biologically active, oxygen-containing free radicals that have the ability to damage DNA and cells. When an imbalance between ROS creation and neutralization occurs, oxidative stress (OS) ensues, leading to damaged lipids, nucleic acids, proteins, and carbohydrates. Spermatozoa are highly susceptible to OS due to their small cytoplasm, the area of the cells that houses repair enzymes and antioxidants. OS can damage sperm quality, leading to lower viability, motility, and fecundity. Along similar lines, reactive nitrogen species (RNS) function in conjunction with ROS to cause nitrosative stress. Common ROS in spermatozoa include superoxide and hydrogen peroxide, while common RNS species consist of nitric oxide and peroxynitrite [36].

It is important to understand that ROS serve both physiological and pathological roles in the context of male fertility. On a physiological level, ROS facilitate chromatin packaging during sperm maturation, the acrosome reaction during capacitation, sperm hyperactivation, and sperm-egg fusion. However, when imbalances occur or when ROS are located in abnormal locations, pathological effects can result. The pathological roles of ROS include lipid peroxidation, apoptosis, and DNA damage. Smoking is one of many exogenous factors that lead to evaluated RNS and ROS levels, causing OS. In fact, studies have shown that smoking is correlated with a 48 % increase in seminal leukocytes and 107 % increase in ROS levels [1]. Given the dangers and effects of increased ROS and RNS levels, the finding that the content of cigarette smoke leads to OS provides strong evidence for the causative link between infertility and cigarette smoke.

Antioxidants, molecules that prevent the oxidation of biological compounds, neutralize the effect of ROS and as a result, prevent OS. Ascorbic acid, a mild reducing agent, is a fundamental antioxidant in human semen; in fact, physiological seminal plasma levels reach 10 mg/dL, more than nine times the concentration of blood plasma [37]. However, smokers have 20–40 % lower ascorbic acid levels in serum, and ascorbic acid supplements given to heavy smokers improve their sperm quality indicative of a causative relationship [37, 38]. Ascorbic acid has also been positively correlated with semen parameters previously discussed such as sperm count, motility, and morphology [39]. Next, superoxide dismutase (SOD), the enzyme responsible for the dismutation of superoxide ROS into hydrogen peroxide, is found in lower concentrations among smokers and has been negatively correlated to both the duration and quantity of cigarette smoking [23, 40]. It is believed that the compounds found in cigarette smoke transverse the blood-testis barrier, causing OS-induced DNA fragmentation and reducing sperm quality [41].

Chromosomal Damage

Studies have postulated that severe DNA damage reduces sperm quality and can even prevent oocyte fertilization [42]. Furthermore, if a DNA-damaged spermatozoa does fertilize an ovum, development could be abnormal or cease altogether. For these reasons, DNA damage to spermatozoa can be a potent cause of male infertility. Relevant experiments found chromosomal DNA damage in Golgi-phase or cap-phase spermatids. During the Golgi phase, spermatids develop polarity and DNA condenses, resulting in transcriptionally inactive chromatin, while in cap phase, the acrosomal cap forms. In these studies, 1.15 % of infertile smokers and 0.82 % of infertile nonsmokers showed DNA-damaged Golgi-phase or cap-phase spermatids [42]. Furthermore, smoking causes an increase in the ratio of single-stranded to double-stranded DNA [43]. Fragmented DNA has also been seen to be higher in male smokers versus nonsmokers although the exact values are variable [41, 44]. However, analysis of the DNA damage after sperm capacitation revealed that tobacco does indeed have a detrimental effect on DNA damage [45], validating the trends found in previous studies. Finally, and perhaps most dangerous, smoking has been demonstrated to induce disomic spermatozoa—sperm with multiple copies of the same chromosome—increasing the risk of aneuploidy [46].

Varicoceles

Varicoceles are abnormal expansions of the veins located in the scrotum that run alongside the spermatic cord and drain a man's testicles. Studies show that when the presence of varicoceles are coupled with cigarette smoke, the incidence of oligozoospermia increased tenfold compared with nonsmoking males with varicoceles [47]. There is speculation that the physiology behind this phenomenon is due to catecholamine secretions from the adrenal medulla due to cigarette smoking. Catecholamines are a class of tyrosine derivatives that circulate in the bloodstream and consist of molecules such as epinephrine, norepinephrine, and dopamine; these compounds arrive at the testes via the spermatic vein through retrograde flow [48], leading to varicoceles, oligospermia, and male infertility problems.

Chewing Tobacco

While chewing (smokeless) tobacco is not the focal point of this chapter, analyzing its effects on male infertility highlights some fundamental points. Overall, chewing tobacco is much less harmful than smoking [49] and does not drastically increase the risk of respiratory tract cancers [50]. Since both forms of tobacco contain similar active compounds, the physical burning of smoking tobacco in a cigarette is thought to initiate deleterious reactions that do not occur with chewing tobacco. In addition, chewing tobacco has a much lower risk of cardiovascular disease compared to smoking [51]. However, its consumption is on the rise and is proving to be more harmful than previously expected. Just in the United States alone, there has been a threefold increase in consumption and the manufacturing output of chewing tobacco has been growing for eight consecutive years [52]. Also, there have been an increasing number of studies that are linking chewing tobacco with infertility, suggesting that even the less harmful form of tobacco can still cause reproductive problems in males. Azoospermia was observed in chewing tobacco groups with 14 % incidence among very frequent users [10]. Furthermore, a statistically significant difference in semen quality (count, motility, morphology, and viability) was seen in tobacco chewers already experiencing infertility evaluation. However, no significant results were obtained regarding semen parameters in men who chewed little to moderate levels of tobacco [10]. These relationships suggest that chewing tobacco, despite being less harmful in many respects compared to cigarette smoke, can still lead to infertility when heavily used. Thus, infertile men who do not smoke but chew tobacco should also be counseled on the adverse effects of their habit on sperm quality.

Prenatal Tobacco Exposure

Cigarette smoking may also have long-term effects on male infertility. Studies have shown that prenatal interaction with cigarette smoke leads to male infertility in adulthood. This correlation was made by counting the number of non-contraception cycles in 600 couples [53]. Thus, not only does cigarette smoke affect a plethora of factors that can lead to male infertility, but also the habit can transcend into the neonatal population as well, comprising the fertility of a generation that is still unborn. A Danish pregnancy cohort also reported an inverse correlation between maternal smoking and total sperm count in adulthood—men exposed to more than 19 cigarettes per day during neonatal development exhibited 19 % reduced semen volume, 38 % lower sperm count, and 17 % lower sperm concentration in relation to men who were unexposed to cigarette smoke in the womb. However, another study found that couples who were prenatally exposed to cigarette smoke displayed no signs of reduced fertility [53].

Contradictory Findings

Although the majority of studies regarding male infertility factors and smoking find statistically significant correlations between the two, there are still some that yield insignificant results. These studies conclude that tobacco consumption does not reduce semen quality [54, 55] and tobacco's effect on infertility is more behavioral (i.e., drug usage, poor socioeconomic status, malnourishment) than biological [56, 57]. In addition, studies found no effect of smoking on semen parameters [57–59], gonadal hormones [48], and DNA distribution [60]. Regarding DNA, a few scientists have shown that there is no significant relationship between smoking and DNA fragmentation (sheared or separated

DNA) when comparing the spermatozoa of smokers (both heavy and light) with nonsmokers [61]. Regarding prenatal tobacco exposure, opposing studies have shown that sons of smokers and nonsmokers of varying degree display no significant differences in sperm count [62].

There are a number of reasons for such variation in associations. First, contradictory data could result from a large variation in sample populations—very different blends of normal, sick, healthy, fertile, and infertile men are included in these experiments. Also, the lines between what is considered light, moderate, and heavy smoking are not consistent across different experiments and clinical trials. Thus, it becomes very difficult to control for confounding factors (such as drug use, sexual lifestyle, socioeconomic status, and varying genital examinations), especially in the smoking sample population, and studies regarding the topic fail to reach a consensus on what background factors to screen for when conducting their clinical prospective studies [1]. For example, in a study done by Saleh's group in 2002, men were screened for drinking and recreational drug use in an effort to eliminate bias. Men were also turned away in this study if they had undergone chemotherapy and radiotherapy or had been exposed to pesticides. However, many of the other studies regarding the same topic failed to use these specific inclusion criteria, partially explaining the disagreement seen in medical literature. This scenario reoccurs in the field of smoking-induced male infertility and calls for the standardization of inclusion criteria, allowing multiple studies across differing sample populations to be compared more effectively. It is also challenging to reach an agreement regarding smoking's effect on male infertility because infertility can present from a multitude of factors and altered parameters, only some of which are affected by the contents of cigarette smoke. Finally, the biological, biochemical, and physiological pathways that connect cigarette smoke to male infertility are unknown, and proposed mechanisms in literature (which will be covered in the following section) have yet to be confirmed.

Mechanisms for Smoking-Induced Male Infertility

Although the exact mechanisms by which cigarette smoke leads to male infertility are unknown, several strong speculations exist in medical literature, laying down the foundation for future basic science experiments. The following section will summarize the major theories (see Fig. 2.2) in literature to date.

ROS Mechanisms

A fundamental principle regarding the relationship between smoking and male infertility is the fact that cigarette smoke causes OS. This fact is of particular importance since spermatozoa are highly susceptible to ROS-induced damage since their plasma membranes contain large quantities of polyunsaturated fatty acids (potentially leading to high levels of lipid peroxidation) [63] and low amounts of protective enzymes [41–44]. To further complicate matters, the intracellular antioxidant enzymes spermatozoa do possess cannot protect the plasma membrane that surrounds

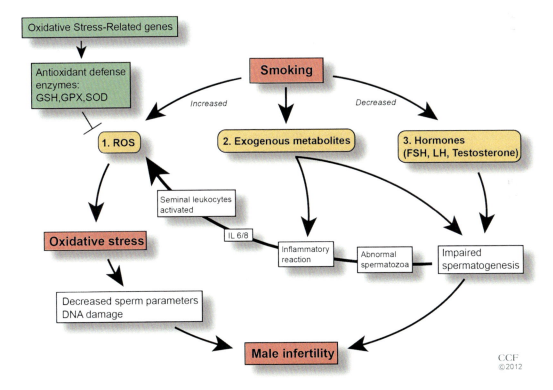

Fig. 2.2 A summary of proposed mechanisms connecting the contents in cigarette smoke to male infertility. (1) Smoking is known to increase ROS which can lead to oxidative stress, DNA damage, morphologically and functionally abnormal sperm, and, eventually, male infertility. (2) Smoking can also increase levels of exogenous metabolites which cause an inflammatory reaction, raising levels of IL6/8, activating seminal leukocytes, which also lead to higher ROS levels. (3) Smoking has also been shown to decrease FSH, LH, and testosterone levels in men, causing impaired spermatogenesis. The increase in abnormal and premature sperm can directly lead to fertility issues and causes a similar inflammatory reaction that increases ROS. (4) Oxidative stress-related genes (*green*) encode enzymes such as GSH, GPX, and SOD which reduce the levels of ROS and impair the pathway leading to oxidative stress and infertility. (*ROS* reactive oxygen species, *FSH* follicle-stimulating hormone, *LH* luteinizing hormone, *GSH* glutathione, *GPX* glutathione peroxidase, *SOD* superoxide dismutase) [Reprinted with permission, Cleveland Clinic Center for Medical Art & Photography © 2012. All Rights Reserved]

the acrosome and tail. As a result, mature spermatozoa are forced to largely rely on seminal plasma for environmental protection. This dependency creates two weaknesses with regard to sperm viability. First, perfectly healthy spermatozoa that reside in poor quality seminal plasma (that is high in ROS levels) can suffer [45]. Second, the small, free-radical scavengers such as uric acid, ascorbate, and ROS-metabolizing enzymes (catalase, glutathione peroxidase, SOD) that lie in seminal plasma constitute the only line of defense between ROS and OS [61].

The epididymal epithelium, also responsible for shielding spermatozoa from ROS, houses antioxidant enzymes. Thus, several OS-related gene families such as epididymal glutathione peroxidases (GPX), glutathione S-transferases (GSTs), and copper-zinc superoxide dismutases (Cozen-SOD) are highly expressed in the epididymis. When ROS levels become elevated in the male reproductive tract, transcription and translation of these protective OS-related genes results. Glutamate cysteine ligase facilitates the biosynthesis of glutathione (GSH), an antioxidant and reducing agent that protects cellular structures from ROS species and peroxides. GPX, another metabolite, protects biological components from oxidative damage by reducing hydroperoxides and hydrogen peroxide to alcohol and water [64]. Finally, CuZn-SODs are copper-zinc-containing enzymes that lower the steady state of the superoxide ion [65]. However, smoking disrupts this delicate balance between antioxidant defense and ROS by adding exogenous ROS in the reproductive tract, leading to OS and male infertility problems. There are several possible ideas about how this pathology occurs at the biological level.

One theory postulates that increased seminal ROS species come from elevated seminal leukocyte concentrations among infertile smokers. Smoking metabolites are thought to induce an inflammatory reaction, releasing interleukins (IL-6 and IL-8) into the male reproductive tract. The interleukins act as immune system mediators, activating leukocytes [28] that produce ROS, overwhelming antioxidant defenses and leading to OS and infertility problems [1, 20]. OS has

been shown repeatedly to have an incredibly damaging effect on spermatozoa membrane quality and DNA integrity [4].

A different mechanism with the same result suggests that the toxic metabolites in smoke impede successful spermatogenesis, increasing the number of abnormal spermatozoa in the male reproductive tract. The presence of these defective cells activates leukocytes that enter the reproductive tract and phagocytose the spermatozoa [13], leading to OS-induced oligospermia and infertility. Finally, increased ROS due to smoking may simply be the result of intrinsic ROS already present in smoke (superoxide anion, hydroxyl radicals, and hydrogen peroxide) [4, 19]. The increased levels of ROS can lead to OS-induced spermatozoa dysfunction, damage to spermatozoa DNA [66], and compromised integrity of the spermatozoa nucleus [67]. The DNA damage that results can facilitate germ cell apoptosis, thereby decreasing sperm counts [68].

On a molecular level, studies have shown that the direct binding of cigarette smoke contents or their metabolic intermediates to DNA can result in chemical DNA adducts [69, 70]. DNA adducts are segments of DNA that are covalently bonded to various chemicals and lead to DNA damage, impaired replication, and even cancer. The ROS in cigarette smoke facilitate the formation of adducts, and this increase has been seen in the embryos of smokers relative to nonsmokers, suggesting the transmission of modified, damaged DNA from parent to offspring due to parental smoking [69].

Toxic Compound and Hormone Mechanisms

In addition to ROS-mediated mechanisms, smoke also contains polycyclic aromatic hydrocarbons (PAHs). PAHs, such as naphthalene and benzopyrene, are highly carcinogenic and have been demonstrated to reduce Sertoli cell function [71] and production of testosterone from Leydig cells [72]. Because the late stages of spermatogenesis are testosterone dependent, spermatozoa formation could be compromised by reduced testosterone concentrations. Also, since the concentrations of testosterone in the testis are 100-fold higher than in blood plasma, even a slight drop of the hormone due to PAHs could lead to a significant reduction in spermatozoa production [71].

Finally, cigarette smoke can lead to male infertility by acting via hormones. For example, nicotine affects reproductive hormone concentrations by changing the hypothalamic-pituitary-gonadal axis via stimulation of growth hormone, vasopressin, and oxytocin. These hormones will then inhibit luteinizing hormone (LH) and prolactin. Studies have also shown that nonsmokers have significantly higher levels of follicle-stimulating hormone (FSH), a molecule secreted by the anterior pituitary gland that acts on the Sertoli cells in males to induce spermatogenesis. Men who smoked more than nine cigarettes a day had 17 % lower FSH concentrations compared to nonsmokers [19].

The relative plausibility of all these theories remains to be determined by scientific experiments. However, because there has been a strong consensus in medical literature that the contents of cigarette smoke causes OS, and OS leads to male infertility, the link between cigarette smoke and infertility seems to follow a logical progression. The majority of results verify this conclusion, but a firm agreement will be difficult to reach until these biochemical mechanisms are tested and verified.

Conclusion

Although the causation between smoking and male infertility has yet to be proven, there is a strong consensus in the literature that smoking is a male infertility risk factor and smokers who are having infertility problems should reduce or preferably stop their tobacco consumption. This conclusion was deduced by two correlations that are well understood and verified in medical literature; (1) cigarette smoke creates ROS species, leading to OS, and (2) OS destroys the quality of spermatozoa, leading to male infertility. Thus, the next logical step would naturally be that the ROS species already present in cigarette

smoke and the new ones induced by seminal leukocytes are causing infertility in males. Currently, there is speculation that if smoking does not directly lead to DNA damage in healthy males, it facilitates the process through OS, resulting in the fertility problems commonly seen in male smokers [1].

However, contradictory studies still exist because of highly variable study design, different patient inclusion criteria, and a lack of agreement as to what is considered low, moderate, and high levels of cigarette use. Thus, even though the majority of studies do find a correlation between cigarette smoke and male infertility, without elucidating a biological mechanism, a final claim cannot be made. This chapter has summarized the major results in studies concerning smoking's effect on male infertility and has demonstrated how there are a myriad of factors from cigarette smoke, outside of just poor semen parameters, that can lead to infertility issues in men.

While there are numerous studies on this topic, further research is needed. First, future studies should aim to stay true to previous inclusion criteria in an effort to develop consistency, making trends easier to ascertain. Next, there is a shortage of reversal studies that clarify whether infertile male smokers who stop their habit will regain their fertility. Lastly, there are several confounding factors in the male smoking population, ranging from drug use to socioeconomic status, that need to be addressed especially when comparing data across various experiments.

Finally, the discussion of cigarette smoke on male infertility presented in this chapter has immediate clinical relevance. Physicians who are advising male smokers with infertility problems should inform them of the consequences of their tobacco consumption (both cigarette and chewing tobacco). Additionally, smoking has been shown to negatively affect assisted reproductive technique (ART) outcomes, and as a result, infertile smokers cannot solely rely on clinical interventions for reproductive success [73]. A daily dose of antioxidants may help neutralize ROS and lessen sperm damage due to OS, but the best option for infertile male smokers remains to quit their use all together.

Key Points

- A third of the world's population over the age of 15 smokes cigarettes daily, and the highest prevalence is among young adult males in their reproductive years.
- The majority of studies find that the spermatozoa of chronic smokers have a decreased fertilization capability and, when coupled to form an embryo, display lower successful implantation rates.
- Cigarette smoke adversely shifts virtually all semen parameters (count, motility, and morphology) away from normal physiological levels. Furthermore, there appears to be no "safe" amount of cigarette smoke intake with regard to semen quality.
- Smoking affects many more elements of fertility besides sperm quality such as seminal plasma, hormones, and accessory sex glands.
- Contradictory studies reporting no significant correlation between cigarette smoke and male infertility do exist in literature, most likely due to an inconsistency in clinical studies with regard to inclusion criteria and controlling for confounding variables.
- Many of the proposed mechanisms explaining smoking-induced male infertility involve an increase in ROS species, leading to OS and reduced sperm quality.
- While there is no firm consensus yet that smoking causes male infertility, it is widely believed that smoking is a male infertility risk factor.
- Infertile male smokers are advised to quit, especially because smoking has also been shown to reduce successful ART outcomes, further reducing the reproductive potential of these men.

References

1. Saleh RA, et al. Effect of cigarette smoking on levels of seminal oxidative stress in infertile men: a prospective study. Fertil Steril. 2002;78(3):491–9.
2. Practice Committee of American Society for Reproductive Medicine. Smoking and infertility. Fertil Steril. 2008;90(5 Suppl):S254–9.
3. Hammond D, et al. Cigarette yields and human exposure: a comparison of alternative testing regimens. Cancer Epidemiol Biomarkers Prev. 2006;15(8): 1495–501.
4. Colagar AH, Jorsaraee GA, Marzony ET. Cigarette smoking and the risk of male infertility. Pak J Biol Sci. 2007;10(21):3870–4.
5. Richthoff J, et al. Association between tobacco exposure and reproductive parameters in adolescent males. Int J Androl. 2008;31(1):31–9.
6. Chia SE, et al. Effect of cadmium and cigarette smoking on human semen quality. Int J Fertil Menopausal Stud. 1994;39(5):292–8.
7. Saaranen M, et al. Human seminal plasma cadmium: comparison with fertility and smoking habits. Andrologia. 1989;21(2):140–5.
8. Keck C, Bramkamp G, Behre HM, Muller C, Jockenhovel F, Nieschlag E. Lack of correlation between cadmium in seminal plasma and fertility status of nonexposed individuals and two cadmium-exposed patients. Reprod Toxicol. 1995;9:35–40.
9. Edwards K, et al. Mainstream and sidestream cigarette smoke condensates suppress macrophage responsiveness to interferon gamma. Hum Exp Toxicol. 1999; 18(4):233–40.
10. Said TM, Ranga G, Agarwal A. Relationship between semen quality and tobacco chewing in men undergoing infertility evaluation. Fertil Steril. 2005;84(3): 649–53.
11. Soares SR, et al. Cigarette smoking affects uterine receptiveness. Hum Reprod. 2007;22(2):543–7.
12. Ramlau-Hansen CH, et al. Parental subfecundity and risk of decreased semen quality in the male offspring: a follow-up study. Am J Epidemiol. 2008;167(12): 1458–64.
13. Gaur DS, Talekar M, Pathak VP. Effect of cigarette smoking on semen quality of infertile men. Singapore Med J. 2007;48(2):119–23.
14. Gornig VM, Schirren C. [Effect of exogenous toxins on fertility]. Fortschr Med. 1996;114(14):169–71.
15. Oyeyipo IP, Raji Y, Emikpe BO, Bolarinwa AF. Effects of nicotine on sperm characteristics and fertility profile in adult male rats: a possible role of cessation. J Reprod Infertil. 2011;12:201–7.
16. Close CE, Roberts PL, Berger RE. Cigarettes, alcohol and marijuana are related to pyospermia in infertile men. J Urol. 1990;144(4):900–3.
17. Ochedalski T, et al. [Evaluating the effect of smoking tobacco on some semen parameters in men of reproductive age]. Ginekol Pol. 1994;65(2):80–6.
18. Kunzle R, et al. Semen quality of male smokers and nonsmokers in infertile couples. Fertil Steril. 2003; 79(2):287–91.
19. Ramlau-Hansen CH, et al. Is smoking a risk factor for decreased semen quality? A cross-sectional analysis. Hum Reprod. 2007;22(1):188–96.
20. Reina Bouvet B, Vicenta Paparella C, Nestor Feldman R. [Effect of tobacco consumption on the spermatogenesis in males with idiopathic infertility]. Arch Esp Urol. 2007;60(3):273–7.
21. Vine MF. Smoking and male reproduction: a review. Int J Androl. 1996;19:323–37.

22. Merino G, Lira SC, Martinez-Chequer JC. Effects of cigarette smoking on semen characteristics of a population in Mexico. Arch Androl. 1998;41(1):11–5.
23. Zhang JP, et al. Effect of smoking on semen quality of infertile men in Shandong, China. Asian J Androl. 2000;2(2):143–6.
24. Shaarawy M, Mahmoud KZ. Endocrine profile and semen characteristics in male smokers. Fertil Steril. 1982;38(2):255–7.
25. Rantala ML, Koskimies AI. Semen quality of infertile couples—comparison between smokers and non-smokers. Andrologia. 1987;19(1):42–6.
26. Saaranen M, et al. Cigarette smoking and semen quality in men of reproductive age. Andrologia. 1987; 19(6):670–6.
27. Chia SE, Ong CN, Tsakok FM. Effects of cigarette smoking on human semen quality. Arch Androl. 1994;33(3):163–8.
28. Hassa H, et al. Effect of smoking on semen parameters of men attending an infertility clinic. Clin Exp Obstet Gynecol. 2006;33(1):19–22.
29. Moskova P, Popov I. Sperm quality in smokers and nonsmokers among infertile families. Akush Ginekol (Sofiia). 1993;32(1):28–30.
30. Mak V, et al. Smoking is associated with the retention of cytoplasm by human spermatozoa. Urology. 2000; 56(3):463–6.
31. Zavos PM, et al. An electron microscope study of the axonemal ultrastructure in human spermatozoa from male smokers and nonsmokers. Fertil Steril. 1998;69(3):430–4.
32. Yeung CH, et al. Coiled sperm from infertile patients: characteristics, associated factors and biological implication. Hum Reprod. 2009;24(6):1288–95.
33. Gerhard I, et al. Relationship of sperm acrosin activity to semen and clinical parameters in infertile patients. Andrologia. 1989;21(2):146–54.
34. Arabi M, Moshtaghi H. Influence of cigarette smoking on spermatozoa via seminal plasma. Andrologia. 2005;37(4):119–24.
35. Pakrashi A, Chatterjee S. Effect of tobacco consumption on the function of male accessory sex glands. Int J Androl. 1995;18(5):232–6.
36. Kothari S, et al. Free radicals: their beneficial and detrimental effects on sperm function. Indian J Exp Biol. 2010;48(5):425–35.
37. Dawson EB, et al. Effect of ascorbic acid supplementation on the sperm quality of smokers. Fertil Steril. 1992;58(5):1034–9.
38. Smith JL, Hodges RE. Serum levels of vitamin C in relation to dietary and supplemental intake of vitamin C in smokers and nonsmokers. Ann N Y Acad Sci. 1987;498:144–52.
39. El-Karaksy A, et al. Seminal mast cells in infertile asthenozoospermic males. Andrologia. 2007;39(6): 244–7.
40. Elshal MF, et al. Sperm head defects and disturbances in spermatozoal chromatin and DNA integrities in idiopathic infertile subjects: association with cigarette smoking. Clin Biochem. 2009;42(7–8):589–94.

41. Sepaniak S, et al. [Negative impact of cigarette smoking on male fertility: from spermatozoa to the offspring]. J Gynecol Obstet Biol Reprod (Paris). 2004;33(5):384–90.
42. Lahdetie J. Micronucleated spermatids in the seminal fluid of smokers and nonsmokers. Mutat Res. 1986; 172(3):255–63.
43. Sokol RZ, Mishell DR, Lobo RA, editors. The year book of infertility and reproductive endocrinology. St. Louis, MO: Mosby Elsevier Health Science; 1996.
44. Sun JG, Jurisicova A, Casper RF. Detection of deoxyribonucleic acid fragmentation in human sperm: correlation with fertilization in vitro. Biol Reprod. 1997;56(3):602–7.
45. Viloria T, et al. Sperm selection by swim-up in terms of deoxyribonucleic acid fragmentation as measured by the sperm chromatin dispersion test is altered in heavy smokers. Fertil Steril. 2007;88(2):523–5.
46. Shi Q, et al. Cigarette smoking and aneuploidy in human sperm. Mol Reprod Dev. 2001;59(4):417–21.
47. Klaiber EL, et al. Interrelationships of cigarette smoking, testicular varicoceles, and seminal fluid indexes. Fertil Steril. 1987;47(3):481–6.
48. Pasqualotto FF, et al. Cigarette smoking is related to a decrease in semen volume in a population of fertile men. BJU Int. 2006;97(2):324–6.
49. Bates C, et al. European Union policy on smokeless tobacco: a statement in favour of evidence based regulation for public health. Tob Control. 2003;12(4): 360–7.
50. Rodu B, Cole P. Smokeless tobacco use and cancer of the upper respiratory tract. Oral Surg Oral Med Oral Pathol Oral Radiol Endod. 2002;93(5):511–5.
51. Asplund K. Smokeless tobacco and cardiovascular disease. Prog Cardiovasc Dis. 2003;45(5):383–94.
52. Lando HA, et al. Smokeless tobacco use in a population of young adults. Addict Behav. 1999;24(3): 431–7.
53. Baird DD, Wilcox AJ. Future fertility after prenatal exposure to cigarette smoke. Fertil Steril. 1986;46(3): 368–72.
54. Dikshit RK, Buch JG, Mansuri SM. Effect of tobacco consumption on semen quality of a population of hypofertile males. Fertil Steril. 1987;48(2):334–6.
55. Goverde HJ, et al. Semen quality and frequency of smoking and alcohol consumption—an explorative study. Int J Fertil Menopausal Stud. 1995;40(3): 135–8.
56. de Mouzon J, Spira A, Schwartz D. A prospective study of the relation between smoking and fertility. Int J Epidemiol. 1988;17(2):378–84.
57. Holzki G, Gall H, Hermann J. Cigarette smoking and sperm quality. Andrologia. 1991;23(2):141–4.
58. Dunphy BC, et al. Male cigarette smoking and fecundity in couples attending an infertility clinic. Andrologia. 1991;23(3):223–5.
59. Osser S, Beckman-Ramirez A, Liedholm P. Semen quality of smoking and non-smoking men in infertile couples in a Swedish population. Acta Obstet Gynecol Scand. 1992;71(3):215–8.

60. Oldereid NB, et al. Cigarette smoking and human sperm quality assessed by laser-Doppler spectroscopy and DNA flow cytometry. J Reprod Fertil. 1989; 86(2):731–6.
61. Sergerie M, et al. Lack of association between smoking and DNA fragmentation in the spermatozoa of normal men. Hum Reprod. 2000;15(6):1314–21.
62. Jensen MS, et al. Lower sperm counts following prenatal tobacco exposure. Hum Reprod. 2005;20(9): 2559–66.
63. Hassan A, et al. Seminal plasma cotinine and insulin-like growth factor-I in idiopathic oligoasthenoteratozoospermic smokers. BJU Int. 2009;103(1): 108–11.
64. Jervis KM, Robaire B. Dynamic changes in gene expression along the rat epididymis. Biol Reprod. 2001;65(3):696–703.
65. Valentine JS, Doucette PA, Zittin Potter S. Copperzinc superoxide dismutase and amyotrophic lateral sclerosis. Annu Rev Biochem. 2005;74:563–93.
66. Aitken RJ, Baker MA. Oxidative stress, sperm survival and fertility control. Mol Cell Endocrinol. 2006;250(1–2):66–9.
67. Agarwal A, Saleh RA. Role of oxidants in male infertility: rationale, significance, and treatment. Urol Clin North Am. 2002;29(4):817–27.
68. Agarwal A, Allamaneni SS. The effect of sperm DNA damage on assisted reproduction outcomes. A review. Minerva Ginecol. 2004;56(3):235–45.
69. Zenzes MT, Bielecki R, Reed TE. Detection of benzo(a)pyrene diol epoxide-DNA adducts in sperm of men exposed to cigarette smoke. Fertil Steril. 1999;72(2):330–5.
70. Fraga CG, et al. Ascorbic acid protects against endogenous oxidative DNA damage in human sperm. Proc Natl Acad Sci U S A. 1991;88(24):11003–6.
71. Raychoudhury SS, Kubinski D. Polycyclic aromatic hydrocarbon-induced cytotoxicity in cultured rat Sertoli cells involves differential apoptotic response. Environ Health Perspect. 2003;111(1):33–8.
72. Inyang F, et al. Disruption of testicular steroidogenesis and epididymal function by inhaled benzo(a) pyrene. Reprod Toxicol. 2003;17(5):527–37.
73. Waylen AL, et al. Effects of cigarette smoking upon clinical outcomes of assisted reproduction: a meta-analysis. Hum Reprod Update. 2009;15(1):31–44.

BMI and Obesity

3

Karishma Khullar, Ashok Agarwal, and Stefan S. du Plessis

Introduction

Obesity, defined by the World Health Organization (WHO) as "abnormal or excessive fat accumulation that may impair health," is a detrimental trend that has been rising worldwide, doubling from 1980 to 2008 [1]. More specifically, the WHO estimates that more than 1.5 billion adults over the age of 20 are overweight and that one in ten adults in the world are obese [1]. It has been suggested that this rising trend of excessive adipose tissue accumulation has not only been caused by an increase in high-sugar and cholesterol-saturated diets, but also by an increase in sedentary lifestyles [1]. While obesity has been associated with a host of cardiovascular disease, the metabolic syndrome, and a wide variety of endocrine abnormalities, recent research has suggested a potential link between obesity and male infertility [2–4]. This association has merited investigation over the past decade because of the concurrent trends of rising obesity, increasing male factor infertility, and declining semen quality [5, 6]. Through comprehensive analysis of studies and reviews on obesity and infertility, this chapter aims to elucidate the hormonal abnormalities caused by obesity, its effect—if any—on semen parameters, and possible lifestyle modifications to alleviate the adverse effects of obesity. Ultimately, this chapter will hopefully serve as a consolidation of important and novel information on the rising concerns of obesity and male infertility.

One most common tool of weight measurement used by both the WHO and researchers alike is body mass index (BMI). Specifically, BMI is a ratio of an individual's weight in kilograms divided by his height squared in meters. The WHO has set forth standards to classify individuals as underweight, normal, overweight or obese. In particular, a BMI of 18.5–24.99 kg/m^2 is classified as normal, 25–29.99 kg/m^2 as overweight, 30–34.99 kg/m^2 as class I obesity, 35–39.99 kg/m^2 as severely obese, and a BMI greater than 40 kg/m^2 as morbidly obese [1]. While BMI is one of the most common methods for measuring body fat, its effectiveness in assessing visceral fat—the type of fat that is thought to contribute the most to the adverse effects of obesity—has been called into question

K. Khullar, BA • A. Agarwal, PhD
Center for Reproductive Medicine,
Cleveland Clinic Foundation/Glickman Urological
and Kidney Institute, 10681 Carnegie Avenue,
Cleveland, OH 44195, USA
e-mail: khullar.karishma@gmail.com;
agarwaa@ccf.org

S.S. du Plessis, BSc (Hons), MSc, MBA,
PhD (Stell) (✉)
Division of Medical Physiology, Department
of Biomedical Sciences, Faculty of Medicine
and Health Sciences, Stellenbosch University,
Tygerberg, Western Cape, South Africa
e-mail: ssdp@sun.ac.za

S.S. du Plessis et al. (eds.), *Male Infertility: A Complete Guide to Lifestyle and Environmental Factors*,
DOI 10.1007/978-1-4939-1040-3_3, © Springer Science+Business Media New York 2014

in recent years. This is likely due to the fact that weight is not directly correlated to fat, since muscle weight differs from fat. As an alternative to utilizing BMI, researchers have started to utilize measures such as waist-to-hip ratio (WHR), waist circumference, abdominal sagittal diameter, computer tomography, magnetic resonance imaging, and ultrasonography [7]. With regard to WHR, a study published by Noble in The Western Journal of Medicine reported that WHR was better correlated than BMI in obese and overweight patients with high cholesterol [8]. Because adipose tissue tends to accumulate around the midsection, it has been suggested that measuring WHR can properly identify the obese and overweight patients better than BMI. However, BMI remains the most popular method of measurement for assessing obesity, since WHR measurement is a relatively new method. Because of the different measurement systems available to classify obesity, this chapter pays special attention to the manner in which each study recorded their results and made sure that the results are comprehensible based on the standards set by the WHO.

Adipose Tissue, Adipocytokines, and Reactive Oxygen Species

Until very recently, adipose tissue had been merely regarded as a passive storage organ for fat. However, recent studies and discoveries of adipose-specific hormones have illuminated its endocrine function. Adipose tissue secretes two main classes of molecules known as adipocytokines and adipose-derived hormones. These substances are especially significant because they have been implicated in creating a chronic state of inflammation and hyperinsulinemia in obese individuals, both of which have been associated with abnormal reproductive function. While interleukin-6 (IL-6) and tumor necrosis factor alpha (TNF-α) are classified as important adipocytokines, which are cell-to-cell signaling proteins, leptin, adiponectin, and resistin are characterized as adipose-derived hormones which are secreted by adipose tissue [9, 10]. While leptin and adiponectin play a role in

increasing insulin sensitivity, resistin, IL-6, and possibly TNF-α are crucial in the development of insulin resistance. Some studies suggest that the insulin resistance promoted by certain adipocytokines is caused by the oxidation of free fatty acids. The oxidation of the fatty acids creates ATP for gluconeogenesis, thereby increasing glucose levels and potentially creating hyperinsulinemia and decreased spermatogenesis [7].

In addition to adipocytokines and adipose-specific hormones compromising male fertility via creating hyperinsulinemia, some play a role in generating reactive oxygen species (ROS). ROS are a group of free radical molecules that contribute to oxidative stress in the body. Oxidative stress, an imbalance between ROS and antioxidant defense mechanisms, has been implicated in adversely affecting semen parameters and male fertility [11]. With regard to adipocytokines and obesity, both IL-6 and TNF-α promote leucocyte production of ROS. Moreover, leptin has also been linked to increased oxidative stress. While further research is needed to substantiate the effect of BMI on ROS and semen quality, Tunc et al. found a small but statistically significant correlation between BMI and seminal macrophage activation. However, the effect of such ROS production on semen parameters is unclear, given that the study found no significant decrease in sperm DNA integrity or motility [12]. Thus, while adipocytokines have important endocrine functions and consequences for the male reproductive system, the effect on eventual reproductive potential remains debatable.

Relationship Between Obesity, Sperm Parameters, and Reproductive Potential

Since the trend in rising obesity has been accompanied by a trend of decreasing sperm quality, many scientists have investigated the effect of obesity on sperm parameters. Some of the sperm characteristics that have been evaluated include motility, morphology, viability, concentration, count, and DNA damage. However, studies conducted over the past decade have not yielded consistent results. For example, while Jensen et al. reported in 2004 a lower sperm concentration, count, and percentage of normal spermatozoa for men with a BMI higher than 25, Fejes et al. only found significant correlations using a different measure of fat merely a year later (Jensen et al.). Specifically, Fejes et al. found that both hip and waist circumference were negatively correlated with total sperm count and motility and that hip circumference was negatively correlated with sperm concentration [13]. While both of these studies reported an association between increased body weight and semen parameters, the difference in measurement methods for body fat demonstrates the difficulty in achieving standardized results. Evidence of body weight affecting semen parameters is furthered by Sallmen et al. and Hammoud et al. who found that BMI has a direct negative correlation to sperm parameters and that BMI is associated with low motile sperm count and low sperm concentration in 2006 and 2008 respectively [5, 14]. Moreover, in 2010, Martini et al. reported no association between sperm concentration and a negative association between BMI and sperm motility, while Hofny et al. found that BMI had a positive correlation with abnormal sperm morphology and a negative correlation with sperm concentration, motility, and testosterone [15, 16]. Additionally, Stewart and Tunc et al. both found that there was a significantly lower sperm concentration in obese men in 2010 [12, 17]. Similarly, a 2011 study by Shayeb et al. suggested that obese men are more likely than those with a normal BMI to have a lower semen volume and a lower amount of morphologically normal spermatozoa [18]. More recently, Fariello et al. found that the progressive motility of sperm was significantly lower in obese and overweight males than in those with a normal BMI. They also found that obese men had a higher percentage of sperm with DNA fragmentation than overweight and normal males [19]. Such results are further substantiated by Hammiche et al. who found that being overweight was negatively associated with progressive motility of sperm and that being obese was negatively associated with ejaculate volume, sperm concentration, and total motile sperm

count using BMI measures. They found similar associations when using waist circumference as a measure, with a waist circumference greater than or equal to 102 cm being inversely associated with sperm concentration and total motile sperm count [20]. Moreover, in their 2012 study, Sermondade et al. reported that overweight and obese men were at significantly higher risk of presenting with oligozoospermia or azoospermia compared to those of normal weight [21]. Finally, La Vignera et al. found that overweight and obese men had a significantly lower amount of spermatozoa with progressive motility and a higher percentage of spermatozoa with decondensed chromatin. They also reported that only obese men showed a lower percentage of normally shaped spermatozoa, a lower percentage of viable spermatozoa, and a higher percentage of spermatozoa with DNA fragmentation [22].

While there are a host of studies that show a negative correlation between increased BMI and sperm parameters, such studies must be treated with caution given the numerous studies that have reported results to the contrary. In particular, Zorn et al. found that BMI was not correlated with BMI in 2006 and Aggerholm et al. reported no significant differences between sperm count and BMI in 2007 [23, 24]. Such evidence was further validated by Pauli et al. who reported that there was no association between BMI and the semen parameters of density, volume, motility, and morphology in 2008 [25]. More recently, Rybar et al. reported that BMI did not significantly affect semen parameters and Chavarro et al. found that obese men had no statistically significant differences in sperm concentration, sperm morphology or sperm motility in 2010 [6, 26]. In fact, Chavarro et al. only found lower sperm count and an increased amount of DNA damage among obese men who had a BMI greater than 35. This suggests that the effect of BMI on semen parameters, if any, is restricted to only the most extreme cases of obesity [26]. Furthermore, while Lotti et al. reported that males with a higher BMI may have signs of prostate inflammation—such as higher prostate volume, higher levels of interleukin-8, and color-Doppler ultrasound features including macro-calcifications, inhomogeneity, and higher arterial peak systolic velocity—no association was found between BMI and semen parameters [27]. Thus, although support exists for the claim that obesity affects reproductive potential, many studies have been published showing no connection between BMI and sperm parameters, thereby making the link between obesity and infertility controversial. The results of studies investigating the relationship between BMI and semen parameters are summarized in Table 3.1.

Hormonal Abnormalities in Obesity

While the effect of obesity on semen parameters remains widely debated, the hormonal abnormalities present in individuals with increased BMI are better understood. In normal males, the hypothalamic-pituitary-gonadal (HPG) axis, a neuroendocrine system, ensures that the reproductive system functions properly. Specifically, the hypothalamus secretes gonadotropin-releasing hormone (GnRH) which binds to receptors connected with G proteins on the plasma membrane of pituitary gonadotrophs. Such interaction between GnRH and the receptors facilitates the release of both luteinizing hormone (LH) and follicle-stimulating hormone (FSH). Subsequently, LH binds to receptors on the plasma membrane of Leydig cells, which results in the formation of enzymes involved in testosterone synthesis. Both testosterone and estrogen control LH secretion through negative feedback [28]. While proper HPG function has been demonstrated in individuals with normal BMI, studies have shown that obesity causes dysregulation of the axis by promoting hormonal abnormalities.

In particular, obesity has been associated with decreased levels of testosterone and increased levels of estrogen in numerous studies, thereby suggesting that obesity has an adverse effect on the male reproductive system [13, 16, 23–26, 29–31]. The suggested mechanism by which this decreased testosterone:estrogen ratio presents in obese individuals is through increased activity of the cytochrome p450 aromatase enzyme, which converts androgens to estrogens [32, 33]. More specifically, aromatase is an enzyme of the cytochrome p450 family and it is produced from the CYP19 gene. The number of tetranucleotide repeats in intron 4 of the gene has been significantly linked to the increased amount of activity thereof. In 2010, Hammoud et al. reported that among severely obese men, increased aromatase activity and estrogen levels were only seen among those who had an increased number of tetranucleotide repeats [34]. Such a finding suggests that genetics, rather than obesity itself, may be the chief contributor to the abnormal levels of testosterone and estrogen in individuals with increased body weight. Nevertheless, since many studies have not yet examined the genetic influence on aromatase, further research is needed to determine the exact mechanism of aromatase activity in obese individuals.

Another hormonal irregularity that has been reported in obese individuals is an increase in leptin levels [16, 23]. Leptin is a protein hormone that is controlled by the Ob-gene and secreted by adipocytes. Its physiological role in the body is to regulate body weight, but the excess levels that have been reported in obese individuals can have adverse effects, particularly on the male reproductive system [9, 23, 33, 35]. Two pathological mechanisms, direct and indirect, have been proposed to account for decreased gonadotropin secretion and spermatogenesis in obese individuals. Normally, Leydig cells stimulate protein kinase A in response to luteinizing hormone and promote steroidogenesis. However, under the direct pathological mechanism, demonstrated most clearly in rats, increased levels of leptin cross the blood–testis barrier. Leptin then acts on Leydig cells to decrease the steroidogenic factor, steroidogenic acute regulatory protein, and steroidogenic mRNAs, thereby inhibiting testosterone secretion. While leptin's site of action in the direct pathological mechanism is the testis, the indirect mechanism involves the hypothalamus. Normally, leptin crosses the blood–brain barrier through a saturable transport system and binds to leptin receptors on kisspeptin neurons in the brain in order to stimulate gonadotropin release. However, in obese individuals, the increased

3 BMI and Obesity

Table 3.1 Research studies of the effects of BMI on the reproductive system

Author	Year published	Findings related to sperm parameters	Findings related to hormones
Chavarro et al.	2010	No statistically significant differences in sperm concentration, sperm morphology or sperm motility for obese males. Only those with a BMI greater than 35 had lower sperm count and higher DNA damage.	There were inverse associations of BMI with serum levels of total testosterone, SHBG, and inhibin B, and a positive association with serum estradiol level.
Winters et al.	2006	–	Inhibin B levels declined with increasing obesity in young men (26 % lower). SHBG and total testosterone were also lower with increasing BMI, but FSH/LH were unaffected.
Zorn et al.	2006	No relationship was found between level of leptin and sperm motility, and morphology. Leptin was correlated negatively with sperm count but this correlation was not present when BMI was used as a control variable.	BMI was negatively correlated with inhibin B, total testosterone, and SHBG.
Martini et al.	2010	Negative association found between BMI and motility and rapid motility. No associations between BMI and sperm concentration or testosterone.	Negative association was found between BMI and NAG levels and a positive correlation between BMI and fructose levels.
Pauli et al.	2008	No correlation between BMI and skinfold thickness with semen parameters (density, volume, motility, and morphology). Men with paternity had lower BMIs and skinfold thickness.	BMI was negatively correlated with testosterone, FSH, and inhibin and testosterone. BMI was also positively correlated with estrogen.
Hofny et al.	2010	BMI had positive correlation with abnormal sperm morphology and negative correlation with sperm concentration and motility.	Obese oligozoospermic had increase in BMI, FSH, LH, estrogen, PRL, and leptin levels. BMI also had a negative correlation with testosterone.
Aggerholm et al.	2007	Overweight had lower sperm count and concentration than normal individuals, but obese did not show reduction in sperm count surprisingly. None of these differences were significant.	Testosterone and inhibin B were lower in obese men compared to normal men, while estrogen was higher.
Fejes et al.	2005	There was a negative correlation between hip circumference and sperm concentration Both hip circumference and waist circumference were negatively correlated with total count and motility. Semen volume was correlated with waist circumference and waist/hip ratio.	BMI and WHR correlated negatively with testosterone, SHBG, and testosterone: estrogen ratio.
Hammond et al.	2008	BMI associated with low sperm concentration and low motile sperm count.	–
Rybar et al.	2010	BMI was not significant in affecting sperm parameters.	–
Sallmen et al.	2006	BMI has a direct negative correlation to sperm parameters.	–
Tunc et al.	2010	Oxidative stress did increase with an increase in BMI due to increase in seminal macrophage activation. But magnitude of increase was small since there was no associated decline in DNA sperm integrity or sperm motility with increasing ROS production. Increased BMI was also found to be linked with a fall in sperm concentration.	Increased BMI was also associated with a fall in testosterone and an increase in estrogen.

(continued)

Table 3.1 (continued)

Author	Year published	Findings related to sperm parameters	Findings related to hormones
Jensen et al.	2004	Men with a BMI higher than 25 had a reduction in sperm concentration and total count compared to men with BMI between 20 and 25. Percentage of normal spermatozoa was reduced in men with high BMI but this was not significant. Volume and percent motility was unaffected.	Serum testosterone, SHBG, inhibin B was decreased with increasing BMI and estrogen was increased.
Stewart	2009	There was a significantly lower sperm concentration in obese men, but this was not accompanied by significant correlations between BMI and any other semen variable.	BMI and obesity had significant inverse correlations with SHBG, inhibin B, and testosterone.
Monti et al.	2006	–	Leptin increases and ghrelin decreases were linear over five BMI groups. There was no threshold of BMI where hormone levels change abruptly.
Lotti et al.	2011	While a higher BMI was associated with indicators of prostate inflammation, no correlation was found between BMI and semen parameters.	–
Shayeb et al.	2011	Obese men are more likely than those with a normal BMI to have a lower semen concentration and a lower amount of spermatozoa with normal morphology.	–
Fariello et al.	2012	Obese and overweight males had lower progressive sperm motility than normal males. Moreover, obese males had a higher percentage of sperm with DNA fragmentation than overweight and normal males.	–
Hammiche et al.	2012	Being overweight was negatively associated with progressive motility of sperm and being obese was negatively associated with ejaculate volume, sperm concentration, and total motile sperm count using BMI measures. Moreover, a waist circumference ≥ 102 cm was inversely associated with sperm concentration and total motile sperm count.	–
Sermondade et al.	2012	Men who were overweight or obese had a significantly increased risk of presenting with oligozoospermia or azoospermia than men of normal weight.	–
La Vignera et al.	2012	Overweight and obese men had a significantly lower amount of spermatozoa with progressive motility and a higher percentage of spermatozoa with decondensed chromatin, but only obese men showed a lower percentage of normally shaped spermatozoa, a lower percentage of viable spermatozoa, and a higher percentage of spermatozoa with DNA fragmentation.	17ß-Estradiol and SHBG were significantly higher in both overweight and obese men compared with those of normal weight.

levels of leptin saturate the blood–brain barrier and do not allow the hypothalamus to be sufficiently activated to release gonadotropins. Thus, at the hypothalamic level, it is actually a deficiency of leptin that inhibits gonadotropin release despite an excess of the hormone being present in the body [33, 36]. More recently, Teerds et al. have also posited consequences for

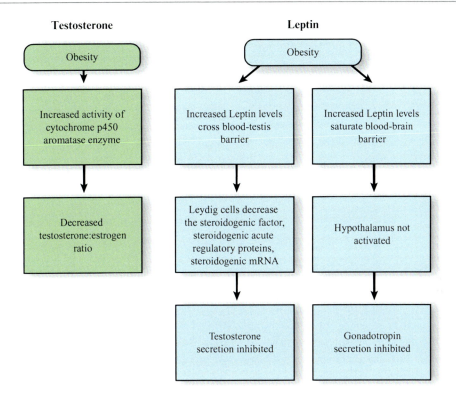

Fig. 3.1 Possible obesity-induced pathological mechanistic pathways for testosterone and leptin

the elevated leptin levels in obese males based upon animal models. Specifically, they suggest that increased leptin levels could result in elevated expression of neuropeptide Y (NPY) and a reduction of the stimulatory effect of leptin on kisspeptin. Both of these consequences combined may adversely affect the HPG axis and male fertility [30]. The possible pathological mechanistic pathways are illustrated in Fig. 3.1.

Not only are leptin levels disrupted as BMI increases, but ghrelin levels are abnormal as well. Ghrelin is a hormone that is produced mainly in the oxyntic glands of the stomach as well as the intestine and, unlike leptin, it plays an important role in increasing appetite. Moreover, it also influences the male reproductive system through its effects on steroidogenesis and testosterone secretion. In particular, ghrelin binds to ghrelin receptors which are more commonly found in the testis than in other locations in the body [37]. It has the ability to decrease testosterone secretion by inhibiting enzymes involved in steroidogenesis such as steroid acute regulatory protein (StAR), the P450 cholesterol side-chain cleavage, the 3β-hydroxysteroid dehydrogenase, and the 17β-hydroxysteroid dehydrogenase type 3 enzymes. In those who are obese, normal function of ghrelin is disrupted and low levels of the hormone have been reported. While further research is needed to determine the precise mechanism responsible for this decrease, it has been suggested in both animal and human studies that testosterone may control the expression of ghrelin receptors. Since low levels of testosterone are well demonstrated in obese men, such an explanation for low ghrelin levels is quite plausible [37, 38].

Along with testosterone, estrogen, leptin, and ghrelin, another hormonal irregularity that has been shown in obese individuals is a decrease in inhibin B levels [24–26, 29, 31]. Generated by Sertoli cells, inhibin B plays a vital role in the inhibition of both FSH and testosterone production. Usually, inhibin B binds to the Activin

Type II receptor in order to inhibin activin, which has a stimulatory effect on FSH. Yet, not all activin tissues are deactivated. Rather, it has been suggested that inhibin acts in the pituitary by binding to p120 and betaglylcan, two newly discovered inhibin receptors [29, 39]. In individuals with an increased BMI, the decreased levels of inhibin B signals an abnormality in the hypothalamic-pituitary-axis (HPA), since the reduced amount of inhibin B does not result in the expected increase in FSH levels. While the exact pathological mechanism is unclear, decreased inhibin B levels in obese men have nevertheless been associated with abnormal spermatogenesis and infertility [25, 40]. More recently, Robeva et al. reported a significant decrease in inhibin B levels in obese males with metabolic syndrome and noted that obesity was independently associated with the hormonal disturbances of the syndrome. They suggested that the decrease in inhibin B was associated with abnormal spermatogenesis, thereby further substantiating the link between obesity-induced abnormalities in inhibin B and male infertility [41].

Another hormone which potentially indicates obesity-induced abnormalities in the hypothalamic-pituitary-testicular axis is resistin. Resistin is a protein that has been linked with both regulating adipogenesis and promoting insulin resistance. Specifically, gene expression is stimulated during adipocyte differentiation and resistin is secreted by mature adipocyte cells. Because resistin is secreted by adipocytes, it is unsurprising that some studies have found increased levels in obese men. Such an increase in resistin levels has been proposed to adversely affect male reproduction primarily because resistin promotes insulin resistance [7, 10]. While the mechanistic pathway of resistin is controversial in humans, Luo et al. suggest that resistin exerts its effect on HepG2 cells by signaling the suppressor of cytokine signaling 3 (SOCS-3) pathway, stimulating the expression of glucose-6-phosphatase and phosphoenolypyruvate carboxykinase, and inhibiting the expressions of insulin receptor substrate 2 and glucose transporter 2. Moreover, resistin suppresses the insulin-induced phosphorylation of Akt though an AMPK-independent mechanism [42]. Not only is hyperinsulinemia associated with infertility and reduced spermatogenesis, but it also affects levels of Sex-Hormone-Binding Globulin (SHBG), which normally binds to estrogen and testosterone to suppress their activity. In obese men, studies have reported a decrease in SHBG, which amounts to a surplus of circulating estrogen. This excess of estrogen further enhances the negative feedback upon gonadotropin release and compromises the efficiency of the male reproductive system [13, 23, 26, 29–31, 43].

Physical Ramifications of Obesity

Not only does obesity adversely affect hormone levels, but it is associated with detrimental physical effects as well. Two significant physical consequences of obesity include increased incidence of erectile dysfunction and increased scrotal temperature. Specifically, erectile dysfunction—the inability to achieve or maintain an erection during sexual activity—is one of the most prominent unfavorable physical manifestations of increased BMI. Obesity has been linked with a 30 % greater risk of erectile dysfunction and 76 % of men with erectile dysfunction or reduced libido are overweight or obese [25, 44]. It contributes to erectile dysfunction through two main pathways. First, obesity promotes increased activation of the renin-angiotensin system. This system promotes vasoconstriction and disrupts the endothelial lining of the penile vasculature, thereby causing erectile dysfunction. Second, as aforementioned, adipocytokines play an instrumental role in creating chronic inflammation in obese individuals and such inflammation can promote erectile dysfunction. In particular, IL-6 and TNF-α disrupt the penile endothelium by creating high levels of ROS, which decrease Nitric Oxide Synthase (NOS) cofactor tetrahydrobiopterin and delay the hydrolysis of NOS inhibitor asymmetric dimethylarginine (ADMA). Obesity-induced interference with such molecules causes erectile dysfunction because nitric oxide has been associated with facilitating a normal erection [45]. The potential obesity-induced

Fig. 3.2 Potential obesity-induced pathways contributing to erectile dysfunction

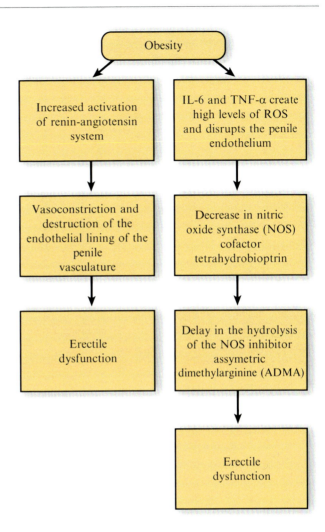

pathways contributing to erectile dysfunction are illustrated in Fig. 3.2.

Not only is erectile dysfunction a detrimental physical manifestation of obesity, but increased scrotal temperature is a negative consequence as well [31]. Normally, testicular temperature is three degrees lower than body temperature and helps to promote spermatogenesis; thus, even small increases in scrotal temperature—denoted as testicular heat stress—can impair male reproductive function [33, 46]. The adverse effects of heat stress on male reproduction is demonstrated by a study conducted by Mieusset et al, which found that an induction of testicular heat stress significantly decreased spermatogenesis, sperm motility, and sperm count [47]. A more recent study which furthered these results was conducted by Hjollund et al. in 2000. This study reported that males who had elevated scrotal temperatures showed decreased sperm concentration and sperm count [46]. While many sources of testicular heat stress have been proposed, obesity has been seen as a major contributor to increased scrotal temperature in recent years. Though no studies report scrotal temperatures in obese populations, obese males nevertheless accumulate fat around the suprapubic region due to their inactive lifestyle and excess adipose tissue, thereby potentially producing a high amount of testicular heat stress. Such stress adversely affects reproductive potential by contributing to abnormally low sperm parameters [33, 48, 49]. The precise pathological mechanism of heat stress on infertility in humans remains unclear, but studies conducted in mice suggest that testicular heat stress affects spermatogenesis by disrupting junctions in the seminiferous tubules and inducing transforming growth factor-beta [50]. Thus, obesity plays an instrumental role in creating physical barriers—erectile dysfunction and testicular heat stress—to successful male reproduction.

Proteomics and Obesity

While hormonal and physical effects of obesity have been investigated heavily in recent years, the effects of increased BMI on a molecular level remain ambiguous. Nevertheless, recent research is starting to elucidate the association between proteins and obesity. In particular, a study of the sperm proteome by Kriegel et al. found that nine sperm proteins were associated with obesity by utilizing the difference gel electrophoresis (DIGE) technique [51]. Evidence of protein involvement in spermatogenesis is furthered by a study conducted by Paasch et al. Specifically, this study reported increased levels of the eppin protein complex (EPC) proteins in obese individuals. The EPC consists of clusterin, lactotransferrin, and semenogelin-1 which are attached to the proteinase inhibitor eppin. These proteins are located on both the surface of ejaculate spermatozoa and in seminal plasma and have a variety of physiological functions in male reproduction. These functions include protection of sperm, regulation of sperm motility, and preparation of sperm for capacitation. In obese individuals, covalently modified versions of clusterin, lactotransferrin, and semenogelin-1 were present. Specifically, semenogelin-1 and clusterin were much smaller in obese individuals and suggested protein degradation, but lactotransferrin did not show much deviation in molecular weight despite existing in a modified form. While the modified forms of clusterin and semenogelin-1 in obese individuals may contribute to disrupted capacitation and inhibited sperm motility respectively, the function of lactotransferrin in spermatogenesis is unclear [52]. Thus, recent proteomic studies in obese individuals have established that increased BMI adversely affects proteins involved in male reproduction. Nevertheless, further studies are necessary in order to both validate the aforementioned studies and discover additional proteins affected by obesity.

Lifestyle Modifications to Avert the Effects of Obesity on Fertility

While the prevalence of obesity continues to increase worldwide and shows no signs of abating, obesity is nevertheless considered a preventable disease. Of the two main contributing factors to obesity—genetic and environmental—the causal effect of environmental factors is easiest to control and modify. Environmental factors contributing to obesity are entrenched in Western culture and are becoming prevalent in many developing countries as well. Such factors include the calorie-dense foods available in fastfood restaurants and decreased amounts of exercise. These factors have all contributed to a sedentary lifestyle that is quickly becoming a norm for many individuals, and the imbalance between physical activity and caloric intake has contributed dramatically to the rise in obesity [4, 53]. Fortunately, the detrimental effects of obesity can be through a variety of lifestyle modifications, including both natural or surgical weight loss and utilization of aromatase inhibitors.

One of the most obvious methods by which obesity's unfavorable effects on the male reproductive system can be averted is through natural or surgical weight loss. Natural weight loss—by means of exercise, decreased caloric intake, and increased nutrition—is considered the optimal method to stem the effects of obesity. In particular, an increase in androgen and inhibin B levels as well as improved semen quality has been reported in obese individuals who used the natural methods of diet and exercise to lose weight [3]. Furthermore, Kaukua et al. reported increases in SHBG and testosterone and decreases in insulin and leptin in obese individuals who followed a very low calorie diet for 4 months. Such hormonal changes through natural weight loss methods have proved successful in enhancing fertility by increasing sperm quality [48, 54]. Not only does natural weight loss alleviate hormonal regularities induced by obesity, but it also plays a role in reversing erectile dysfunction. Specifically, Esposito et al. reported that a third of the obese men in their study who had erectile dysfunction regained sexual function following a 2-year weight loss regimen of increased physical activity [44]. Thus, while presumably more difficult than other methods of weight loss, natural weight loss can be achieved and can yield favorable results with regard to male reproductive potential.

While natural weight loss as demonstrated is the most favored lifestyle modification to alleviate obesity, surgical methods can be utilized as well when natural weight loss is not feasible. A surgical method which has been demonstrated to be effective is removal of fat from the testicular area and restoring testicular temperature to normal levels is scrotal lipectomy. This is demonstrated by a study conducted by Shafik and Olfat of infertile and fertile male scrotal fat patterns. In particular, they found that scrotal lipectomy improved sperm quality for 65 % of patients and helped 20 % achieve pregnancies [55]. Not only is scrotal lipectomy a potential lifestyle modification that can reduce the adverse effects of obesity on fertility, but gastric bypass is an effective surgical weight loss technique as well. While studies of gastric bypass in obese individuals have been limited, Bastounis et al. found positive results of gastric bypass surgery in 1998 when they studied a group of morbidly obese patients for a year after they had a vertical banded gastroplasty. In particular, they found an increase in FSH, testosterone, and SHBG levels and a decrease in estradiol levels [56]. Although these results indicate that normal HPA function is restored, gastric bypass surgery causes rapid weight loss, which can shock the body and halt spermatogenesis [57]. In fact, a 2012 study by Lazaros et al. alludes to the negative effects of gastric bypass through their study of two male patients. These two men had been obese and had achieved fertility through assistive reproductive technology (ART).

However, following bariatric surgery, the patients presented with severe oligoasthenospermia and azoospermia respectively upon examination for a second fertility treatment. Such results indicate that bariatric surgery may adversely affect male fertility and reduce sperm parameters for up to 18 months following surgery, but further studies are needed to confirm these results [58]. Negative effects of bariatric surgery are further suggested in a recent study by Sermondade et al. In particular, their study found that three obese patients who underwent bariatric surgery showed signs of severe oligoasthenoteratozoospermia, cryptozoospermia, and oligozoospermia up to a year following the surgery [59]. Possible mechanisms for such alterations in sperm parameters include a disruption of normal GnRH secretion, nutritional deficiencies in iron, calcium, and vitamins B_1, B_{12}, and B_9, and a massive release of liposoluble toxic substances after surgery. Yet, Sermondade et al. further reported that the negative results may be reversible and that intracytoplasmic sperm injection with fresh spermatozoa may be successful in restoring fertility [59]. Thus, many studies have demonstrated positive effects of surgical techniques in combating obesity-induced male infertility, thereby making it a plausible lifestyle modification. Ultimately, however, further studies are needed to determine whether the positive hormonal effects outweigh the negative effects of gastric bypass on male fertility that have been reported in patients shortly after the procedure [31].

Although attempting surgical or natural weight loss is a prominent lifestyle modification that can alleviate the obesity and its potential adverse effects on infertility, utilizing aromatase inhibitors is another relatively new method that has been proposed. As aforementioned, the aromatase cytochrome p450 functions in adipose tissue to convert androgen to estrogen [32, 49]. The overactivity of this enzyme disrupts the HPG axis by creating large amounts of estrogen and altering spermatogenesis by negatively regulating the release of GnRH from the hypothalamus [60]. By contrast, aromatase inhibitors—such as anastrozole, letrozole, and testolactone—counteract the effects of aromatase and the decreased testosterone:estrogen ratio [32]. For instance, a study by Zumoff et al. found that in obese patients who were treated with testolactone, the effects of hypogonadotropic hypogonadism were alleviated and normal HPA function and spermatogenesis were restored [61]. More recently, Elkhiat et al. made further suggestions about the role of aromatase inhibitors in alleviating obesity-induced male infertility. Specifically, they posited that while high doses of aromatase inhibitors may not improve semen parameters, low doses may be advantageous due to the minimal threshold of estrogen required for spermatogenesis. They furthered that aromatase inhibitors were particularly beneficial for inducing spermatogenesis in nonobstructive azoospermia and may help those males who are obese and have low testosterone, high estradiol, or a reduced testosterone-estradiol ratio [62]. Hence, while aromatase inhibitors have not been widely studied in males, there have nevertheless been indications that such pharmacological interventions may be useful in treating the effects of obesity that are mediated through increased aromatase activity [61].

Conclusion

Thus, the rise of obesity worldwide combined with the trend of decreasing semen quality has caused researchers to posit a potential link between obesity and male infertility. Yet, research has not yielded consistent results regarding the extent to which obesity affects male reproductive potential. While investigation of the mechanisms for obesity-induced hormonal abnormalities is ongoing, numerous studies have nevertheless substantiated that decreased testosterone, ghrelin, inhibin B as well as increased estrogen, resistin, and leptin levels are present in obese males [10, 16, 23, 25, 26, 29, 37]. Some of the better understood hormonal mechanisms that may negatively impact spermatogenesis include aromatase overactivity, hypothalamic-based leptin insufficiency and direct leptin saturation in the testis, ghrelin-induced inhibition of StAR and β-hydroxysteroid dehydrogenases, and the stimulation of the SOCS-3 pathway by resistin

[33, 34, 36, 37, 42]. Although such abnormalities alter the HPA, these changes do not necessarily alter sperm potential, as demonstrated by studies such as those conducted by Pauli et al., Rybar et al., and Martini et al. [6, 15, 25].

While obesity-induced hormonal abnormalities may not affect sperm quality, increased BMI can nevertheless inhibit male reproduction by its adverse physical and proteomic effects. With regard to detrimental physical ramifications, both erectile dysfunction and increased testicular temperature cause infertility and have been associated with obesity [31]. While obesity promotes erectile dysfunction through both stimulation of the renin-angiotensin system and disruption of proper nitric oxide function, it also may lead to increased scrotal temperature due to accumulation of adipose tissue around the suprapubic region [33, 45, 48]. Not only does obesity have unfavorable physical effects that contribute to infertility, but its effects on the sperm proteome may impair male reproductive potential as well. While further investigations are needed, increased levels of modified clusterin, lactotransferrin, and semenogelin-1—which are part of the EPC—have been implicated in decreasing sperm quality [52]. Because obesity-induced hormonal abnormalities, physical alterations, and proteomic changes have been reported to adversely affect male reproductive potential, it is important to elucidate methods by which the detrimental effects of obesity can be averted. Fortunately, there are three main lifestyle modifications—natural weight loss, surgical weight loss, and the aromatase inhibitors—that have been implicated in restoring normal hormone levels and improving reproductive potential. In particular, natural weight loss is considered the most favorable to combat obesity and has led to increases in testosterone, SHBG, and inhibin B as well as decreases in leptin and insulin [3, 54]. Moreover, natural weight loss and increased physical exercise can also help reverse erectile dysfunction [44]. Similarly, studies report that surgical weight loss techniques, such as scrotal lipectomy and gastric bypass, improve semen quality and normalize FSH, testosterone, SHBG, and estradiol levels respectively. While both natural and surgical weight loss have demonstrated positive results in alleviating the effects of obesity, natural weight loss is able to avoid the potential inhibition of spermatogenesis and the adverse effects on sperm parameters that are caused by rapid weight loss ensuing from some of the surgical techniques [55, 56, 58, 59]. Not only is weight loss an important lifestyle modification that can be made to mitigate the detrimental effects of obesity, but pharmacological interventions can be made as well. Although studies have been limited, researchers have nevertheless have made progress in demonstrating the favorable effects of aromatase inhibitors [32, 62]. Hence, while there have not been consistent reports about the effects of obesity on infertility, a detailed understanding and continued investigation of the adverse effects to obesity, underlying mechanisms, and lifestyle modifications may have important clinical implications, such as improving semen quality and decreasing the burgeoning rates of male factor infertility [48].

References

1. World Health Organization. Office of health communications and public relations. Obesity and overweight. Geneva: World Health Organization; 2006.
2. Pasquali R. Obesity, fat distribution and infertility. Maturitas. 2006;54(4):363–71.
3. Kasturi SS, Tannir J, Brannigan RE. The metabolic syndrome and male infertility. J Androl. 2008;29(3):251–9.
4. Ferris WF, Crowther NJ. Once fat was fat and that was that: our changing perspectives on adipose tissue. Cardiovasc J Afr. 2011;22(3):147–54.
5. Hammoud AO, Wilde N, Gibson M, Parks A, Carrell DT, Meikle AW. Male obesity and alteration in sperm parameters. Fertil Steril. 2008;90(6):2222–5.
6. Rybar R, Kopecka V, Prinosilova P, Markova P, Rubes J. Male obesity and age in relationship to semen parameters and sperm chromatin integrity. Andrologia. 2011;43(4):286–91.
7. Bulcao C, Ferreira SR, Giuffrida FM, Ribeiro-Filho FF. The new adipose tissue and adipocytokines. Curr Diabetes Rev. 2006;2(1):19–28.
8. Noble RE. Waist-to-hip ratio versus BMI as predictors of cardiac risk in obese adult women. West J Med. 2001;174(4):240–1.
9. Gong D, Yang R, Munir KM, Horenstein RB, Shuldiner AR. New progress in adipocytokine research. Curr Opin Endocrinol Diabetes. 2003;10(2):115–21.
10. Pittas AG, Joseph NA, Greenberg AS. Adipocytokines and insulin resistance. J Clin Endocrinol Metab. 2004;89(2):447–52.

11. Ramya T, Misro MM, Sinha D, Nandan D. Sperm function and seminal oxidative stress as tools to identify sperm pathologies in infertile men. Fertil Steril. 2010;93(1):297–300.
12. Tunc O, Bakos HW, Tremellen K. Impact of body mass index on seminal oxidative stress. Andrologia. 2011;43(2):121–8.
13. Fejes I, Koloszar S, Szollosi J, Zavaczki Z, Pal A. Is semen quality affected by male body fat distribution? Andrologia. 2005;37(5):155–9.
14. Sallmen M, Sandler DP, Hoppin JA, Blair A, Baird DD. Reduced fertility among overweight and obese men. Epidemiology. 2006;17(5):520–3.
15. Martini AC, Tissera A, Estofan D, Molina RI, Mangeaud A, de Cuneo MF, et al. Overweight and seminal quality: a study of 794 patients. Fertil Steril. 2010;94(5):1739–43.
16. Hofny ER, Ali ME, Abdel-Hafez HZ, Kamal Eel D, Mohamed EE, Abd El-Azeem HG, et al. Semen parameters and hormonal profile in obese fertile and infertile males. Fertil Steril. 2010;94(2):581–4.
17. Stewart TM, Liu DY, Garrett C, Jorgensen N, Brown EH, Baker HW. Associations between andrological measures, hormones and semen quality in fertile Australian men: inverse relationship between obesity and sperm output. Hum Reprod. 2009;24(7):1561–8.
18. Shayeb AG, Harrild K, Mathers E, Bhattacharya S. An exploration of the association between male body mass index and semen quality. Reprod Biomed Online. 2011;23(6):717–23.
19. Fariello RM, Pariz JR, Spaine DM, Cedenho AP, Bertolla RP, Fraietta R. Association between obesity and alteration of sperm DNA integrity and mitochondrial activity. BJU Int. 2012;110(6):863–7.
20. Hammiche F, Laven JSE, Twigt JM, Boellaard WPA, Steegers EAP, Steegers-Theunissen RP. Body mass index and central adiposity are associated with sperm quality in men of subfertile couples. Hum Reprod. 2012;27(8):2365–72.
21. Sermondade N, Faure C, Fezeu L, Lévy R, Czernichow S, Group O-FC. Obesity and increased risk for oligozoospermia and azoospermia. Arch Intern Med. 2012;172(5):440–2.
22. La Vignera S, Condorelli RA, Vicari E, Calogero AE. Negative effect of increased body weight on sperm conventional and nonconventional flow cytometric sperm parameters. J Androl. 2012;33(1):53–8.
23. Zorn B, Osredkar J, Meden-Vrtovec H, Majdic G. Leptin levels in infertile male patients are correlated with inhibin B, testosterone and SHBG but not with sperm characteristics. Int J Androl. 2007;30(5):439–44.
24. Aggerholm AS, Thulstrup AM, Toft G, Ramlau-Hansen CH, Bonde JP. Is overweight a risk factor for reduced semen quality and altered serum sex hormone profile? Fertil Steril. 2008;90(3):619–26.
25. Pauli EM, Legro RS, Demers LM, Kunselman AR, Dodson WC, Lee PA. Diminished paternity and gonadal function with increasing obesity in men. Fertil Steril. 2008;90(2):346–51.
26. Chavarro JE, Toth TL, Wright DL, Meeker JD, Hauser R. Body mass index in relation to semen quality,

sperm DNA integrity, and serum reproductive hormone levels among men attending an infertility clinic. Fertil Steril. 2010;93(7):2222–31.

27. Lotti F, Corona G, Colpi GM, Filimberti E, Degli Innocenti S, Mancini M, et al. Elevated body mass index correlates with higher seminal plasma interleukin 8 levels and ultrasonographic abnormalities of the prostate in men attending an andrology clinic for infertility. J Endocrinol Invest. 2011;34(10):336–42.

28. Mah PM, Wittert GA. Obesity and testicular function. Mol Cell Endocrinol. 2010;316(2):180–6.

29. Winters SJ, Wang C, Abdelrahaman E, Hadeed V, Dyky MA, Brufsky A. Inhibin-B levels in healthy young adult men and prepubertal boys: is obesity the cause for the contemporary decline in sperm count because of fewer Sertoli cells? J Androl. 2006;27(4):560–4.

30. Teerds KJ, de Rooij DG, Keijer J. Functional relationship between obesity and male reproduction: from humans to animal models. Hum Reprod Update. 2011;17(5):667–83.

31. Reis LO, Dias FG. Male fertility, obesity, and bariatric surgery. Reprod Sci. 2012;19(8):778–85.

32. Roth MY, Amory JK, Page ST. Treatment of male infertility secondary to morbid obesity. Nat Clin Pract Endocrinol Metab. 2008;4(7):415–9.

33. Phillips KP, Tanphaichitr N. Mechanisms of obesity-induced male infertility. Expert Rev Endocrinol Metab. 2010;5(2):229–51.

34. Hammoud AO, Griffin J, Meikle AW, Gibson M, Peterson CM, Carrell DT. Association of aromatase (TTTAn) repeat polymorphism length and the relationship between obesity and decreased sperm concentration. Hum Reprod. 2010;25(12):3146–51.

35. Wozniak SE, Gee LL, Wachtel MS, Frezza EE. Adipose tissue: the new endocrine organ? A review article. Dig Dis Sci. 2009;54(9):1847–56.

36. Barash IA, Cheung CC, Weigle DS, Ren H, Kabigting EB, Kuijper JL, et al. Leptin is a metabolic signal to the reproductive system. Endocrinology. 1996;137(7):3144–7.

37. Pasquali R. Obesity and androgens: facts and perspectives. Fertil Steril. 2006;85(5):1319–40.

38. Monti V, Carlson JJ, Hunt SC, Adams TD. Relationship of ghrelin and leptin hormones with body mass index and waist circumference in a random sample of adults. J Am Diet Assoc. 2006;106(6):822–8; quiz 9–30.

39. Meachem SJ, Nieschlag E, Simoni M. Inhibin B in male reproduction: pathophysiology and clinical relevance. Eur J Endocrinol. 2001;145(5):561–71.

40. Pierik FH, Burdorf A, de Jong FH, Weber RF. Inhibin B: a novel marker of spermatogenesis. Ann Med. 2003;35(1):12–20.

41. Robeva R, Tomova A, Kirilov G, Kumanov P. Anti-Müllerian hormone and inhibin B levels reflect altered Sertoli cell function in men with metabolic syndrome. Andrologia. 2012;44(1):329–34.

42. Luo Z, Zhang Y, Li F, He J, Ding H, Yan L, et al. Resistin induces insulin resistance by both AMPK-dependent and AMPK-independent mechanisms in HepG2 cells. Endocrine. 2009;36(1):60–9.

43. Jensen TK, Andersson AM, Jorgensen N, Andersen AG, Carlsen E, Petersen JH, et al. Body mass index in relation to semen quality and reproductive hormones among 1,558 Danish men. Fertil Steril. 2004;82(4):863–70.

44. Esposito K, Giugliano F, Di Palo C, Giugliano G, Marfella R, D'Andrea F, et al. Effect of lifestyle changes on erectile dysfunction in obese men: a randomized controlled trial. JAMA. 2004;291(24):2978–84.

45. Tamler R. Diabetes, obesity, and erectile dysfunction. Gend Med. 2009;6 Suppl 1:4–16.

46. Hjollund NH, Bonde JP, Jensen TK, Olsen J. Diurnal scrotal skin temperature and semen quality. The Danish First Pregnancy Planner Study Team. Int J Androl. 2000;23(5):309–18.

47. Mieusset R, Bujan L, Mansat A, Pontonnier F, Grandjean H. Hyperthermia and human spermatogenesis: enhancement of the inhibitory effect obtained by 'artificial cryptorchidism'. Int J Androl. 1987;10(4):571–80.

48. Hammoud AO, Gibson M, Peterson CM, Meikle AW, Carrell DT. Impact of male obesity on infertility: a critical review of the current literature. Fertil Steril. 2008;90(4):897–904.

49. Cabler S, Agarwal A, Flint M, du Plessis SS. Obesity: modern man's fertility nemesis. Asian J Androl. 2010;12(4):480–9.

50. Cai H, Ren Y, Li XX, Yang JL, Zhang CP, Chen M, et al. Scrotal heat stress causes a transient alteration in tight junctions and induction of TGF-beta expression. Int J Androl. 2011;34(4):352–62.

51. Kriegel TM, Heidenreich F, Kettner K, Pursche T, Hoflack B, Grunewald S, et al. Identification of diabetes- and obesity-associated proteomic changes in human spermatozoa by difference gel electrophoresis. Reprod Biomed Online. 2009;19(5):660–70.

52. Paasch U, Heidenreich F, Pursche T, Kuhlisch E, Kettner K, Grunewald S, et al. Identification of increased amounts of eppin protein complex components in sperm cells of diabetic and obese individuals by difference gel electrophoresis. Mol Cell Proteomics. 2011;10(8):M110 007187.

53. James PT, Leach R, Kalamara E, Shayeghi M. The worldwide obesity epidemic. Obes Res. 2001;9 Suppl 4:228S–33S.

54. Kaukua J, Pekkarinen T, Sane T, Mustajoki P. Sex hormones and sexual function in obese men losing weight. Obes Res. 2003;11(6):689–94.

55. Shafik A, Olfat S. Scrotal lipomatosis. Br J Urol. 1981;53(1):50–4.

56. Bastounis EA, Karayiannakis AJ, Syrigos K, Zbar A, Makri GG, Alexiou D. Sex hormone changes in morbidly obese patients after vertical banded gastroplasty. Eur Surg Res. 1998;30(1):43–7.

57. di Frega AS, Dale B, Di Matteo L, Wilding M. Secondary male factor infertility after Roux-en-Y

gastric bypass for morbid obesity: case report. Hum Reprod. 2005;20(4):997–8.

58. Lazaros L, Hatzi E, Markoula S, Takenaka A, Sofikitis N, Zikopoulos K, et al. Dramatic reduction in sperm parameters following bariatric surgery: report of two cases. Andrologia. 2012;44(6):428–32.

59. Sermondade N, Massin N, Boitrelle F, Pfeffer J, Eustache F, Sifer C, et al. Sperm parameters and male fertility after bariatric surgery: three case series. Reprod BioMed Online. 2012;24:206–10.

60. Hammoud AO, Gibson M, Peterson CM, Hamilton BD, Carrell DT. Obesity and male reproductive potential. J Androl. 2006;27(5):619–26.

61. Zumoff B, Miller LK, Strain GW. Reversal of the hypogonadotropic hypogonadism of obese men by administration of the aromatase inhibitor testolactone. Metabolism. 2003;52(9):1126–8.

62. Elkhiat Y, Fahmy I. Aromatase inhibitors in the treatment of male infertility. Hum Androl. 2011;1(2): 35–8.

The Impact of Physical Exercise on Male Fertility

4

Diana Maria Vaamonde Martin, Marzo Edir Da Silva-Grigoletto, Asghar Abbasi, and Juan Manuel García Manso

Introduction

While there is an increasing trend in engaging in physical exercise activities, not having adequate knowledge on how to perform these activities might, on occasion, lead to negative side effects (lesions, pathologies, etc.) that may even result in a wide variety of problems relating to several systemic processes such as osteomuscular injuries, blood pressure, and overtraining syndrome. On the contrary, with an adequate knowledge, physical exercise may promote many benefits when performed on a regular and adequate basis.

While it is known that the effects of lifestyle such as smoking, poor diet, alcohol abuse, obesity, psychological stress, and sedentary habits are important factors affecting male reproductive performance and fertility and may have an impact on the fertility of their offspring [1], little is known about the beneficial and deleterious effects of physical exercise and sports on reproductive performance. While several investigators have demonstrated that prolonged exhaustive exercise may lead to adverse effects on physiological systems and particularly the reproductive system and fertility [2–5], others believe that regular exercise affects an individual's general health and well-being. Researchers have emphasized during the last decade the deleterious effect of exercise on reproductive functions in males [6, 7]. It has been observed that particularly exhaustive endurance exercise may exert a negative effect on reproductive hormones [5, 7–9] and semen parameters [3, 5, 7, 10, 11]. It has been recently demonstrated that intensified exercise can cause oxidative stress and DNA damage in spermatozoa of male athletes [12, 13].

While exercise volume was firstly hypothesized to be the variable most affecting reproduction [10, 14], later studies suggested that the effects of exercise intensity on male fertility were, at least, comparable with regard the deleterious effects induced [7, 15]. Depending on the exercise modalities, there may be other parameters adding to this equation as can be bike saddles

D.M. Vaamonde Martin, BS, MS, PhD (✉)
Department of Morphological Sciences, University of Cordoba, Avda. Menendez Pidal sn, Cordoba 14004, Spain
e-mail: fivresearch@yahoo.com

M.E. Da Silva-Grigoletto, PhD
Department of Physical Education, Federal University of Sergipe, Rua Napoleao Dorea, 165, Aracaju, Sergipe 49037-460, Brazil
e-mail: pit_researcher@yahoo.es; editor.ramd.ccd@juntadeandalucia.es

A. Abbasi
Division of Exercise Immunology & Genetics, Institute of Clinical and Experimental Transfusion Medicine (IKET)/University Hospital Tübingen, Otfried-Mueller-Str. 4/1, Tuebingen 72076, Germany
e-mail: Ashgar.Abbasi@med.uni-tuebingen.de

J.M. Garcia Manso, BS, MS, PhD
Department of Physical Education, Universidad de Las Palmas de GranCanaria, Campus Universitario de Tafira (Edificio de Educación Física), Las Palmas de Gran Canaria, Islas Canarias (Gran Canaria) 35017, Spain
e-mail: jgarciamanso@gmail.com

S.S. du Plessis et al. (eds.), *Male Infertility: A Complete Guide to Lifestyle and Environmental Factors*, DOI 10.1007/978-1-4939-1040-3_4, © Springer Science+Business Media New York 2014

which impose great deal of friction [16]. Some others just seem to consider exercise as potentially harmful in the case of a previous existing pathology related to the reproductive system [17, 18]. However, from a scientific standpoint, it is extremely complex to establish a clear and unequivocal affirmation of this interrelation due to the fact that male reproductive parameters are, "per se," the subject of ample variety [19]. The reproductive system is, without any doubt, a complex system on which many factors act upon. So, the notorious lack of consensus about the aforementioned relationship or interdependence is probably due to the fact that different parameters were used during the training sessions that athletes underwent.

Yet, some research exists in relation to potential beneficial effect of physical fitness on reproduction. In this sense, Vaamonde and colleagues have recently reported better semen parameters and hormonal levels in physically active subjects when compared to sedentary people [20].

Therefore, the aim of the present chapter is to review the impact of physical exercise on male fertility.

Physical Activity and Exercise

It is necessary to have a basic understanding regarding physical activity and exercise as well as the different parameters and types of exercise in order to more easily follow the information offered in the chapter. We must bear in mind that physical activity and physical exercise and sports training have different connotations, requirements, development, and objectives. Physical activity is any type of movement that requires muscle contraction. This includes daily activities, such as gardening, walking, going up and down the stairs, housework, and everything else done throughout the day. Exercise, while it is a physical activity, is a very specific form of it. It is a purposeful and planned form of activity and is performed with the intention of acquiring health benefits and increasing fitness level. Exercise includes activities such as swimming, running, cycling, as well as other types of sports. Most of the papers to be discussed in this chapter will deal with sports training and to a lesser extent with physical exercise. The main two types of exercise which differ in several aspects, primarily the metabolic route used, are endurance exercise and strength exercise.

Endurance training is based on increasing stamina and the ability to endure a sports activity. It predominantly trains the aerobic system instead of the anaerobic. It involves many systemic processes and events as it induces many central and peripheral physiological adaptations. Catabolic and oxidation events are crucial in these types of athletes so as to increase the capacity to use fat and glycogen to meet energetic demands (glycogenolysis, glycolysis, and lipolysis) as well as greater efficiency in oxygen transport and distribution. Typical examples of endurance sports are long-distance running events, cycling, and swimming. Combinations of these sports such as duathlon and triathlon are also endurance sports [21].

Strength training deals with using some sort of resistance (weights, body weight, rubber bands, etc.) with the objective of producing muscular contractions for increasing strength, anaerobic endurance, and muscle size. It is primarily an anaerobic activity which provides significant functional benefits and thus promotes health improvement, especially related to bone and muscle metabolism and hormonal responses. Typical sports based on strength training are bodybuilding, weight lifting, and powerlifting.

Parameters

There are several parameters that are important to take into account with regard to sports training. These will be discussed subsequently.

Training load is the quantitative amount of work developed during training. It mainly implies the degree of stimulation imposed on the body and that will lead to a series of changes and adaptations. Training load entails physical and mental activities performed by the sportsman in order to develop capacities and the addition of all training effects on organism.

Training volume is the amount of work performed (kilometers covered, kilograms lifted, number of repetitions, etc.). Training volume is a key element to be defined for further training planning (number of sessions, number of exercises per trained muscle group, sets per each exercise, repetitions per set, duration of recovery phases, etc.) [22].

Training intensity on the other hand refers to the qualitative element of physical work. It is how "hard" the athlete will perceive the exercise. It is normally expressed as percentage of variables such as maximal oxygen uptake (VO_{2max}), heart rate (HR), and one repetition maximum (1RM).

Training density expresses the relation between effort duration and recovery duration [23]. This applies to intra-session (taking recovery times between repetitions) density or inter-session density (recovery time between different training sessions or sets) [24]. Training density will affect both acute and chronic responses induced by exercise.

Effect of Exercise on Male Fertility

The hypothalamic-pituitary-gonadal (HPG) axis, which is regulated by a negative feedback system, is central to male reproduction. The male gonads, namely, the testes, are responsible for production of steroid hormones, mainly testosterone and sperm production. Testosterone, in turn, is the major regulatory hormone [25]. Gonadotropin-releasing hormone (GnRH) is secreted in a pulsatile manner by the hypothalamus and stimulates the release of the following hormone: luteinizing hormone (LH) and follicle-stimulating hormone (FSH). LH is responsible for testosterone secretion by the Leydig cells, while FSH is fundamental for proper spermatogenesis. Any alteration in this system may have an impact on fertility. With regard to the effect of exercise on male fertility, much controversy still exist as many studies have resulted contradictory; some have not reported any changes in semen parameters [26, 27], while significant changes have been reported by others [3, 5, 10, 15, 28, 29]. Both the negative and positive effects of exercise on male fertility will be subsequently discussed.

Negative Effects

Regardless of the many known health benefits of exercise, there is growing evidence and concern that exercise, especially when excessively practiced, may lead to adverse effects on physiological systems and in particular the reproductive system and fertility [2, 4]. Research has linked sports activities to a condition referred to as "exercise-related female reproductive dysfunction," characterized by luteal phase defects, amenorrhea, anovulation, and infertility in females [30]. In males, research has resulted in controversial results as semen samples show much variation and study designs have not always been proper. Yet, it seems possible that exercise could be an underlying cause in male infertility, especially in cases of idiopathic infertility. The pathological aspects of physical exercise on male reproduction are summarized in the remainder of this section.

Resistance Exercise

Steroids
It must be noted that this modality of exercise is specifically the one closely related to anabolic steroid use, and therefore, one should be cautious about it. While there are many doping substances that may be used by athletes and exercising people to increase performance and physical fitness and appearance, anabolic steroids are used in resistance training as the goal of this type of training is to increase muscle strength and size. The anabolic effects of steroids are intimately linked to androgenic effects.

Due to the fact that their use is rather extensive among many athletes, the dangerous side effects they pose to fertility and reproductive potential must be explained. Therefore, the effects of these compounds will be included throughout the different sections of this part of the chapter.

Hormonal Effects

The effect of resistance training on hormonal parameters is of anabolic nature; therefore, as expected there is an increase in testosterone. In fact, testosterone mediates anabolic responses through two pathways: one directly stimulating protein synthesis and muscle growth and the other (indirect one) by increasing GH release and increasing muscle force through interactions with the nervous system [31]. The acute effects of a single session of resistance training are generally an increase in testosterone. Resistance training seems to induce an increase in both frequency and amplitude of testosterone secretion [31]. This increase in testosterone is related to recruitment and activation of large muscle groups or to moderate-to-high volume training [32]. As part of chronic adaptations, there is also an increase in testosterone, unless training becomes excessive, and such increase accompanies greater muscle and strength development [33].

Although most studies report an increase in testosterone secretion after resistance training, Arce and colleagues found lower levels of total and free testosterone both in endurance- and resistance-trained athletes when compared to sedentary controls; therefore, these authors postulated that both training types similarly produce modifications on male reproductive hormones [10].

When anabolic steroids come into play (i.e., oxandrolone, methandienone, stanozolol, nandrolone decanoate, and boldenone undecylenate), the result is clearly a hindered secretion of endogenous testosterone precisely due to the negative feedback that regulates the reproductive hormones [34].

Seminological Effects

Although to date, to the best of our knowledge, there is only one study reporting sperm quality as a result of resistance training under physiological (nonsteroid taking) conditions, there are some reports on the effect of concomitant use of androgenic-anabolic steroids (AAS) along with resistance training. Arce and colleagues showed that, contrary to what happened with endurance athletes, no alterations were found for sperm density, motility, and morphology or in vitro cervical mucus sperm penetration [10].

In the case of AAS use, first we need to be aware that many AAS abusers do not disclose taking them and that they normally take other substances along with AAS (aromatase inhibitors, antiestrogens, and human chorionic gonadotropin (hCG)) in hopes of counteracting the undesirable effects of AAS abuse, such as hypogonadotropic hypogonadism and gynecomastia, and to avoid detection of their use [35, 36]. Moreover, hCG and clomiphene are sometimes concurrently used as they stimulate endogenous testosterone production and prevent testicular atrophy [37].

Nevertheless, when intake of AAS reaches supraphysiologic levels, they cause a decrease in FSH, LH, and endogenous testosterone as they exert negative feedback on the HPG axis. This in turn may result in alterations in the testes (atrophy, hypogonadotropic hypogonadism) and spermatogenesis (azoospermia, oligozoospermia, mobility alterations, and increased number of morphological anomalies, especially of the head and midpiece) [34, 36, 38–40]. In rats, testes weights and other sperm parameters were decreased, while apoptosis in cells of the male germ line was increased when nandrolone decanoate was administered concurrently with exercise [41]. Although the exercise model employed was swimming which is a typical endurance activity, it was worth including the study under this section as endurance athletes rarely ever take AAS in supraphysiologic doses, which would be needed for a negative effect.

Some studies have reported the spontaneous recovery of spermatogenesis within 4–6 months following termination of AAS use [42], while others have reported a period of 3 years or longer [43]. This difference in time could possibly be due to the different AAS and combinations used. Therefore, it is easily understood that it is difficult to clearly determine the effects of AAS use and especially regarding time and outcome or recovery of spermatogenesis [34].

Endurance and Ultra-endurance Exercise

Hormonal Effects

It has been reported that both hypothalamic and testicular endocrine functions may be suppressed during acute and prolonged physical exercise. The exercise-induced suppression of serum testosterone is associated with suppressed endogenous GnRH stimulation of gonadotropin release during exercise [44]. Qualitatively and quantitatively normal spermatogenesis is critically dependent on an intact HPG axis as androgens are essential for the initiation and maintenance of normal spermatogenesis.

It must be highlighted that the different parameters of exercise training may have a different impact on hormonal behavior. As such, we begin discussing the different studies with regard to training volume. We shall begin with studies in which athletes were covering low-to-medium training volume.

With regard to running, of the many studies assessing hormonal behavior in endurance sports, many of them reported changes in either free testosterone (FT) or total testosterone (TT) that were not significant [6, 27, 45]. On the other hand, another set of studies have found a significant decrease in total testosterone [26, 46, 47] and in free testosterone [47].

From the studies performed with runners with a high training volume, the following ones should be highlighted.

TT was diminished in the studies by Roberts and colleagues [48] and De Souza et al. [6], the latter also finding decreased FT. In a study by Arce and colleagues, endurance-trained and resistance-trained athletes presented with significantly lower levels of total and free testosterone, compared with sedentary controls [10]. Several studies used serial sampling in assessing hormonal behavior with contradictory results; while MacConnie and colleagues [49] found lowered LH but normal TT, Hackney and colleagues [50] found lowered FT and TT but no differences in either pulse frequency or amplitude in LH secretion.

Later on, Hackney and colleagues [51] reported that endurance training produces an increased response of prolactin (PRL) and an attenuated release of LH from the pituitary gland. Such alterations may have a direct effect on the functional status of the HPT axis, resulting in the suppression of testosterone basal levels in the group of trained subjects. However, in their study PRL and LH responses were produced by exogenous dopamine and GnRH administration, and thus, this exogenous administration may interfere with the effects of exercise itself.

Most of the studies have not assessed LH; the studies that have assessed it have shown that this hormone stays unaltered or slightly varies with changes that do not reach statistical significance [47, 50, 51]; other studies have shown that there are significant changes but either just in amplitude [52] or just in frequency [49].

In cycling, results have also been vague and controversial; while Lucia and colleagues [11] found no significant differences in hormonal profiles of cyclists, a study by Fernández-Garcia and colleagues [53] showed decreased T values in relation to the competition period.

On the other hand, in elite swimmers, differences in hormonal levels (T and C) have not been observed when increasing training load for a 4-week period [54]; other authors observe a decrease in the hormone during exercise reverting to initial values during recovery phase [55].

When taking intensity as the main differential parameter, it can be observed that this parameter may exert an influence on hormonal profiles.

In one of the most comprehensive and controlled studies to date on the effect of exercise on the reproductive hormones and semen quality, 286 subjects were submitted to either a moderate-intensity exercise (60 % of VO_{2max}) or a high-intensity exercise (80 % of VO_{2max}) group [5]. Exercise duration was 60 weeks with 5 weekly sessions of 120 min of treadmill running; afterwards, a 36-week low-intensity recovery period followed. In both exercise conditions, testosterone, LH, and FSH began to decrease from 12 weeks onwards, while sex hormone-binding

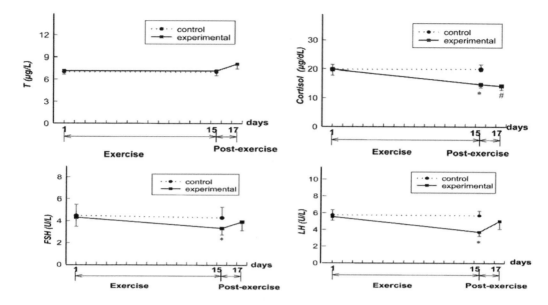

Fig. 4.1 The most relevant hormones analyzed related to the effect of intensive endurance exercise over a 2-week period. [Reprinted from Vaamonde D, Da Silva ME, Poblador MS, Lancho JL. Reproductive profile of physically active men after exhaustive endurance exercise. Int J Sports Med. 2006;27:680-9. With permission from Thieme]

globulin (SHBG) increased. LH and FSH responses to a GnRH stimulation test were blunted [5]. It must be noted that hormones returned to baseline values after the recovery period.

In a previous study, physically active subjects were submitted to maximal-intensity exercise for a short period of time (2 weeks) observing altered values of FSH, LH, PRL, DHEA, and cortisol though no significant changes were observed for testosterone, progesterone, or estradiol. After 3 days into recovery, hormones returned to pre-training values [7] (Fig. 4.1).

Although it could be seen in this study, as well as in the Safarinejad study [5], that the observed change in hormonal values was transient and returned to normal ranges, if exercise does not include enough recovery periods or becomes chronic instead of acute in nature, then changes may be non-reversible, especially when dealing with athletes that start training at a pre- or peripubertal age.

Ultra-endurance exercise can manifest positive physiological adaptations in the cardiovascular and hematopoietic systems and body composition, but can also adversely affect the neuroendocrine system and reproductive health [9, 56].

Although most research assessing the effects of exercise on reproductive health has focused on endurance-trained athletes, some of the most recent studies have looked at male ultra-endurance-trained athletes. For example, men exposed to chronic ultra-endurance training for competition by running or cycling 10–20 h a week have been shown to present a hypogonadal state with low basal-resting testosterone levels [57]. Literature describing male endocrine status across a range of exercise durations and intensities is sparse, but would be important to better characterize the point at which adverse effects on the neuroendocrine system and male reproductive health might occur. More recently, the work by Fitzgerald and colleagues showed that triathletes have significantly lower amounts of estradiol and testosterone as compared with cyclists and recreationally active men [8], although previous studies by Lucia and colleagues [11] did not find differences. As a conclusion, testosterone levels have been found to be lower among highly trained endurance athletes than among resistance-trained or control subjects, introducing the possibility of exercise-related sex hormone dysfunction [58, 59]. We must not forget

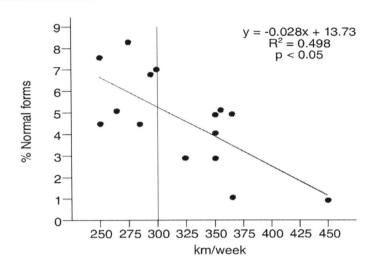

Fig. 4.2 Correlation between sperm morphology and weekly training volume of cycling. [Reprinted from Vaamonde D, Da Silva-Grigoletto ME, García-Manso JM, Cunha-Filho JS, Vaamonde-Lemos R. Sperm morphology normalcy is inversely correlated to cycling kilometers in elite triathletes. Rev Andal Med Deporte. 2009;02:43-6. With permission from Elsevier]

that glucocorticoids, which may be increased in athletes, provoke direct inhibitory actions on the number of LH receptors in the Leydig cells, thus altering steroidogenesis [60].

It seems clear that both intensity and volume may affect the hormonal response. When observing the disparity in results, it is clear that a consensus in the study design needs to be reached as there is much heterogeneity in the sample chosen or the type of intervention, etc. At any rate, we must not forget that hormones are integrated in a complex inhibitory and stimulatory loop.

Seminological Effects

With regard to semen, there is no clear consensus either regarding the effects that endurance exercise produces upon sperm production yet evidence exists that it can alter spermatogenesis and sperm output. It seems clear that long-term exhaustive exercise can lower sperm quality and the potential for reproduction [3, 28].

In runners, some studies report alterations in seminal quality, with even up to 10 % of the subjects from the study exhibiting severe oligospermia [26]; on the other hand, other authors postulate that there is no alteration or, if any alteration exists, it would not reach clinical significance despite the existing difference between runners and control subjects [10, 14, 27, 46]. Some authors have reported an increase in non-sperm cell elements, such as round cells [10], which would be indicative of possible infection and/or inflammation. It seems evident that subjects with a higher training volume showed greater differences than those undergoing a lower volume when compared to control subjects [14]. A minimum running volume of 100 km/week for athletes to exhibit differences in semen parameters has been hypothesized [10]. Yet, some have reported that intensified training during 6 weeks (gradual increase to 186 % of normal training) followed by 2 weeks of detraining (50 % of normal training) does not seem to alter sperm count, motility, and morphology [61]. Another study reported alteration in sperm density, motility, and morphology as well as in the in vitro cervical mucus sperm penetration test [10]. Consistently, Safarinejad and colleagues observed significant decline in semen parameters in high-intensity exercise group compared to those athletes exercising at moderate intensity. Interestingly enough, all of the above-mentioned parameters improved to their pre-exercise levels during the recovery period [5].

When dealing with high-level athletes that have been training for years (those regularly involved in competitions), it would be, at least, difficult to estimate the threshold to start observing abnormal semen parameters. Nevertheless, high cycling volume relates to sperm morphology alterations [28, 62]. A volume of 300 km/week in cycling correlates with serious alterations in sperm morphology [28] (Fig. 4.2).

In cyclists, lower sperm motility ($46.2 \pm 19.5\%$) has been observed during periods of competition when compared to other groups (recreational marathon runners and sedentary subjects) during their respective competition periods ($P<0.05$) or with themselves during the other two periods of study ($P<0.01$) [11]. Another study highlighted the fact that long-distance competitive cyclists had a significantly lower proportion of spermatozoa with normal morphology and a significantly higher proportion of morphologically abnormal tapered forms compared to controls (no significant difference in semen volume and sperm motility, viability, and concentration was observed) [29]. Even recreational athletes who modify training and exercise to the point of exhaustion showed altered seminological and hormonal values [7]. Exercise seems to act as an aggravating factor in the case of men who present with a previous pathology, such as varicocele, and whose sperm parameters may be already affected by such pathology [17].

In a study using rats, the authors have observed that, after submitting them to a swimming stress, their reproductive capacity is maintained; likewise, the morphology of the newborns is kept unaltered; however, the number of spermatids is reduced [63]. A study by Manna and colleagues [64], using also rats as study subjects, shows not only a decrease in spermatids but also a decrease in other sperm cells in different stages. The same authors report also a decrease in serum hormones, enzymes involved in the processes of hormone conversion, and protective agents against oxidative stress such as catalase and others. Vaamonde's group has also observed, in mice submitted to forced swimming stress, that there is alteration in morphology in the exercising group although this can be prevented by antioxidant supplementation with trans-resveratrol [65].

In ultra-endurance, a study comparing men participating in three different training modalities (physically active men, water polo players, and triathletes) showed that sperm concentration/number, velocity, and morphology were significantly different among the different groups. Morphology showed the greatest difference among the groups ($<5\%$ normal forms in the triathlete group) [3].

Moreover, Ironman triathletes have been shown to exhibit systemic oxidative damage as a result of training and competition [66].

Erectile dysfunction (ED) or impotence, greatly associated with cycling, has also been attributed to continuous strenuous exercise [16] as friction from the bike saddle may induce microtrauma and compression.

It is easily understandable that inherent parameters of exercise such as type, volume, and intensity seem to play a role, alone or in combination in the equation of exercise and fertility; therefore, they must be carefully analyzed.

As in the case of the studies assessing hormones, training volume and intensity were variable in the studies assessing seminal quality. Despite this inconvenience, it seems evident that subjects with a higher training load (volume and/or intensity) showed greater differences. As already stated the deleterious effects may not be reversible if athletes have been training for many years or started training at a pre-or peripubertal age.

Oxidative Stress Biomarkers and DNA Damage

There is only little information regarding the pathological effects of exercise on oxidative stress biomarkers in male individuals. Just recently it was shown that elite athletes have significantly higher resting seminal 8-isoprostane, reactive oxygen species (ROS), malondialdehyde (MDA), and sperm DNA fragmentation and lower SOD, catalase, and TAC levels, as compared with recreationally active and nonactive men. A significantly positive correlation was reported between sperm DNA fragmentation with VO_{2max}, seminal 8-isoprostane, ROS, and MDA levels by these investigators. This suggests that elite athletes are more vulnerable to sperm dysfunction as compared to men who are exercising recreationally as well as sedentary people [13]. Vaamonde's group, in a preliminary study, has found that, as happened with sperm morphology, cycling volume directly correlates to sperm DNA damage. Therefore, athletes showing the greatest sperm DNA damage had systematically undergone higher annual mean weekly training volume [12]. Moreover, some authors report altered leukocyte number in athletes, especially in overtrained subjects, and changes in immune response [67].

It must be noted that there are some sports (soccer, basketball, rugby, handball, etc.) that are mixed modalities. In these cases, there have been reports of both hormones and semen parameters and that exercise may act as aggravating factor when there is a previous pathology [17, 18]. However, in these sports it is difficult to establish clear relationships between the different parameters and even with regard to the metabolic route employed. Therefore, more studies are needed in these sports to clarify the relationship.

It seems clear that intensity, as well as volume, may affect the hormonal and seminological response. Moreover, the other parameters and characteristics inherent to training may also play a role. In line with this, the subjects' own characteristics and how their adaptive systems are prepared for the challenge will determine the final response. Due to the fact that exercise may produce or aggravate previously existing, reproductive profile pathologies, such as hormonal and seminological alterations, it would be appropriate to further assess this relationship.

Positive Effect

It is widely known that regular exercise promotes beneficial effects on the cardiorespiratory system, immune system, endocrine system, brain, muscle, and other organs and provides protection from several diseases including obesity, cardiovascular disease, diabetes, osteoporosis, and chronic systemic inflammation. It seems that the reproductive system may also benefit from exercise as well.

Resistance Exercise

There are a number of reasons why it could be beneficial to manipulate the concentrations of circulating anabolic hormones and the anabolic-to-catabolic hormone ratio in men. From the perspective of an athlete, an increase in anabolic-androgenic hormones can improve performance by decreasing body fat and increasing lean body mass and muscular strength [68]. Muscle adaptation to exercise is strongly influenced by anabolic endocrine hormones and local load-sensitive autocrine/paracrine growth factors. GH, IGF-I, and testosterone (T) are directly involved in muscle adaptation to exercise because they promote muscle protein synthesis, whereas T and locally expressed IGF-I have been reported to activate muscle stem cells [69]. In fact, administration of T improves lean body mass and maximal voluntary strength in healthy older men [69].

Heavy resistance training can actually increase the production of testosterone, which can exhibit a secondary effect on other hormones that contribute to fertility in men. The acute testosterone (T) response to resistance exercise is characterized by a brief increase followed by a decline to resting (or even below resting) concentrations [70, 71].

A study by Tremblay and colleagues showed an increase in total testosterone levels after a bout of resistance exercise followed by a pronounced decline in total testosterone during recovery from resistance exercise. Free testosterone was significantly greater during the resting session than during the run or resistance exercise session. As seen with total testosterone, there was a significant decline in free testosterone during recovery from resistance exercise, despite an initial increase after exercise. Testosterone increased back to baseline levels by time 4 (4.5 h) after resistance exercise [72]. In the same study, the resistance exercise session resulted in greater LH concentrations than either the resting or the run sessions. Moreover, in the resistance-trained subjects there was a significant increase in LH that was maintained during the recovery period after performing a resistance training session. An acute bout of low-intensity resistance exercise significantly increased blood testosterone levels in male subjects [73]. Resistance-trained subjects have been shown to have higher basal testosterone levels [74, 75]. Testosterone concentrations have been shown to increase after an acute bout of resistance [76]. One season of resistance exercise has also been shown to increase immunoreactive growth hormone (iGH) in recreationally resistance-trained men [77].

Endurance and Ultra-endurance Exercise

Hormonal Effects
The majority of studies exploring the effects of exercise on androgens have focused on acute effects in short-term exercise protocols, and most of these demonstrate that exercise bouts are associated with an initial increase followed by a decline to or below the baseline levels in testosterone, with variable effects on other androgens when these are measured [55, 78–80]. The effect of long-term, moderate-intensity, aerobic exercise on hormonal levels in men has not been well studied. Therefore, it may be important to differentiate between the acute and chronic effects of exercise, as acute changes may relate more to muscle growth and tissue remodeling, whereas chronic changes may mediate exercise effects on long-term health [71, 81]. Some cross-sectional studies conducted in middle-aged and older men indicate that circulating testosterone concentrations may be higher in men who regularly exercise [82, 83]. Prospective, nonrandomized studies of resistance exercise over a few weeks either increased testosterone [84] or not [85, 86], whereas one study of daily aerobic exercise together with a low-fat diet increased SHBG, which could counteract the biological activity of testosterone [87]. A higher amount of SHBG has also been reported for men who have engaged in long-term exercise versus those who have not [88]. A randomized clinical study of a 12-month, moderate-intensity, aerobic exercise intervention on serum hormones in sedentary men showed an increase in serum dihydrotestosterone (DHT) and SHBG levels at 3 months and at 12 months during exercise intervention in exercisers compared to control group [58]. Recently, Vaamonde and colleagues [20] reported higher amounts of FSH, LH, testosterone as well as the T/C ratio (index of anabolic versus catabolic status) in physically active men compared to sedentary people, which further supports the possibility of an improved hormonal environment [20].

Seminological Effects
Semen Parameters
There is not much data about the beneficial effect of exercise or physical activity on seminal status of athletes or recreationally active men. However, a new finding of Vaamonde and colleagues [20] showed that physically active men (PA) have better semen parameters when compared to sedentary (SE) counterparts. Statistically significant differences were found for several semen parameters such as total progressive motility (PA: 60.94 ± 5.03; SE: 56.07 ± 4.55) and morphology (PA: 15.54 ± 1.38, SE: 14.40 ± 1.15). The seminological values observed were supported by differences in hormones [20]. Palmer and colleagues also reported an improvement in sperm motility (1.2-fold) and morphology (1.1-fold, $P<0.05$) following 8 week of swimming in C57BL6 male mice [89].

Oxidative Stress and DNA Damage
The reduction in sperm DNA damage (1.5-fold), ROS (1.1-fold), and mitochondrial membrane potential (1.2-fold, $P<0.05$) has been recently reported in male mice following 8 week of swimming exercise [89] (Table 4.1).

Conclusions and Final Recommendations

Although exercising reduces the risk of developing diseases and promotes many health benefits, exhaustive exercise and overtraining may alter male fertility and the HPG axis. High-load exercise seems to be able to negatively impact male fertility as observed by seminal or hormonal alterations which may lead to subfertility or infertility. Though many studies show full recovery upon cessation of the exercise stimulus, we must be aware that exercise is a potential cause for male fertility disorders. Moreover, we need to be careful with how many years athletes have been training or at which age they started training. On the other hand, it has also been observed

Table 4.1 Exercise (chronic effect)[a]

Endurance		Resistance		
Positive effects (moderate exercise)	Negative effects (intensive exercise)	Positive effects (moderate exercise)	Resistance + AAS	Negative effects (intensive exercise)
Hormones	Hormones	Hormones	Hormones	Hormones
↑T, DHT, FSH, LH, T/C	↓GnRH, FSH, LH, T, E₂, DHEA, T/C	↑T, LH, T/C, GH	↓FSH, LH, T	↓T, T/C
	↑PRL, C	↓Myostatin		↑C
Semen	Semen	Semen	Semen	Semen
Mobility	Oligospermia		Azoospermia	
↓Morphology anomalies, DNA fragmentation	↑Morphology anomalies, round cells, DNA fragmentation		Oligozoospermia	
	↓Sperm count, mobility, germ cell line		↑Apoptosis in germ cell line, morphology anomalies	
			↓Mobility	
Oxidative stress	Oxidative stress	Oxidative stress	Oxidative stress	Oxidative stress
↓ROS	↑ROS, MDA			
	↓SOD, CAT, TAC			
Erectile dysfunction	Erectile dysfunction	Erectile dysfunction	Erectile dysfunction	Erectile dysfunction
	↑ED in modalities including cycling			

Abbreviations: *AAS* androgenic-anabolic steroids, *T* testosterone, *DHT* dihydrotestosterone, *FSH* follicle-stimulating hormone, *LH* luteinizing hormone, *T/C* testosterone to cortisol ratio, *GnRH* gonadotropin-releasing hormone, *E2* estradiol, *DHEA* dehydroepiandrosterone, *PRL* prolactin, *C* cortisol, *GH* growth hormone, *ROS* reactive oxygen species, *MDA* malondialdehyde, *SOD* superoxide dismutase, *CAT* catalase, *TAC* total antioxidant capacity, *ED* erectile dysfunction
[a]The above mentioned effects are load-dependent

that regular exercise may improve both hormone and semen profiles.

Further research should therefore be undertaken to clarify this relationship.

References

1. Homan GF, Davies M, Norman R. The impact of lifestyle factors on reproductive performance in the general population and those undergoing infertility treatment: a review. Hum Reprod Update. 2007;13:209–23.
2. Mastaloudis A, Yu TW, O'Donnell RP, Frei B, Dashwood RH, Traber MG. Endurance exercise results in DNA damage as detected by the comet assay. Free Radic Biol Med. 2004;36:966–75.
3. Vaamonde D, Da Silva-Grigoletto ME, Garcia-Manso JM, Vaamonde-Lemos R, Swanson RJ, Oehninger SC. Response of semen parameters to three training modalities. Fertil Steril. 2009;92:1941–6.
4. Olive DL. Exercise and fertility: an update. Curr Opin Obstet Gynecol. 2010;22:259–63.
5. Safarinejad MR, Azma K, Kolahi AA. The effects of intensive, long-term treadmill running on reproductive

hormones, hypothalamus-pituitary-testis axis, and semen quality: a randomized controlled study. J Endocrinol. 2009;20:259–71.
6. De Souza MJ, Arce JC, Pescatello LS, Scherzer HS, Luciano AA. Gonadal hormones and semen quality in male runners. A volume threshold effect of endurance training. Int J Sports Med. 1994;15:383–91.
7. Vaamonde D, Da Silva ME, Poblador MS, Lancho JL. Reproductive profile of physically active men after exhaustive endurance exercise. Int J Sports Med. 2006;27:680–9.
8. Fitzgerald LZ, Robbins WA, Kesner JS, Xun L. Reproductive hormones and interleukin-6 in serious leisure male athletes. Eur J Appl Physiol. 2012; 112:3765–73.
9. Maimoun L, Lumbroso S, Manetta J, Paris F, Leroux JL, Sultan C. Testosterone is significantly reduced in endurance athletes without impact on bone mineral density. Horm Res Paediatr. 2003;59:285–92.
10. Arce JC, De Souza MJ, Pescatello LS, Luciano AA. Subclinical alterations in hormone and semen profile in athletes. Fertil Steril. 1993;59:398–404.
11. Lucia A, Chicharro JL, Perez M, Serratosa L, Bandres F, Legido JC. Reproductive function in male endurance athletes: sperm analysis and hormonal profile. J Appl Physiol. 1996;81:2627–36.

12. Vaamonde D, Da Silva-Grigoletto ME, Garcia-Manso JM, Vaamonde-Lemos R. Differences in sperm DNA fragmentation between high- and low-cycling volume triathletes: preliminary results. Fertil Steril. 2012;98(3 Suppl):S85.
13. Tartibian B, Maleki BH. Correlation between seminal oxidative stress biomarkers and antioxidants with sperm DNA damage in elite athletes and recreationally active men. Clin J Sport Med. 2012;22:132–9.
14. De Souza MJ, Miller BE. The effect of endurance training on reproductive function in male runners. A 'volume threshold' hypothesis. Sports Med. 1997; 23:357–74.
15. Jensen CE, Wiswedel K, McLoughlin J, van der Spuy Z. Prospective study of hormonal and semen profiles in marathon runners. Fertil Steril. 1995;64:1189–96.
16. Brock G. Erectile function of bike patrol officers. J Androl. 2002;23:758–9.
17. Di Luigi L, Gentile V, Pigozzi F, Parisi A, Giannetti D, Romanelli F. Physical activity as a possible aggravating factor for athletes with varicocele: impact on the semen profile. Hum Reprod. 2001;16:1180–4.
18. Naessens G, De Slypere JP, Dijs H, Driessens M. Hypogonadism as a cause of recurrent muscle injury in a high level soccer player. A case report. Int J Sports Med. 1995;16:413–7.
19. WHO. WHO laboratory manual for the examination of human semen and sperm-cervical mucus interaction. 4th ed. Cambridge, UK: Cambridge University Press; 1999.
20. Vaamonde D, Da Silva-Grigoletto ME, García-Manso JM, Barrera N, Vaamonde-Lemos R. Physically active men show better semen parameters and hormone values than sedentary men. Eur J Appl Physiol. 2012; 112:3267–73.
21. Wilmore JH, Costill DL, Kenney WL. Physiology of sport and exercise. 4th ed. Champaign, IL: Human Kinetics; 2008.
22. Pradet M. La Preparación Física. INDE: Barcelona, Spain; 1999.
23. Nacleiro F. Entrenamiento de la fuerza y prescripción del ejercicio. In: Jiménez A, editor. Entrenamiento Personal. Bases, fundamentos y aplicaciones. Barcelona, Spain: INDE; 2005. p. 99.
24. Heredia JR, Isidro F, Peña G, Moral S, Mata F, Martín M, Segarra V, Da Silva ME. Criterios básicos para el diseño de programas de acondicionamiento neuromuscular saludable en centros de fitness. Revista Digital 2012;17:170. EFDeportes.com, Buenos Aires.
25. Hackney AC. Endurance training and testosterone levels. Sports Med. 1989;8:117–27.
26. Ayers JW, Komesu Y, Romani T, Ansbacher R. Anthropomorphic, hormonal, and psychologic correlates of semen quality in endurance-trained male athletes. Fertil Steril. 1985;43:917–21.
27. Bagatell CJ, Bremner WJ. Sperm counts and reproductive hormones in male marathoners and lean controls. Fertil Steril. 1990;53:688–92.
28. Vaamonde D, Da Silva-Grigoletto ME, García-Manso JM, Cunha-Filho JS, Vaamonde-Lemos R. Sperm morphology normalcy is inversely correlated to cycling kilometers in elite triathletes. Rev Andal Med Deporte. 2009;2:43–6.
29. Gebreegziabher Y, Marcos E, McKinon W, Rogers G. Sperm characteristics of endurance trained cyclists. Int J Sports Med. 2004;25:247–51.
30. Mastorakos G, Pavlatou M, Diamanti-Kandarakis E, Chrousos GP. Exercise and the stress system. Hormones. 2005;4:73–89.
31. McArdle WD, Katch FI, Katch VL. Essentials of exercise physiology. 3rd ed. Philadelphia, PA: Williams and Wilkins; 2006.
32. Kraemer WJ. Endocrine responses to resistance exercise. Med Sci Sport Exerc. 1988;20(5 Suppl):S152–7.
33. Hakkinen K, Pakarinen A, Kraemer WJ, Newton RU, Alen M. Basal concentrations and acute responses of serum hormones and strength development during heavy resistance training in middle-aged and elderly men and women. J Gerontol A Biol Sci Med Sci. 2000;55:B95–105.
34. Fronczak CM, Kim ED, Barqawi AB. The insults of illicit drug use on male fertility. J Androl. 2012; 33:515–28.
35. Kanayama G, Brower KJ, Wood RI, Hudson JI, Pope Jr HG. Anabolic-androgenic steroid dependence: an emerging disorder. Addiction. 2009;104:1966–78.
36. Karila T, Hovatta O, Seppala T. Concomitant abuse of anabolic androgenic steroids and human chorionic gonadotrophin impairs spermatogenesis in power athletes. Int J Sports Med. 2004;25:257–63.
37. Hoffman JR, Kraemer WJ, Bhasin S, Storer T, Ratamess NA, Haff GG, Willoughby DS, Rogol AD. Position stand on androgen and human growth hormone use. J Strength Cond Res. 2009;23(5 Suppl):S1–59.
38. Schurmeyer T, Knuth UA, Belkien L, Nieschlag E. Reversible azoospermia induced by the anabolic steroid 19-nortestosterone. Lancet. 1984;1:417–20.
39. Torres-Calleja J, Gonzalez-Unzaga M, DeCelis-Carrillo R, Calzada-Sanchez L, Pedron N. Effect of androgenic anabolic steroids on sperm quality and serum hormone levels in adult male bodybuilders. Life Sci. 2001;68:1769–74.
40. Bonetti A, Tirelli F, Catapano A, Dazzi D, Dei Cas A, Solito F, Ceda G, Reverberi C, Monica C, Pipitone S, Elia G, Spattini M, Magnati G. Side effects of anabolic androgenic steroids abuse. Int J Sports Med. 2008;29:679–87.
41. Shokri S, Aitken RJ, Abdolvahhabi M, Abolhasani F, Ghasemi FM, Kashani I, Ejtemaeimehr S, Ahmadian S, Minaei B, Naraghi MA, Barbarestani M. Exercise and supraphysiological dose of nandrolone decanoate increase apoptosis in spermatogenic cells. Basic Clin Pharmacol Toxicol. 2010;106:324–30.
42. Knuth UA, Maniera H, Nieschlag E. Anabolic steroids and semen parameters in bodybuilders. Fertil Steril. 1989;52:1041–7.
43. Schurmeyer Menon DK. Successful treatment of anabolic steroid-induced azoospermia with human chorionic gonadotropin and human menopausal

gonadotropin. Fertil Steril. 2003;79 Suppl 3: 1659–61.

44. Kujala UM, Alen M, Huhtaniemi IT. Gonadotrophin-releasing hormone and human chorionic gonadotrophin tests reveal that both hypothalamic and testicular endocrine functions are suppressed during acute prolonged physical exercise. Clin Endocrinol. 1990;33:219–25.

45. Mathur DN, Toriola AL, Dada OA. Serum cortisol and testosterone levels in conditioned male distance runners and nonrunners after maximal exercise. J Sports Med Phys Fitness. 1986;26:245–50.

46. Griffith RO, Dressendorfer RH, Fullbright CD, Wade CE. Testicular function during exhaustive endurance training. Phys Sports Med. 1990;18:54–64.

47. Wheeler GD, Singh M, Pierce WD, Epling WF, Cumming DC. Endurance training decreases serum testosterone levels in men without change in luteinizing hormone pulsation release. J Clin Endocrinol Metab. 1991;72:422–5.

48. Roberts AC, McClure RD, Weiner RI, Brooks GA. Overtraining affects male reproductive status. Fertil Steril. 1993;60:686–92.

49. MacConnie SE, Barkan A, Lampman RM, Schork MA, Beitins IZ. Decreased hypothalamic gonadotropin-releasing hormone secretion in male marathon runners. N Engl J Med. 1986;315:411–7.

50. Hackney AC, Sinning WE, Bruot BC. Reproductive hormonal profiles of endurance-trained and untrained males. Med Sci Sports Exerc. 1988;20:60–5.

51. Hackney AC, Sinning WE, Bruot BC. Hypothalamic-pituitary-testicular axis function in endurance-trained males. Int J Sports Med. 1990;11:298–303.

52. McColl EM, Wheeler GD, Gomes P, Bhambhani Y, Cumming DC. The effects of acute exercise on pulsatile LH release in high-mileage male runners. Clin Endocrinol. 1989;68:402–11.

53. Fernández-Garcia B, Lucía A, Hoyos J, Chicharro JL, Rodriguez-Alonso M, Bandrés F, Terrados N. The response of sexual and stress hormones of male procyclists during continuous intense competition. Int J Sports Med. 2002;23:555–60.

54. Mackinnon LT, Hooper SL, Jones S, Gordon RD, Bachmann AW. Hormonal, immunological, and hematological responses to intensified training in elite swimmers. Med Sci Sports Exerc. 1997;29:1637–45.

55. Bonifazi M, Bela E, Carli G, et al. Influence of training on the response of androgen plasma concentrations to exercise in swimmers. Eur J Appl Physiol Occup Physiol. 1995;70:109–14.

56. Izquierdo M, Ibáñez J, Häkkinen K, Kraemer WJ, Ruesta M, Gorostiaga EM. Maximal strength and power, muscle mass, endurance and serum hormones in weightlifters and road cyclists. J Sports Sci. 2004;22:465–78.

57. Hackney AC, Moore AW, Brownlee KK. Testosterone and endurance exercise: development of the exercise-hypogonadal male condition. Acta Physiol Hung. 2005;92:121–37.

58. Hawkins VN, Foster-Schubert K, Chubak J, Sorensen B, Ulrich CM, Stancyzk FZ, Plymate S, Stanford J, White E, Potter JD, McTiernan A. Effect of exercise on serum sex hormones in men: a 12-month randomized clinical trial. Med Sci Sports Exerc. 2008; 40:223–33.

59. Hackney AC. Endurance exercise training and reproductive endocrine dysfunction in men: alterations in the hypothalamic-pituitary-testicular axis. Curr Pharm Des. 2001;7:261–73.

60. Bambino TH, Hsueh AJ. Direct inhibitory effect of glucocorticoids upon testicular luteinizing hormone receptor and steroidogenesis in vivo and in vitro. Endocrinology. 1981;108:2142–8.

61. Hall HL, Flynn MG, Carroll KK, Brolinson PG, Shapiro S, Bushman BA. Effects of intensified training and detraining on testicular function. Clin J Sport Med. 1999;9:203–8.

62. Du Plessis S, Kashou A, Vaamonde D, Agarwal A. Is there a link between exercise and male factor infertility? Open Reprod Sci J. 2011;3:105–13.

63. Mingoti GZ, Pereira RN, Monteiro CM. Fertility of male adult rats submitted to forced swimming stress. Braz J Med Biol Res. 2003;36:677–81.

64. Manna I, Jana K, Samanta PK. Effect of different intensities of swimming exercise on testicular oxidative stress and reproductive dysfunction in mature male albino Wistar rats. Indian J Exp Biol. 2004; 42:816–22.

65. Vaamonde D, Diaz A, Rodriguez I. Preliminary results of trans-resveratrol as an effective protector against exercise-induced morphology abnormalities on mice sperm. Fertil Steril. 2011;96(3 Suppl):S166–7.

66. Knez WL, Jenkins DG, Coombes JS. Oxidative stress in half and full Ironman triathletes. Med Sci Sports Exerc. 2007;39:283–8.

67. Lehmann M, Dickhuth HH, Gendrisch G, Lazar W, Thum M, Kaminski R, Aramendi JF, Peterke E, Wieland W, Keul J. Training-overtraining. A prospective, experimental study with experienced middle- and long-distance runners. Int J Sports Med. 1991;12(5):444–52.

68. Myhal M, Lamb DR. Hormones as performance enhancing drugs. In: Warren MP, Constantini NW, editors. Sport endocrinology. Totowa, NJ: Humana; 2000. p. 433–76.

69. Giannoulis MG, Martin FC, Nair KS, Umpleby AM, Sonksen P. Hormone replacement therapy and physical function in healthy older men. Time to talk hormones? Endocr Rev. 2012;33:314–77.

70. Bloomer RJ, Sforzo GA, Keller BA. Effects of meal form and composition on plasma testosterone, cortisol, and insulin following resistance exercise. Int J Sport Nutr Exerc Metab. 2000;10:415–24.

71. Kraemer WJ, Ratamess NA. Hormonal responses and adaptations to resistance exercise and training. Sports Med. 2005;35:339–61.

72. Tremblay MS, Copeland JL, Van Helder W. Effect of training status and exercise mode on endogenous steroid hormones in men. J Appl Physiol. 2004;96:531–9.

73. Kon M, Ikeda T, Homma T, Suzuki Y. Effects of low-intensity resistance exercise under acute systemic

73. hypoxia on hormonal responses. J Strength Cond Res. 2012;26:611–7.

74. Hakkinen K, Pakarinen A, Alen M, Kauhanen H, Komi PV. Neuromuscular and hormonal adaptations in athletes to strength training in two years. J Appl Physiol. 1988;65:2406–12.

75. Kraemer WJ, Hakkinen K, Newton RU, Nindl BC, Volek JS, McCormick M, Gotshalk LA, Gordon SE, Fleck SJ, Campbell WW, Putukian M, Evans WJ. Effects of heavy-resistance training on hormonal response patterns in younger vs. older men. J Appl Physiol. 1999;87:982–92.

76. Pullinen T, Mero A, Huttunen P, Pakarinen A, Komi PV. Resistance exercise-induced hormonal responses in men, women, and pubescent boys. Med Sci Sports Exerc. 2002;34:806–13.

77. Migiano MJ, Vingren JL, Volek JS, Maresh CM, Fragala MS, Ho JY, Thomas GA, Hatfield DL, Häkkinen K, Ahtiainen J, Earp JE, Kraemer WJ. Endocrine response patterns to acute unilateral and bilateral resistance exercise in men. J Strength Cond Res. 2010;24:128–34.

78. Hackney AC, Premo MC, McMurray RG. Influence of aerobic versus anaerobic exercise on the relationship between reproductive hormones in men. J Sports Sci. 1995;13:305–11.

79. Kraemer WJ, Hakkinen K, Newton RU, et al. Acute hormonal responses to heavy resistance exercise in younger and older men. Eur J Appl Physiol Occup Physiol. 1998;77:206–11.

80. Willoughby DS, Taylor L. Effects of sequential bouts of resistance exercise on androgen receptor expression. Med Sci Sports Exerc. 2004;36:1499–506.

81. Herbst KL, Bhasin S. Testosterone action on skeletal muscle. Curr Opin Clin Nutr Metab Care. 2004;7:271–7.

82. Ari Z, Kutlu N, Uyanik BS, Taneli F, Buyukyazi G, Tavli T. Serum testosterone, growth hormone, and insulin-like growth factor-1 levels, mental reaction time, and maximal aerobic exercise in sedentary and long-term physically trained elderly males. Int J Neurosci. 2004;114:623–37.

83. Muller M, den Tonkelaar I, Thijssen JH, Grobbee DE, van der Schouw YT. Endogenous sex hormones in men aged 40–80 years. Eur J Endocrinol. 2003; 149:583–9.

84. Sallinen J, Hoglund I, Engstrom M, et al. Pharmacological characterization and CNS effects of a novel highly selective alpha2C-adrenoceptor antagonist JP-1302. Br J Pharmacol. 2007;150:391–402.

85. Izquierdo M, Hakkinen K, Ibanez J, et al. Effects of strength training on muscle power and serum hormones in middle-aged and older men. J Appl Physiol. 2001;90:1497–507.

86. Nicklas BJ, Ryan AJ, Treuth MM, et al. Testosterone, growth hormone and IGF-I responses to acute and chronic resistive exercise in men aged 55–70 years. Int J Sports Med. 1995;16:445–50.

87. Tymchuk CN, Tessler SB, Aronson WJ, Barnard RJ. Effects of diet and exercise on insulin, sex hormone-binding globulin, and prostate-specific antigen. Nutr Cancer. 1998;31:127–31.

88. Cooper CS, Taaffe DR, Guido D, Packer E, Holloway L, Marcus R. Relationship of chronic endurance exercise to the somatotropic and sex hormone status of older men. Eur J Endocrinol. 1998;138:517–23.

89. Palmer NO, Bakos HW, Owens JA, Setchell BP, Lane M. Diet and exercise in an obese mouse fed a high-fat diet improve metabolic health and reverse perturbed sperm function. Am J Physiol Endocrinol Metab. 2012;302:E768–80.

The Importance of Diet, Vitamins, Malnutrition, and Nutrient Deficiencies in Male Fertility

5

Landon W. Trost, Ahmet Gudeloglu, Edmund Y. Ko, and Sijo J. Parekattil

Introduction

Male-factor infertility/subfertility is a relatively common condition, affecting up to 1 in 20 men and accounting for an estimated 80 million cases worldwide [1, 2]. Among couples attempting to conceive, 15 % will experience infertility, with a male factor implicated in 50 % of cases [3, 4].

Temporal changes to the prevalence of sub-/infertility remain a controversial topic, with some authors suggesting an increasing prevalence in recent decades [5]. As numerous societal changes occurred concurrent with this time period, including environmental, dietary, and lifestyle alterations, some investigators have sought to find associations among these conditions. Although the true prevalence of infertility and its change over time remain unknown, the possibility of identifying and treating modifiable risk factors for male infertility remains an important subject for ongoing research.

The underlying etiologies of male-factor infertility are numerous and include congenital, hormonal, iatrogenic, and infectious causes, among others. Despite these recognized factors, up to 20–40 % of infertile males are classified as idiopathic [6, 7]. Similarly, among males undergoing infertility evaluation, only 50 % are found to have abnormal semen analyses [8]. This suggests that in addition to known causes, several unidentified factors likely have a significant impact on overall fertility status.

Reactive Oxygen Species

One potential etiology contributing towards male-factor infertility is an elevated level of reactive oxygen species (ROS). ROS are the product of, and are required for, normal spermatogenesis, including capacitation, acrosomal reaction, and fertilization [9]. Excessive production of ROS, however, results in lipid peroxidation of the spermatozoal membrane, DNA damage, reduced sperm motility, disrupted membrane integrity, and impaired fertilization [10–15]. As abnormal sperm are associated with a higher rate of ROS production, this further contributes towards the ROS imbalance and leads to additional spermatic impairment [16, 17].

ROS are normally counterbalanced in seminal plasma and spermatozoa through the natural excretion/production of endogenous (enzymatic)

L.W. Trost, MD
Department of Urology, Mayo Clinic,
200 First Street SW, Rochester, MN 55905, USA
e-mail: trost.landon@mayo.edu

A. Gudeloglu, MD • S.J. Parekattil, MD (✉)
Department of Urology, University of Florida &
Winter Haven Hospital, 199 Avenue B North West
Suite 310, Winter Haven, FL 33881, USA
e-mail: sijo.parekattil@winterhavenhospital.org

E.Y. Ko, MD
Department of Urology, Loma Linda University,
11234 Anderson Street, A560, Loma Linda, CA
92354, USA
e-mail: edko05@gmail.com

S.S. du Plessis et al. (eds.), *Male Infertility: A Complete Guide to Lifestyle and Environmental Factors,*
DOI 10.1007/978-1-4939-1040-3_5, © Springer Science+Business Media New York 2014

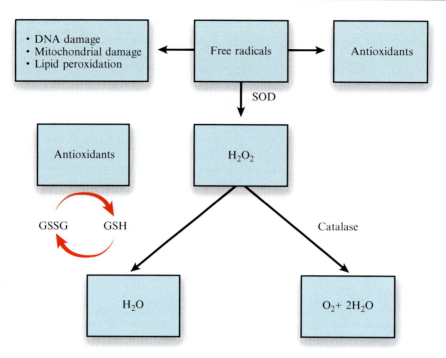

Fig. 5.1 Graphical representation of the interaction between endogenous and exogenous antioxidants in the metabolism of reactive oxygen species. GSH—reduced (active) form of glutathione peroxidase; GSSG—oxidized (inactive) form of glutathione peroxidase; SOD—superoxide dismutase

and exogenous (vitamin) antioxidants, such as Vitamins C and E, superoxide dismutase (SOD), glutathione peroxidase, catalase, and thioredoxin, among others [1, 18]. Antioxidants act as free radical scavengers to reduce oxidative damage and may be supplemented through dietary sources [17]. See Fig. 5.1 for graphical representation of antioxidant conversion of free radical compounds. Increased seminal antioxidant levels have been repeatedly linked with improved semen parameters and fertility outcomes [1, 17, 19–21].

Numerous studies have evaluated the efficacy of dietary supplementation on improving male-factor fertility. Several vitamins, minerals, and fatty acids with antioxidant properties have been studied to date and include alpha-lipoic acid (ALA), anthocyanins, L-arginine, astaxanthin, beta-carotene, biotin, L-carnitine (LC)/L-acetyl carnitine (LAC), cobalamin, co-enzyme Q10 (CoQ10), ethylcysteine, folic acid, glutathione, inositol, lycopene, magnesium, N-acetyl cysteine (NAC), pentoxifylline, phosphodiesterase (PDE) 5 inhibitors, polyunsaturated fatty acids (PUFAs), selenium, Vitamins A, C, D, and E, and zinc. In addition to these supplements, several authors have evaluated the impact of dietary patterns and obesity on fertility outcomes.

In reviewing the currently available literature, it is important to recognize several important limitations, which restrict potential conclusions. The majority of studies available are non-randomized by design, lack placebo groups, include small populations with short-term follow-up, lack standardization of dose or defined end points, involve varied numbers of agents studied, lack controls for other infertility-relevant male and/or female pathologies, and have varied baseline nutritional status/dietary intake. Regarding these limitations, a recent Cochrane meta-analysis of randomized, controlled trials (RCTs) concluded that findings were only able to achieve their lowest rating for overall quality of evidence [22]. As such, the astute reader should interpret any outcomes and conclusions with significant caution and recognize the need for larger RCTs with strict methodology prior to the definitive recognition of efficacy.

The current review is structured to identify the role of diet in general on male infertility and compare outcomes among several published dietary programs. The impact of obesity and weight loss will be briefly discussed, followed by a more detailed review of available literature on the various individual and combined supplements for the treatment of male infertility. The proposed mechanisms and classifications of the supplements as well as available data reporting outcomes on male-factor infertility are also discussed. To perform the review, a PubMed search was performed of all English-language publications from 1970 to present using the search items male fertility, subfertility, infertility, supplement, diet, vitamin, nutrition, and antioxidant. Preference was given towards more recent publications, meta-analyses, and RCTs, when available.

Role of Nutrition in Male Fertility

Despite an abundance of research on the role of nutrition, exercise, and body composition with female fecundity, there is limited data available regarding male fertility [23, 24]. Although the impact of lifestyle modifications, including exercise and exogenous substance use (tobacco, alcohol, testosterone supplementation, etc.), is beyond the scope of this chapter, the impact of diet on obesity and maintaining appropriate nutritional status is relevant and will be reviewed.

Diet and Obesity

Several studies have identified associations between impaired male-factor fertility and dietary patterns. Among 701 young Danish men undergoing routine screening prior to entry into military service, those with higher intakes of saturated fat were found to have lower sperm counts, with the highest quartile experiencing a 41 % lower count than those in the lowest quartile [25]. This is supported by Gaskin and colleagues who

reported on 188 men aged 18–22 from the University of Rochester [26]. In comparing semen analysis (SA) outcomes of patients with a "Western" pattern diet (high intake of red meat, refined grains, pizza, snacks, high-energy drinks, sweets) to those with a "prudent" diet (high intake of fish, chicken, fruit, vegetables, legumes, whole grains), the authors noted a positive association with progressively motile sperm among those eating a "prudent" diet. Further studies have confirmed lower risks of asthenospermia with higher intakes of fruits, vegetables, poultry, skim milk, and seafoods and increased risks among those consuming the highest levels of processed meats and sweets (OR 2.0, CI 1.7–2.4 and OR 2.1, CI 1.1–2.3, respectively) [27, 28].

Outcomes of assisted reproductive techniques (ART) have similarly demonstrated a nonsignificant trend towards higher rates of pregnancy among couples adhering to a Mediterranean diet compared to a "health conscious-low processed" diet (OR 1.4, CI 1.0–1.9 versus OR 0.8, CI 0.6–1.0, respectively) [29].

In addition to specific diets, semen quality has been associated with overall body mass index (BMI). In reviewing the outcomes of 250 couples undergoing intracytoplasmic sperm injection (ICSI), sperm motility and concentration were negatively influenced by BMI, while those undergoing a weight-loss diet experienced improved sperm counts [30]. Semen parameters were positively influenced by the higher consumption of cereals and legumes.

Animal studies have repeatedly confirmed the role of diet on maintaining optimal semen characteristics and fertility. Rato and colleagues evaluated fertility parameters in rats fed with high-energy (high fat) diets and demonstrated increases in abnormal sperm morphology and elevated markers of oxidative stress [31]. Similar reductions in sperm quality, motility, capacitation, and acrosomal reaction have been demonstrated in obese and hypercholesterolemic animal models [32–34]. Impairments in fertility may be improved through a combination of diet and/or exercise. One study of obese animals showed significant improvements in sperm motility (1.2-fold), morphology (1.1-fold), reduced sperm

DNA damage (1.5-fold), ROS (1.1-fold), and sperm binding (1.4-fold) following treatment with a standard diet [35].

Obesity may impair host defenses against toxic exposures in addition to its direct effects on fertility. Obese mice treated with acrylamide (reproductive toxin) experienced fewer successful pregnancies compared to lean mice receiving acrylamide [34]. Although this may be due, in part, to the observed higher rate of DNA damage sustained with obesity, underlying mechanisms remain unknown [36].

Fullston and colleagues recently reported perhaps the most intriguing findings on the impact of obesity on male fertility [37]. In their analysis of rats fed high-fat diets, they noted that two subsequent generations of both sexes experienced impaired fertility rates, despite being fed a standard diet. These findings suggest that obesity may impair fertility in future progeny, as well as in the obese animal itself. Potential mechanisms to account for this result include alteration of epigenetic profiles, which are influenced by environmental factors and can negatively affect implantation, placentation, and fetal growth [38]. Certainly these results have several potential significant implications regarding the importance of diet and obesity on both current and future generational fertility.

Malnutrition/Nutrient Deficiencies

Appropriate nutrition likely has a significant role in maintaining optimal fertility. Although little data is currently available, several observational studies and animal models have identified associations between sub-/infertility and reduced vitamin/mineral concentrations [39–44]. As many vitamins and minerals have potent indirect or direct antioxidant activity, reduced levels may result in an altered ROS to antioxidant ratio with subsequent reduction in total antioxidant capacity (TAC) [39, 45].

Several studies have identified an optimal range for select vitamin/mineral administration, with impairments in fertility noted with both under- and over-supplementation. Two studies evaluating the role of selenium in mice demonstrated reduced fertility among animals receiving either under- or over-supplementation, with resultant oxidative stress causing germ cell apoptosis [43, 46]. Other studies have reported similar optimal ranges for Vitamin D, with impairments in fertility at high and low serum levels [44, 47].

Although data regarding the toxicity of over-supplementation is limited, all nutrients likely have a certain threshold above which their impact is negated or detrimental. This is particularly relevant given that many studies use varying doses and/or combinations of vitamins/minerals in their patient cohorts. Similarly, as individual populations likely experience varying degrees of nutrient deficiencies, select groups may benefit more from supplementation than others. This may also account (in part) for contradictory findings of studies examining the effect of individual nutrients.

Nutrient Supplementation in Male Infertility

A comprehensive listing of every study performed on nutrients associated with infertility is beyond the scope of any one publication. As the quality of evidence for each study varies, this chapter attempts to highlight studies with the highest level of evidence available. In the absence of human RCTs, all available literature is reviewed, with an emphasis on higher quality studies. However, findings from non-RCT should not be interpreted as equivalent to the higher quality trials. The current listing also does not represent a complete listing of every nutrient or supplement, but rather those with the most abundant literature available. Each nutrient will be presented in alphabetic order, with a brief description as to its classification and mechanism if available. Data will be provided supporting or contradicting its use with male fertility as well as the authors' interpretation as to a consensus of evidence. See Table 5.1 for a brief summary of nutrient supplements with data

Table 5.1 Summary of effects of nutrient supplementation on male-factor infertility

Agent	Class/function	Proposed mechanism of action	Summary of effect on infertility
Antioxidants (in general)	Reduction of reactive oxygen species	Improved sperm function, DNA integrity, fertilization capacity	May improve live birth and pregnancy rates, DNA fragmentation, sperm motility
L-Arginine	Amino acid; precursor to NO	Precursor for putrescine, spermidine, spermine, and required for sperm capacitation	Conflicting and inadequate data
L-Carnitine, L-acetyl carnitine	Quaternary ammonium compounds; transport fatty acids to mitochondria	Antioxidant; assists with sperm maturation and motility	May result in improved pregnancy rates
Cobalamin	Form of vitamin B12	Functions in combination with folic acid in DNA synthesis	Deficiency associated with infertility; insufficient data to suggest benefit to supplementation
Coenzyme Q10	Vitamin-like substance in mitochondria; produces adenosine triphosphate through electron transport chain	Lipid-soluble antioxidant; may enhance motility through mitochondrial activity	Improves markers of oxidative stress; insufficient data to suggest benefit to supplementation
Folic acid	Vitamin B9	Functions in DNA synthesis, repair, methylation; required for normal spermatogenesis; indirectly functions as antioxidant	Deficiency associated with infertility; insufficient data to suggest benefit to supplementation
Glutathione	Endogenous antioxidant	Endogenous antioxidant; replenishes other antioxidants; detoxifies foreign compounds and carcinogens	May improve sperm motility, morphology, DNA integrity; may be used adjunctively in ART sperm media
Lycopene	Nonessential carotenoid pigment	Antioxidant; functions in genetic expression, cell regulation, immunomodulation	Conflicting results on antioxidant capacity; no RCTs available
N-Acetyl cysteine	Derivative of the amino acid cysteine	Antioxidant; helps regenerate glutathione	Conflicting and inadequate data
Pentoxifylline	Methylated xanthine derivative; nonselective PDEI	Possibly reduces inflammation through PDEI	May improve sperm motility; may be used adjunctively in ART sperm media
Polyunsaturated fatty acids	Triglyceride compounds (omega-3, -6, -9)	Modulates inflammation; required for sperm capacitation and spermatogenesis	Conflicting and inadequate data
Selenium	Chemical element required for cellular function	Essential for normal function of endogenous antioxidants	Deficiency associated with infertility; combination therapy with vitamin E may improve motility
Vitamin C	Vitamin cofactor for enzymatic reactions (e.g., collagen synthesis)	Indirect and direct antioxidant	Deficiency associated with infertility; may improve DNA fragmentation; conflicting data on impact on sperm
Vitamin E	Fat-soluble vitamin, which encompasses tocopherols and tocotrienols	Antioxidant; restores other antioxidants to reduced state	May improve pregnancy and live birth rates
Zinc	Metallic element; cofactor in enzymatic processes	Required for reproductive gland growth and spermatic function	Deficiency associated with infertility; may benefit semen parameters, pregnancy, and birth rates

ART assisted reproductive techniques, *NO* nitric oxide, *PDEI* phosphodiesterase inhibitor, *RCT* randomized, controlled trial available, including class of agent, proposed mechanisms of action, and efficacy with improving infertility.

L-Arginine

Class and Mechanism

L-Arginine is an amino acid, which serves as a precursor of nitric oxide (NO) via nitric oxide synthase. NO subsequently functions as an endogenous ROS and is required for routine signal transduction during sperm capacitation [48]. L-Arginine is also utilized in the synthesis of putrescine, spermidine, and spermine, which regulate various cellular processes and are thought to function in sperm motility [49].

Data Supporting Use

Very limited data is available on the use of L-arginine for male fertility. Initial human studies of supplemental L-arginine administered up to 4 g/day reported improved sperm concentration and motility [50–52]. A placebo-controlled, crossover, RCT comparing the supplement Prelox (combination of L-arginine and the antioxidant pycnogenol) in 50 men similarly reported improved sperm concentration, volume, and motility in the treatment group [53, 54]. However, as the study used combination therapy, it is unclear which agent accounted for the improvements noted.

Data Contradicting Use

Several human and animal studies have reported no improvements or impaired fertility with L-arginine directly, or through its downstream product, NO. Two early human studies failed to identify any improvements in SA parameters or pregnancy rates, with more recent studies demonstrating impaired fertility, decreased sperm motility, spermatic toxicity, and reduced sperm-zona binding following L-arginine administration [55–59].

Consensus of Opinion

Inadequate and contradictory data exist regarding the effect of L-arginine on SA parameters and pregnancy rates.

L-Carnitine and L-Acetyl Carnitine

Class and Mechanism

L-Carnitine (LC) and its acetylated form (LAC) are quaternary ammonium compounds, which serve to transport fatty acids to the mitochondria. From a fertility standpoint, carnitine assists with sperm maturation and motility and functions as an antioxidant [60].

Data Supporting Use

LC and LAC are among the most studied nutrients in male fertility, with deficiencies in seminal carnitine previously associated with reduced sperm concentration, motility, and DNA integrity among infertile males [61]. Similarly, compared to normal controls, infertile males have been shown to have lower levels of seminal free LC [62]. Multiple RCTs are available comparing its efficacy to placebo and other agents, with a recent Cochrane meta-analysis performed to summarize results [22, 63–71]. Combined outcomes of the RCTs demonstrated significantly improved pregnancy outcomes with LC or combination of LC+LAC versus placebo (OR 4.5 and 5.1; CI 1.5–17.1 and 1.8–11.4, respectively) [63–66, 68]. Comparing LC+LAC to Vitamin E+C supplementation, the carnitine group demonstrated improved motility and concentration at 3 months compared to vitamins (OR 23.1; CI 20.2–25.9 and OR 15.5; CI 12.5–18.5, respectively) [67].

A less-stringent meta-analysis performed in 2007 of clinical and RCTs comparing LC and/or LAC to placebo, reported improved pregnancy rates (OR 4.1; CI 2.1–8.1), motility (weighted mean difference [WMD] 7.43; CI 1.7–13.1), and morphology (WMD 5.7; CI 3.6–7.9) [72]. No significant differences were noted on sperm concentration or semen volume.

Individual studies demonstrated varied improvements in semen characteristics. Among men with no, small, or moderate-sized varicoceles, Cavallini and colleagues noted that supplementation with carnitine and cinnoxicam (nonsteroidal anti-inflammatory) resulted in improved sperm concentration, motility, and morphology, although

5 The Importance of Diet, Vitamins, Malnutrition, and Nutrient Deficiencies in Male Fertility

similar improvements were not found among patients with higher-grade varicoceles [64]. A similar combination study of carnitine and cinnoxicam in men with prostato-vesiculo-epididymitis demonstrated selective improvements in motility in men with <1 million/mL seminal WBCs [69]. Among patients with oligo-asthenoteratospermia (OAT) undergoing ICSI, combination of LC+LAC and cinnoxicam resulted in improved sperm morphology and reduced aneuploidy with resultant higher rates of pregnancies and live births [73].

One study by de Rosa and colleagues supplemented oligospermic infertile males with motilities <50 % and demonstrated improvements in motility, live sperm count, and cervical penetration capacity compared to baseline [61]. In comparing LC+Vitamin E versus Vitamin E alone, patients receiving combination therapy demonstrated improved motility (45 % versus 28 % pretreatment, $p < 0.01$) and higher pregnancy rates (31.1 % [combination] versus 3.8 % [Vitamin E alone], $p < 0.01$), with otherwise unchanged sperm concentrations and morphology [71].

Data Contradicting Use

The effect of LC and/or LAC on sperm motility is inconclusive, with 3- and 6-month data from a Cochrane meta-analysis demonstrating conflicting findings [22]. Data ≥ 9 months on LC versus placebo demonstrated significant improvements with a wide confidence interval for motility (OR 11.5; CI 1.7–21.4) and no significant improvements with LC or combination of LC+LAC [63]. The Cochrane meta-analysis similarly demonstrated no significant differences in sperm concentration among two included studies at 6- and ≥ 9-month time points with LC, LAC, or combination therapy [63, 66]. When comparing LC+LAC to Vitamin E+C supplementation, no significant differences were noted with pregnancies achieved (OR 2.9; CI 0.9–9.5) [67]. A separate RCT not included in the Cochrane review similarly demonstrated a lack of improvement with LC on seminal volume, sperm concentration, motility, or morphology [70].

Consensus of Opinion

Although the data remain inconclusive as to the benefits of LC±LAC on individual semen characteristics, significant improvements in pregnancy rates have been reported. However, as the confidence intervals remain very wide, this finding requires larger, well-controlled trials to validate.

Cobalamin (Vitamin B12)

Class and Mechanism

Cobalamin represents one of several forms of B12 and may be considered equivalent physiologically to B12. The underlying mechanism for the role of B12 in fertility is unclear, although it may relate to its role in DNA synthesis, activation of antioxidant enzymes, or methyl group donation.

Data Supporting Use

Cobalamin deficiency has long been recognized to be associated with sub-/infertility, with observational studies confirming reduced levels in cases of non-obstructive azoospermia [40, 74, 75]. Among men undergoing in vitro fertilization (IVF)/ICSI, sperm concentrations have been shown to positively correlate with cobalamin levels [76].

Multiple early Japanese studies were performed to evaluate the efficacy of methylcobalamin supplementation on fertility and SA parameters [77–80]. The majority of trials reported significant improvements in sperm concentration and motility; however, the criteria for success were loosely defined. Since these early reports, no additional human trials have been reported.

Data Contradicting Use

Although the majority of studies demonstrate an association between cobalamin deficiency and sub-/infertility, cobalamin concentrations beyond a minimal threshold may not result in improvement in semen parameters [41]. One multi-institution, double-blinded, placebo-controlled, RCT performed on cobalamin supplementation demonstrated no overall impact of therapy on sperm motility or concentration [77].

Consensus of Opinion

Cobalamin deficiency (resulting in clinical pernicious anemia) is linked with infertility. The impact of cobalamin supplementation beyond minimum requirements lacks sufficient data to suggest a proven benefit on male fertility.

Co-enzyme Q10

Class and Mechanism

CoQ10 is a vitamin-like substance present in the mitochondria, which functions to produce adenosine triphosphate through the electron transport chain. From a fertility standpoint, CoQ10 may provide benefit through lipid-soluble antioxidant properties and/or through enhancing motility via mitochondrial activity [81].

Data Supporting Use

CoQ10 concentrations in seminal plasma have been correlated with total sperm counts and motility, while ratios of its reduced (ubiquinol) to oxidized (ubiquinone) state are associated with alterations in the percentage of abnormal sperm morphology [82].

A Cochrane meta-analysis and review of RCTs summarized outcomes from two RCTs utilizing CoQ10 [22, 81, 83]. It is noteworthy that one of the trials reported results of questionable validity and reliability, suggesting that conclusions must be interpreted with caution [83]. Combined results demonstrated significant improvements in motility at 6 months (OR 4.5; CI 3.9–5.1), which was not sustained at $\geq$9 months (OR −0.0; CI −1.1 to 6.2). Two additional RCTs, which were not included in the Cochrane review, demonstrate significant improvements in markers of oxidative stress with CoQ10 supplementation among patients with OAT, including elevated catalase, SOD, and TAC [84, 85]. Additionally, one trial identified a positive correlation between CoQ10 concentrations and normal sperm morphology [85].

Data Contradicting Use

The previously cited Cochrane review demonstrated no significant improvements with CoQ10 supplementation on the rate of pregnancies (OR 2.2; CI 0.5–8.8) or sperm concentration at 6 or $\geq$9 months (OR 3.9; CI −2.1 to 9.8 and OR 1.5; CI 0.5–2.6, respectively). Similarly, two RCTs performed on CoQ10 administration among OAT patients failed to demonstrate improvements in sperm concentration or motility despite demonstrably higher levels of TAC [84, 85].

Consensus of Opinion

CoQ10 supplementation appears to improve markers of oxidative stress and improve TAC. However, its impact on semen parameters and pregnancy rates remains unproven.

Folic Acid (Vitamin B9)

Class and Mechanism

Folic acid is a water-soluble B Vitamin, which has roles in DNA synthesis, repair, and methylation and is an essential cofactor. Folic acid is required for normal spermatogenesis and may function as an indirect antioxidant through creation of methyl donor compounds [86, 87].

Data Supporting Use

Folic acid levels have been associated with sperm characteristics, including chromosomal aneuploidy and total sperm concentration, with low levels correlating with infertility [20, 41, 88]. Several RCTs have demonstrated beneficial effects of folic acid on semen parameters and pregnancy rates. The earliest RCT was performed by Wong and colleagues, who compared folic acid, zinc, folic acid + zinc, or placebo among 211 men of mixed fertility [89]. Results demonstrated a 74 % increase in total sperm count and improved morphology in the combination group. Subsequent RCTs by Ebisch and colleagues confirmed improved sperm concentrations among patients (regardless of fertility status) supplemented with folic acid and zinc compared to controls [90, 91].

Data Contradicting Use

With limited data available, the previously cited RCT by Wong and colleagues failed to demonstrate significant improvements in concentration, motility, or morphology with folic acid or zinc supplementation alone, despite significant improvements noted in the combination group [89]. This may be a reflection of limited statistical power or indicate a need for combined mechanisms of action to achieve improved semen characteristics. A prior study similarly demonstrated no significant improvements on sperm counts, motility, or DNA content among normo- and oligospermic men treated with folic acid [92].

Consensus of Opinion

Currently available data is insufficient to demonstrate improved outcomes with folic acid supplementation in regard to SA characteristics or pregnancy rates.

Glutathione

Class and Mechanism

Glutathione is an endogenous antioxidant and is one of the most abundant found in the body. It has important roles in maintaining supplementary antioxidants (i.e., Vitamins C and E) in their reduced (active) states and in detoxifying carcinogens and foreign compounds [93, 94].

Data Supporting Use

Multiple studies have associated reduced glutathione levels and infertility, including decreased sperm motility and morphology [95]. However, as glutathione is an endogenous antioxidant, lower levels signify a higher rate of oxidative stress and may not relate to inadequate production. When provided as an adjunctive compound in ART sperm media, sperm motility, plasma membrane integrity, overall viability, fertility success, and DNA integrity are all improved [96, 97].

An initial pilot study examining intramuscular supplementation with glutathione in 11 men resulted in improved sperm motility [98]. A subsequent placebo-controlled, blinded, crossover study of 20 infertile patients with varicoceles ($n = 10$) or non-bacterial genitourinary inflammatory conditions ($n = 10$) confirmed improved sperm motility, progression, and morphology [99]. An additional pilot study of infertile males

identified a higher rate of sperm DNA damage, which was significantly improved with intramuscular glutathione administration [100]. No studies have evaluated the impact of glutathione supplementation on pregnancy outcomes in non-ART settings.

Data Contradicting Use

None.

Consensus of Opinion

Limited data suggests a potential benefit of glutathione supplementation on improving sperm motility, morphology, and DNA integrity as well as its adjunctive use in sperm media with ART. Due, in part, to the need for intramuscular administration, the widespread adoption of glutathione has been limited [101].

Lycopene

Class and Mechanism

Lycopene is a nonessential, carotenoid pigment with no Vitamin A activity. It has received increasing attention as a potential anticarcinogenic agent due to its antioxidant properties and role in genetic expression, cell regulation, and immunomodulation [102].

Data Supporting Use

Lycopene is highly concentrated in reproductive organs, including the testes and seminal fluid, with decreased levels associated with male sub-/infertility [103]. In a placebo-controlled, crossover trial evaluating the effect of lycopene on advanced glycation end products in seminal fluid (marker of oxidative stress), Oborna and colleagues noted significant improvements in lycopene-supplemented men [104].

Currently, no human placebo-controlled RCTs have evaluated the efficacy of lycopene supplementation on fertility and SA parameters. A pilot study of infertile males with OAT undergoing lycopene supplementation demonstrated significant improvements in sperm count (66 % with median 22 million increase) and motility (53 % with median 25 % improvement) [103].

Minimal changes were noted in men with severe oligospermia (<5 million/mL). Among men presenting for IVF, higher arachidonic acid (AA) to docosahexaenoic acid (DHA) ratios (indicating oxidative stress) have been reported when compared to control subjects [105]. When patients were treated with lycopene, these levels returned to baseline in patients without SA abnormalities, while nonsignificant improvements were noted among those with SA abnormalities. Results further demonstrated an observed increased rate of spontaneous pregnancies (16 %) and successful IVF outcomes (42 %) in treatment patients (control results not reported).

Data Contradicting Use

One trial found no increase in TAC among men undergoing supplementation, despite elevated blood and semen levels of lycopene [45].

Consensus of Opinion

Currently available data are insufficient to suggest any potential benefits with lycopene supplementation on SA parameters or pregnancy rates.

N-Acetyl Cysteine

Class and Mechanism

NAC is a derivative of cysteine and is commonly utilized as a mucolytic agent and in the management of acetaminophen overdose. Its role in infertility is likely due to antioxidative properties through regeneration of endogenous glutathione levels [106].

Data Supporting Use

A Cochrane review of two RCTs performed demonstrated significant improvements with NAC administration on sperm motility at 3- and 6-month time points (OR 11.0; CI 7.9–14.0 and OR 1.9; CI 1.0–2.8, respectively) [22, 107, 108]. Sperm concentration was unchanged at 3 months (OR −0.5; CI −6.7 to 5.8) and increased at 6 months (OR 3.3; CI 1.2–5.4); however, as previously noted, the reliability of results from the study author involved at the 6-month time period has previously been called into question [22, 107–110].

One non-RCT performed by Comhaire and colleagues supplemented 27 men with AA/DHA and either NAC or Vitamins E+C [111]. Following treatment, men with oligospermia were found to have increased sperm counts from 7.4 to 12.5 million, with additional improvements in ROS noted. The overall pregnancy rate was 4.5 % at 134 months follow-up. However, these findings are of limited benefit due to the lack of a control group and an undefined number of patients receiving NAC compared to Vitamins E+C.

One animal study of diabetic rats demonstrated an upregulation of endogenous antioxidants and attenuation of diabetes-induced testicular cell death among NAC-treated animals [112]. Similarly, an in vitro study of semen samples incubated with or without supplementary NAC demonstrated a dose-dependent decrease in ROS [113]. Sperm additionally had improved motility, without changes in acrosome reaction.

Data Contradicting Use

In the RCT previously described by Ciftci and colleagues, among the 120 patients randomly divided to receive NAC or placebo, no changes were noted in total sperm counts or morphology [107]. Similarly, in their prospective trial of 27 men treated with NAC or Vitamins E+C and AA/DHA, Comhaire and colleagues demonstrated no effect on sperm motility, morphology, WBC, or round cells in semen among all patients, and no improvement in sperm counts in non-oligospermic men [111].

Consensus of Opinion

Limited data suggests a possible benefit of NAC supplementation on sperm motility, without improvements in other SA parameters. No information is available regarding its impact on pregnancy rates or live deliveries.

Pentoxifylline

Class and Mechanism

Pentoxifylline is a methylated xanthine derivative and is a nonselective PDE inhibitor. Its mechanism

5 The Importance of Diet, Vitamins, Malnutrition, and Nutrient Deficiencies in Male Fertility

for improving fertility has not been defined, although it may be secondary to downstream effects of PDE inhibition, including reduced inflammation [114].

Data Supporting Use

Two placebo-controlled RCTs have evaluated the efficacy of pentoxifylline on improving semen parameters [22, 115, 116]. Compared to no treatment, pentoxifylline resulted in significant improvements in sperm motility (OR 12.8; CI 9.2–16.3) and morphology at 3 months [22, 115].

One in vitro study comparing pentoxifylline to the hypoosmotic swelling test for selection of appropriate sperm for ART demonstrated improved fertilization (62.1 % versus 41.1 %) and pregnancy rates (32 % versus 16 %) with pentoxifylline [117]. These data are consistent with other studies, which suggest a potential role for pentoxifylline as an adjunctive therapy with ART [118–120].

Data Contradicting Use

In the previously described RCT by Wang and colleagues, the authors found no significant improvements in sperm concentration at the 3- and 6-month time points (OR 4.3; CI −0.7 to 9.3 and OR 2.8; CI −2.6 to 8.2) [116].

Consensus of Opinion

With limited data available, pentoxifylline supplementation may result in improved sperm motility and may have benefits as an in vitro adjunct in couples undergoing ART.

Polyunsaturated Fatty Acids

Class and Mechanism

PUFAs (alternatively named highly unsaturated fatty acids) represent a class of triglyceride compounds, which include the omega-3, -6, and -9 fatty acids. Two commonly reported PUFAs are AA (omega-6) and DHA (omega-3), which have been shown to have pro- and anti-inflammatory effects, respectively [121]. AA is required for normal sperm capacitation, and the ratio of AA:DHA is hypothesized to affect the

functional capacity of spermatozoa [122–124]. DHA additionally functions as an indirect anti-oxidant through regeneration of glutathione levels [125].

Data Supporting Use

The proposed benefit of PUFA supplementation is based on the association between reduced omega-3 levels and an altered omega-6:omega-3 ratio and impaired fertility [105, 124]. One double-blinded, placebo-controlled, RCT performed by Safarinejad and colleagues reported significant improvements in sperm count (38.7–61.7 million, $p = 0.001$), with positive associations noted between DHA concentrations and seminal SOD and catalase activities (markers of oxidative stress) [126]. However, as previously mentioned, the validity and reliability of results from this author are suspect, with a prior retracted article and several authors noting discrepancies in reported findings [22, 109, 110].

Data Contradicting Use

One double-blind, placebo-controlled, RCT of 28 men with asthenospermia evaluated the efficacy of varying dosages of DHA on semen characteristics [127]. Results demonstrated elevated levels of DHA and DHA:AA ratio, without evidence for DHA incorporation into the spermatic membrane. Additionally, no significant differences were noted on sperm motility (OR −15.2; CI −34.3 to 3.9) or concentration (OR 1.5; CI −35.2 to 38.2) at 3 months (higher dosage ORs listed).

The impact of DHA supplementation on pregnancy outcomes is unknown. Among infertile men undergoing IVF therapy, altered DHA:AA ratios were identified. Following supplementation with lycopene, this ratio returned to control levels among normospermic infertile males; however, when comparing successful versus unsuccessful pregnancies achieved, no differences were noted with DHA:AA ratios between groups [105].

Consensus of Opinion

Available data on the efficacy of DHA supplementation on sperm characteristics is contradictory and inconclusive.

Selenium

Class and Mechanism

Selenium is a chemical element required for normal cellular function. It is an essential component of the endogenous antioxidants glutathione peroxidase and thioredoxin reductase and thus functions indirectly to enhance intrinsic antioxidant capacity [128].

Data Supporting Use

Selenium deficiency is associated with decreased sperm motility, altered midpiece stability, and abnormal sperm morphology [129, 130]. Two placebo-controlled RCTs have evaluated the efficacy of selenium supplementation on improving sperm characteristics. Scott and colleagues reported on 69 patients randomized to placebo, selenium, or combination of selenium with Vitamins A, C, and E [131]. Although individual groupings failed to achieve significant results, when both treatment groups were combined, significantly improved motility was noted without any benefits on sperm concentration. An 11 % rate of paternity was observed in the treatment group versus 0 % in the placebo arm. Safarinejad and colleagues reported significant improvements in sperm motility (OR 3.2; CI 2.3–4.1) and concentration (OR 4.1; CI 1.9–6.3) at 6 months. However, as previously indicated, these results are suspect (given the uniquely narrow confidence intervals when compared to all other available antioxidant RCTs, the author's prior inconsistencies, and redacted manuscript) and are therefore of questionable validity and reliability [22, 109, 110].

A head-to-head randomized comparison of 20 patients receiving Vitamin E and selenium versus Vitamin B demonstrated improved sperm motility and oxidative stress markers among those receiving selenium and Vitamin E [132]. Similarly, in comparing selenium to selenium+Vitamins A, C, and E, no difference in sperm motility was noted [131].

Two studies evaluated the efficacy of combination of selenium and Vitamin E compared to baseline SA levels [133, 134]. Moslemi and colleagues reported on a large series of 690 infertile males with asthenoteratospermia [134]. Following 100 days of supplementation, 43 % experienced improved motility, 9 % improved morphology, and 10.8 % achieved spontaneous pregnancies. A second, smaller study evaluated nine men with OAT treated with combination of selenium and Vitamin E [133]. Compared to baseline values, results demonstrated significant improvements in motility (19 %), morphology (28.6 %), and sperm viability (27.9 %), which returned to baseline levels following therapy discontinuation.

Data Contradicting Use

One trial of 33 subfertile men treated patients with selenium alone over a period of 3 months [135]. Results demonstrated no significant improvements in sperm count, motility, or morphology, with weak correlations between selenium seminal levels and glutathione peroxidase activity noted.

Of interest, two animal studies evaluating variable dosages of selenium noted impaired fertility, increased ROS, and germ cell apoptosis, among animals receiving either too high or too low levels of selenium [43, 46]. These findings suggest a specific range of selenium required for optimal function.

Consensus of Opinion

Data is lacking on solitary administration of selenium; however, combination therapy of selenium with other vitamins (particularly Vitamin E) may result in improved motility. The effect of combined selenium and vitamins on pregnancy remains unclear.

Vitamin C

Class and Mechanism

Vitamin C (L-ascorbic acid) is a nutrient cofactor in several enzymatic reactions, including those involved with collagen synthesis. In the reproductive tract, Vitamin C is highly concentrated in seminal fluid and is required for normal reproductive function [136]. It exerts antioxidant effects both directly and indirectly through reduction of oxidized Vitamin E [137, 138].

Data Supporting Use

Several placebo-controlled RCTs have evaluated the efficacy of Vitamin C alone or in combination with other antioxidants on male fertility. Dawson and colleagues administered Vitamin C at 200 mg/day versus 1,000 mg/day and demonstrated significant improvements in sperm motility only at the higher dosage (OR 45.0; CI 15.3–74.8) [139]. In comparing Vitamin C (1,000 mg) + Vitamin E to placebo, Greco and colleagues noted significant decreases in DNA fragmentation (22.1 % versus 9.1 %; OR −13.8; CI −17.5 to −10.1) in the treatment group [140]. One trial comparing zinc, zinc + Vitamin E, zinc + Vitamins C and E, or placebo in 45 men with asthenospermia demonstrated no significant differences among treatment groups and improved motility in the combined group (OR 26.0; CI 8.9–43.2) [18]. As with any combination therapy trial, it is difficult to elucidate if findings are due to any single agent or the synergistic effect of multiple therapies.

Vitamin C supplementation may reduce the extent of damage sustained from environmental gonadotoxins. An observational study of 120 men exposed to lead from a battery-manufacturing industry experienced improvements in sperm concentration, motility, and morphology following prophylactic Vitamin C administration [141]. A similar animal study evaluating the effect of electromagnetic radiation on rat testes showed a protective effect and reduced oxidative stress in animals treated with combination of Vitamins C + E [142].

Data Contradicting Use

Two placebo-controlled RCTs of combined Vitamin C (1,000 mg) + Vitamin E have demonstrated no improvements in sperm motility, morphology, or concentration [140, 143]. A meta-analysis of the two studies resulted in no significant difference in sperm concentration in the treatment group compared to placebo (OR 1.4; CI −10.0 to 12.7) [22, 140, 143].

Consensus of Opinion

Available RCTs demonstrate conflicting results on sperm motility and no benefits on concentration or morphology with Vitamin C alone, or in combination with Vitamin E. Vitamin C 1,000 mg daily may improve sperm DNA fragmentation.

Vitamin E

Class and Mechanism

Vitamin E encompasses several fat-soluble compounds, including tocopherols and tocotrienols. As a potent antioxidant, it functions to reduce seminal ROS and restore other antioxidants to their functional (reduced) state [144, 145].

Data Supporting Use

Several placebo-controlled RCTs have been performed evaluating the efficacy of Vitamin E alone or in combination with other antioxidants on improving male-factor infertility. A meta-analysis of two RCTs comparing Vitamin E alone to placebo demonstrate significant improvements with live birth rates (OR 6.4; CI 1.7–24.0), pregnancy rate (OR 6.6; CI 1.8–23.9), and sperm motility (OR 13.0; CI 7.0–19.0), without significant differences noted in the rate of miscarriage (OR 5.4; CI 0.3–93.3) [22, 145, 146].

Similar to other vitamins, several studies evaluate Vitamin E in combination with other antioxidants. Greco and colleagues demonstrated significant improvements in DNA fragmentation indices (OR −13.8; CI −17.5 to −10.1) following supplementation with Vitamins C + E [140]. One study comparing Vitamin E + zinc (OR 26.0; CI 9.0–43.0) or Vitamins C + E + zinc (OR 26.0; CI 8.9–43.2) showed improvements in sperm motility at 3 months compared to no treatment [18].

Two uncontrolled studies of selenium and Vitamin E demonstrated improvements in motility, morphology, sperm viability, and pregnancy rate, when compared to baseline SA levels [133, 134].

As with other antioxidants, low Vitamin E levels have been associated with sub-/infertility [39, 147]. Similarly, animal studies of Vitamin E suggest a possible role for prevention of damage in conditions of high oxidative stress (e.g., radiation, cryptorchidism) [142, 148].

Data Contradicting Use

The previously cited study by Greco and colleagues demonstrated no significant change in sperm motility (OR 2.9; CI −7.8 to 13.6) with Vitamins C+E, despite the observed improvement in DNA fragmentation indices [140]. Similarly, in combining the two available RCTs of Vitamins C+E, no significant improvements on sperm concentration were observed (OR 1.4; CI −10.0 to 12.7) [22, 140, 143].

Several RCTs have also compared Vitamin E alone or in combination with other antioxidants to other agents. Akiyama and colleagues reported no differences in sperm motility (OR −1.9; CI −42.0 to 38.2) or concentration (OR 2.2; CI −16.7 to 21.1) between patients supplemented with Vitamin E or ethylcysteine [149]. In comparing Vitamins C+E to LC and LC+LAC, Li and colleagues noted superiority of LC with or without LAC in regard to motility (OR 23.1; CI 20.2–25.9) and concentration (OR 15.5; CI 12.5–18.5) at 3 months [67]. No differences were noted on sperm motility with Vitamin E+selenium versus Vitamin B (OR 0.0; CI −10.7 to 10.7), Vitamin E+zinc versus zinc (OR 1.0; CI −13.0 to 15.0), or Vitamins E+C+zinc versus zinc (OR 1.0; CI −17.7 to 19.7) [18, 22, 132].

Consensus of Opinion

Although Vitamin E has not been shown to consistently improve semen parameters, limited results suggest a potential benefit on improving overall pregnancy and live birth rates.

Zinc

Class and Mechanism

Zinc is a metallic element and essential cofactor in multiple enzymatic processes. Zinc is highly concentrated in the semen and is essential for normal reproductive gland growth and spermatic function [87].

Data Supporting Use

One placebo-controlled RCT evaluating the efficacy of zinc on markers of oxidative stress and fertility has been reported [18]. A combined 45

men with asthenospermia (defined as ≥40 % immotile sperm) were randomized to zinc, zinc+Vitamin E, zinc+Vitamins C+E, or placebo over a treatment period of 3 months. Results demonstrated significant improvements in live birth (OR 3.7; CI 1.0–13.5, $p=0.05$) and pregnancy rates (OR 4.8; CI 1.5–15.2), with no change in miscarriage rates (OR 7.2; CI 0.1–364.9). Zinc administered alone or in combination with Vitamins E±C resulted in improved motility at 3 months and further reduced the DNA fragmentation index and markers of oxidative stress. No difference in sperm parameters was noted among the three zinc treatment groups.

Animal models of zinc deficiency have demonstrated impaired spermatogenesis, semen parameters, and a higher sensitivity towards oxidative damage and testicular cell death [112, 150]. Zinc is commonly included in multi-supplement trials and will be discussed in this context later in the chapter [151–153].

Data Contradicting Use

An observational study by Young and colleagues evaluated sperm samples from 89 healthy men who completed questionnaires on food intake [20]. Data was extrapolated from questionnaires to estimate levels of zinc, folate, Vitamins C and E, and beta-carotene intake. In comparing estimated nutrient levels against sperm aneuploidy testing, no association was noted among high or low levels of zinc and overall sperm aneuploidy. Given the nature of the study design and methodology, limited conclusions may be drawn from the results presented.

Consensus of Opinion

Limited data suggests a potential benefit for zinc supplementation on semen parameters, pregnancy, and birth rates.

Other Supplements

Several additional nutritional supplements have been evaluated for their potential beneficial effects on male fertility, including but not limited to ALA, anthocyanins, astaxanthin, beta-carotene, biotin, ethylcysteine, inositol, magnesium, PDE5 inhibitors, and Vitamins A and D, among others. Given the relatively limited amount of data currently available on the efficacy of these compounds in male fertility, only brief mention will be made of selected studies for each nutrient. The proposed mechanisms for the compounds vary, with several purported to function via antioxidant pathways either directly or indirectly through reduced inflammation or restoration of endogenous antioxidant levels.

Individual RCTs are available on five of the above listed compounds [70, 149, 154–156]. Pawlowicz and colleagues performed a placebo-controlled RCT of anthocyanins and demonstrated significant improvements in seminal fructose levels and markers of oxidative stress [154]. Similarly, a double-blinded, placebo-controlled, RCT of the carotenoid astaxanthin noted improvements in ROS, inhibin B levels, sperm linear velocity, and pregnancy rates (54.5 % versus 10.5 %, $p = 0.03$) compared to placebo [155]. In comparing the efficacy of Vitamin E to ethylcysteine, Akiyama and colleagues found no difference in regard to sperm density and motility, although ROS were significantly lower among ethylcysteine-treated patients [149]. In a placebo-controlled RCT of two PDE5 inhibitors (vardenafil, sildenafil), Dimitriadis and colleagues reported improved sperm concentration, motility, and morphology following treatment with either agent compared to pretreatment levels [70]. An additional placebo-controlled RCT evaluating magnesium orotate demonstrated no significant improvements in sperm concentration, motility, or pregnancy rates compared to placebo [156].

Vitamin A is commonly utilized in combination supplement trials due to its antioxidant activity [131, 151]. Given the combined use with other agents, individual efficacy on semen parameters and fertility cannot be determined. Vitamin D has also been associated with infertility; however, similar to selenium, both high and low levels have been associated with decreased SA parameters, with one study suggesting an optimal level of 20–50 ng/mL [44, 47, 157, 158]. ALA has been shown in animal models to both attenuate

oxidative stress and improve sperm concentration, motility, and testicular histologic features [159, 160]. Low levels of beta-carotene, as an inactive precursor to Vitamin A, have also been associated with infertility [161]. Biotin (Vitamin B7), inositol, and ALA have shown efficacy in improving semen parameters when used as adjunctive agents to sperm media [120, 162, 163].

Each of the above agents has demonstrated some potential for improving SA parameters and overall male-factor fertility. However, due to the limited data available, further studies are required to assess their individual efficacy.

Combined Supplementation and Overall Antioxidant Efficacy

Several studies have evaluated the efficacy of combination supplements on male-factor fertility. Two RCTs compared multiple supplements to placebo: Galatioto and colleagues (NAC, Vitamins C, E, and A, thiamine, riboflavin, pyridoxine, nicotinamide, pantothenate, biotin, cyanocobalamin, ergocalciferol, calcium, magnesium, phosphate, iron, manganese, copper, and zinc) and Tremellen and colleagues (Vitamins C and E, zinc, folic acid, lycopene, garlic oil, selenium) [151, 152]. Combined results from these studies demonstrated a significant improvement in pregnancy rate (OR 4.0; CI 1.4–11.3) and unchanged risk of miscarriage (OR 0.48; CI 0.1–4.0). Numerous additional studies, which evaluate the efficacy of combined nutrients, are reviewed in the individual nutrient sections previously listed.

To evaluate the overall effect of nutrient supplementation on male-factor fertility, a Cochrane meta-analysis was performed of all RCTs meeting strict inclusion criteria [22]. Combined results demonstrated a significantly increased rate of live births (OR 4.9; CI 1.9–12.2) and pregnancy rate (OR 4.2; CI 2.7–6.6), with no impact on miscarriage rates (OR 1.5; CI 0.3–7.3). Antioxidants further improved DNA fragmentation rates (OR −13.8; CI −17.5 to −10.1) and sperm motility (6 months—OR 5.5; CI 3.8–7.2; ≥9-month time point not significant). No significant difference was noted among combined trials on sperm concentration (3 months—OR 6.0; CI −5.4 to 17.5). In reviewing results, the authors concluded that antioxidants might be recommended for subfertile men whose partners are undergoing ART. They additionally note that the current data is inconclusive and assigned a very low grade to the quality of evidence included.

Summary

Male-factor infertility has long been recognized to be associated with markers of oxidative stress and elevated ROS. Numerous studies have demonstrated reduced levels of both exogenous and endogenous antioxidants among infertile patients. Given these associations, several investigators have sought to evaluate the efficacy of antioxidant and nutrient supplementation on improving direct (pregnancy, live births) and indirect (SA parameters, DNA damage) measures of male fertility. Nutrients demonstrating some beneficial effects on male fertility parameters include ALA, anthocyanins, L-arginine, astaxanthin, beta-carotene, biotin, LC/LAC, cobalamin, CoQ10, ethylcysteine, folic acid, glutathione, inositol, lycopene, magnesium, NAC, pentoxifylline, PDE5 inhibitors, PUFAs, selenium, Vitamins A, C, D, and E, and zinc.

Numerous studies, including RCTs, have been performed evaluating the efficacy of nutrients alone or in combination on improving male sub-/infertility. Although individual studies report varying efficacies, antioxidant supplementation as a whole likely results in improvements in pregnancy rate, live births, DNA fragmentation indices, and sperm motility. Antioxidant supplementation does not likely impact sperm concentration, and the optimal combination of supplements is unknown, with insufficient data available to suggest superiority of any single nutrient. Despite the lack of definitive data, given the relative minimal risks of nutrient supplementation and potential benefits herein discussed, routine use of supplementation in infertile males is reasonable. Further well-designed, placebo-controlled trials reporting main outcome measures of pregnancy and live birth are mandated.

References

1. Tremellen K. Oxidative stress and male infertility—a clinical perspective. Hum Reprod Update. 2008;14(3):243–58. Epub 2008/02/19.
2. Tournaye H. Evidence-based management of male subfertility. Curr Opin Obstet Gynecol. 2006;18(3):253–9. Epub 2006/06/01.
3. Thonneau P, Marchand S, Tallec A, Ferial ML, Ducot B, Lansac J, et al. Incidence and main causes of infertility in a resident population (1,850,000) of three French regions (1988-1989). Hum Reprod. 1991;6(6):811–6. Epub 1991/07/01.
4. Attia AM, Al-Inany HG, Farquhar C, Proctor M. Gonadotrophins for idiopathic male factor subfertility. Cochrane Database Syst Rev. 2007;(4): CD005071. Epub 2007/10/19.
5. Swan SH, Elkin EP, Fenster L. The question of declining sperm density revisited: an analysis of 101 studies published 1934-1996. Environ Health Perspect. 2000;108(10):961–6. Epub 2000/10/26.
6. Jungwirth A, Giwercman A, Tournaye H, Diemer T, Kopa Z, Dohle G, et al. European Association of Urology guidelines on male infertility: the 2012 update. Eur Urol. 2012;62(2):324–32.
7. Anderson K, Nisenblat V, Norman R. Lifestyle factors in people seeking infertility treatment—a review. Aust N Z J Obstet Gynaecol. 2010;50(1): 8–20. Epub 2010/03/12.
8. Hirsh A. Male subfertility. BMJ. 2003; 327(7416):669–72. Epub 2003/09/23.
9. Griveau JF, Le Lannou D. Reactive oxygen species and human spermatozoa: physiology and pathology. Int J Androl. 1997;20(2):61–9. Epub 1997/04/01.
10. Lopes S, Jurisicova A, Sun JG, Casper RF. Reactive oxygen species: potential cause for DNA fragmentation in human spermatozoa. Hum Reprod. 1998;13(4):896–900. Epub 1998/06/10.
11. Aitken RJ, De Iuliis GN, Finnie JM, Hedges A, McLachlan RI. Analysis of the relationships between oxidative stress, DNA damage and sperm vitality in a patient population: development of diagnostic criteria. Hum Reprod. 2010;25(10):2415–26. Epub 2010/08/19.
12. Kao SH, Chao HT, Chen HW, Hwang TI, Liao TL, Wei YH. Increase of oxidative stress in human sperm with lower motility. Fertil Steril. 2008;89(5):1183–90. Epub 2007/08/03.
13. Aitken RJ, Clarkson JS, Fishel S. Generation of reactive oxygen species, lipid peroxidation, and human sperm function. Biol Reprod. 1989; 41(1):183–97. Epub 1989/07/01.
14. Agarwal A, Saleh RA, Bedaiwy MA. Role of reactive oxygen species in the pathophysiology of human reproduction. Fertil Steril. 2003;79(4):829–43. Epub 2003/05/17.
15. Tarozzi N, Bizzaro D, Flamigni C, Borini A. Clinical relevance of sperm DNA damage in assisted reproduction. Reprod Biomed Online. 2007;14(6):746–57. Epub 2007/06/21.

16. Henkel R, Kierspel E, Stalf T, Mehnert C, Menkveld R, Tinneberg HR, et al. Effect of reactive oxygen species produced by spermatozoa and leukocytes on sperm functions in non-leukocytospermic patients. Fertil Steril. 2005;83(3):635–42. Epub 2005/03/08.
17. Sikka SC, Rajasekaran M, Hellstrom WJ. Role of oxidative stress and antioxidants in male infertility. J Androl. 1995;16(6):464–8. Epub 1995/11/01.
18. Omu AE, Al-Azemi MK, Kehinde EO, Anim JT, Oriowo MA, Mathew TC. Indications of the mechanisms involved in improved sperm parameters by zinc therapy. Med Princ Pract. 2008;17(2):108–16. Epub 2008/02/22.
19. Eskenazi B, Kidd SA, Marks AR, Sloter E, Block G, Wyrobek AJ. Antioxidant intake is associated with semen quality in healthy men. Hum Reprod. 2005;20(4):1006–12. Epub 2005/01/25.
20. Young SS, Eskenazi B, Marchetti FM, Block G, Wyrobek AJ. The association of folate, zinc and antioxidant intake with sperm aneuploidy in healthy non-smoking men. Hum Reprod. 2008;23(5):1014–22. Epub 2008/03/21.
21. Saleh RA, Agarwal A, Nada EA, El-Tonsy MH, Sharma RK, Meyer A, et al. Negative effects of increased sperm DNA damage in relation to seminal oxidative stress in men with idiopathic and male factor infertility. Fertil Steril. 2003;79 Suppl 3:1597–605. Epub 2003/06/13.
22. Showell MG, Brown J, Yazdani A, Stankiewicz MT, Hart RJ. Antioxidants for male subfertility. Cochrane Database Syst Rev. 2011;(1):CD007411. Epub 2011/01/21.
23. Dupont C, Cordier AG, Junien C, Mandon-Pepin B, Levy R, Chavatte-Palmer P. Maternal environment and the reproductive function of the offspring. Theriogenology. 2012;78(7):1405–14. Epub 2012/08/29.
24. Mmbaga N, Luk J. The impact of preconceptual diet on the outcome of reproductive treatments. Curr Opin Obstet Gynecol. 2012;24(3):127–31. Epub 2012/04/11.
25. Jensen TK, Heitmann BL, Jensen MB, Halldorsson TI, Andersson AM, Skakkebaek NE, et al. High dietary intake of saturated fat is associated with reduced semen quality among 701 young Danish men from the general population. Am J Clin Nutr. 2013;97(2):411–8. Epub 2012/12/28.
26. Gaskins AJ, Colaci DS, Mendiola J, Swan SH, Chavarro JE. Dietary patterns and semen quality in young men. Hum Reprod. 2012;27(10):2899–907. Epub 2012/08/14.
27. Eslamian G, Amirjannati N, Rashidkhani B, Sadeghi MR, Hekmatdoost A. Intake of food groups and idiopathic asthenozoospermia: a case-control study. Hum Reprod. 2012;27(11):3328–36. Epub 2012/09/04.
28. Mendiola J, Torres-Cantero AM, Moreno-Grau JM, Ten J, Roca M, Moreno-Grau S, et al. Food intake and its relationship with semen quality: a case-control study. Fertil Steril. 2009;91(3):812–8. Epub 2008/03/04.
29. Vujkovic M, de Vries JH, Lindemans J, Macklon NS, van der Spek PJ, Steegers EA, et al. The preconception Mediterranean dietary pattern in couples undergoing in vitro fertilization/intracytoplasmic sperm injection treatment increases the chance of pregnancy. Fertil Steril. 2010;94(6):2096–101. Epub 2010/03/02.
30. Braga DP, Halpern G, Figueira Rde C, Setti AS, Iaconelli Jr A, Borges Jr E. Food intake and social habits in male patients and its relationship to intracytoplasmic sperm injection outcomes. Fertil Steril. 2012;97(1):53–9. Epub 2011/11/15.
31. Rato L, Alves MG, Dias TR, Lopes G, Cavaco JE, Socorro S, et al. High-energy diets may induce a prediabetic state altering testicular glycolytic metabolic profile and male reproductive parameters. Andrology. 2013;1(3):495–504. Epub 2013/03/16.
32. Fernandez CD, Bellentani FF, Fernandes GS, Perobelli JE, Favareto AP, Nascimento AF, et al. Diet-induced obesity in rats leads to a decrease in sperm motility. Reprod Biol Endocrinol. 2011;9:32. Epub 2011/03/15.
33. Saez Lancellotti TE, Boarelli PV, Monclus MA, Cabrillana ME, Clementi MA, Espinola LS, et al. Hypercholesterolemia impaired sperm functionality in rabbits. PLoS One. 2010;5(10):e13457. Epub 2010/10/27.
34. Ghanayem BI, Bai R, Kissling GE, Travlos G, Hoffler U. Diet-induced obesity in male mice is associated with reduced fertility and potentiation of acrylamide-induced reproductive toxicity. Biol Reprod. 2010;82(1):96–104. Epub 2009/08/22.
35. Palmer NO, Bakos HW, Owens JA, Setchell BP, Lane M. Diet and exercise in an obese mouse fed a high-fat diet improve metabolic health and reverse perturbed sperm function. Am J Physiol Endocrinol Metab. 2012;302(7):E768–80. Epub 2012/01/19.
36. Palmer NO, Fullston T, Mitchell M, Setchell BP, Lane M. SIRT6 in mouse spermatogenesis is modulated by diet-induced obesity. Reprod Fertil Dev. 2011;23(7):929–39. Epub 2011/08/30.
37. Fullston T, Palmer NO, Owens JA, Mitchell M, Bakos HW, Lane M. Diet-induced paternal obesity in the absence of diabetes diminishes the reproductive health of two subsequent generations of mice. Hum Reprod. 2012;27(5):1391–400. Epub 2012/02/24.
38. Dada R, Kumar M, Jesudasan R, Fernandez JL, Gosalvez J, Agarwal A. Epigenetics and its role in male infertility. J Assist Reprod Genet. 2012;29(3):213–23. Epub 2012/02/01.
39. Benedetti S, Tagliamonte MC, Catalani S, Primiterra M, Canestrari F, De Stefani S, et al. Differences in blood and semen oxidative status in fertile and infertile men, and their relationship with sperm quality. Reprod Biomed Online. 2012;25(3):300–6. Epub 2012/07/24.
40. Pront R, Margalioth EJ, Green R, Eldar-Geva T, Maimoni Z, Zimran A, et al. Prevalence of low

serum cobalamin in infertile couples. Andrologia. 2009;41(1):46–50. Epub 2009/01/16.

41. Murphy LE, Mills JL, Molloy AM, Qian C, Carter TC, Strevens H, et al. Folate and vitamin B12 in idiopathic male infertility. Asian J Androl. 2011;13(6):856–61. Epub 2011/08/23.

42. Clagett-Dame M, Knutson D. Vitamin A in reproduction and development. Nutrients. 2011;3(4):385–428. Epub 2012/01/19.

43. Kaushal N, Bansal MP. Diminished reproductive potential of male mice in response to selenium-induced oxidative stress: involvement of HSP70, HSP70-2, and MSJ-1. J Biochem Mol Toxicol. 2009;23(2):125–36. Epub 2009/04/16.

44. Hammoud AO, Meikle AW, Peterson CM, Stanford J, Gibson M, Carrell DT. Association of 25-hydroxy-vitamin D levels with semen and hormonal parameters. Asian J Androl. 2012;14(6):855–9. Epub 2012/10/09.

45. Goyal A, Chopra M, Lwaleed BA, Birch B, Cooper AJ. The effects of dietary lycopene supplementation on human seminal plasma. BJU Int. 2007;99(6):1456–60. Epub 2007/05/09.

46. Kaushal N, Bansal MP. Dietary selenium variation-induced oxidative stress modulates CDC2/cyclin B1 expression and apoptosis of germ cells in mice testis. J Nutr Biochem. 2007;18(8):553–64. Epub 2007/02/27.

47. Ramlau-Hansen CH, Moeller UK, Bonde JP, Olsen J, Thulstrup AM. Are serum levels of vitamin D associated with semen quality? Results from a cross-sectional study in young healthy men. Fertil Steril. 2011;95(3):1000–4. Epub 2010/12/03.

48. Thundathil J, de Lamirande E, Gagnon C. Nitric oxide regulates the phosphorylation of the threonine-glutamine-tyrosine motif in proteins of human spermatozoa during capacitation. Biol Reprod. 2003;68(4):1291–8. Epub 2003/02/28.

49. Sinclair S. Male infertility: nutritional and environmental considerations. Altern Med Rev. 2000;5(1):28–38. Epub 2000/03/01.

50. Schachter A, Goldman JA, Zukerman Z. Treatment of oligospermia with the amino acid arginine. J Urol. 1973;110(3):311–3. Epub 1973/09/01.

51. De Aloysio D, Mantuano R, Mauloni M, Nicoletti G. The clinical use of arginine aspartate in male infertility. Acta Eur Fertil. 1982;13(3):133–67. Epub 1982/09/01.

52. Tanimura J. Studies on arginine in human semen. II. The effects of medication with L-arginine-HCL on male infertility. Bull Osaka Med Sch. 1967;13(2):84–9. Epub 1967/10/01.

53. Nikolova V, Stanislavov R, Vatev I, Nalbanski B, Punevska M. [Sperm parameters in male idiopathic infertility after treatment with prelox]. Akush Ginekol. 2007;46(5):7–12. Epub 2007/11/03.

54. Stanislavov R, Nikolova V, Rohdewald P. Improvement of seminal parameters with Prelox: a randomized, double-blind, placebo-controlled, cross-over trial. Phytother Res. 2009;23(3):297–302. Epub 2009/01/15.

55. Miroueh A. Effect of arginine on oligospermia. Fertil Steril. 1970;21(3):217–9. Epub 1970/03/01.

56. Pryor JP, Blandy JP, Evans P, Chaput De Saintonge DM, Usherwood M. Controlled clinical trial of arginine for infertile men with oligozoospermia. Br J Urol. 1978;50(1):47–50. Epub 1978/02/01.

57. Wu TP, Huang BM, Tsai HC, Lui MC, Liu MY. Effects of nitric oxide on human spermatozoa activity, fertilization and mouse embryonic development. Arch Androl. 2004;50(3):173–9. Epub 2004/06/19.

58. Ratnasooriya WD, Dharmasiri MG. L-arginine, the substrate of nitric oxide synthase, inhibits fertility of male rats. Asian J Androl. 2001;3(2):97–103. Epub 2001/06/19.

59. Rosselli M, Dubey RK, Imthurn B, Macas E, Keller PJ. Effects of nitric oxide on human spermatozoa: evidence that nitric oxide decreases sperm motility and induces sperm toxicity. Hum Reprod. 1995;10(7):1786–90. Epub 1995/07/01.

60. Palmero S, Bottazzi C, Costa M, Leone M, Fugassa E. Metabolic effects of L-carnitine on prepubertal rat Sertoli cells. Horm Metab Res. 2000;32(3):87–90. Epub 2000/04/29.

61. De Rosa M, Boggia B, Amalfi B, Zarrilli S, Vita A, Colao A, et al. Correlation between seminal carnitine and functional spermatozoal characteristics in men with semen dysfunction of various origins. Drugs R&D. 2005;6(1):1–9. Epub 2005/04/02.

62. Ahmed SD, Karira KA, Jagdesh, Ahsan S. Role of L-carnitine in male infertility. J Pak Med Assoc. 2011;61(8):732–6. Epub 2012/02/24.

63. Balercia G, Regoli F, Armeni T, Koverech A, Mantero F, Boscaro M. Placebo-controlled double-blind randomized trial on the use of L-carnitine, L-acetylcarnitine, or combined L-carnitine and L-acetylcarnitine in men with idiopathic asthenozoospermia. Fertil Steril. 2005;84(3):662–71. Epub 2005/09/20.

64. Cavallini G, Ferraretti AP, Gianaroli L, Biagiotti G, Vitali G. Cinnoxicam and L-carnitine/acetyl-L-carnitine treatment for idiopathic and varicocele-associated oligoasthenospermia. J Androl. 2004;25(5):761–70; discussion 71–2; Epub 2004/08/05.

65. Lenzi A, Lombardo F, Sgro P, Salacone P, Caponecchia L, Dondero F, et al. Use of carnitine therapy in selected cases of male factor infertility: a double-blind crossover trial. Fertil Steril. 2003;79(2):292–300. Epub 2003/02/06.

66. Lenzi A, Sgro P, Salacone P, Paoli D, Gilio B, Lombardo F, et al. A placebo-controlled double-blind randomized trial of the use of combined l-carnitine and l-acetyl-carnitine treatment in men with asthenozoospermia. Fertil Steril. 2004;81(6):1578–84. Epub 2004/06/15.

67. Li Z, Chen GW, Shang XJ, Bai WJ, Han YF, Chen B, et al. [A controlled randomized trial of the use of combined L-carnitine and acetyl-L-carnitine treatment in men with oligoasthenozoospermia]. Zhonghua Nan Ke Xue. 2005;11(10):761–4.

68. Sigman M, Glass S, Campagnone J, Pryor JL. Carnitine for the treatment of idiopathic asthenospermia: a randomized, double-blind, placebo-controlled trial. Fertil Steril. 2006;85(5):1409–14. Epub 2006/04/08.

69. Vicari E, Calogero AE. Effects of treatment with carnitines in infertile patients with prostato-vesiculo-epididymitis. Hum Reprod. 2001;16(11):2338–42. Epub 2001/10/27.

70. Dimitriadis F, Tsambalas S, Tsounapi P, Kawamura H, Vlachopoulou E, Haliasos N, et al. Effects of phosphodiesterase-5 inhibitors on Leydig cell secretory function in oligoasthenospermic infertile men: a randomized trial. BJU Int. 2010;106(8):1181–5. Epub 2010/02/27.

71. Wang YX, Yang SW, Qu CB, Huo HX, Li W, Li JD, et al. [L-carnitine: safe and effective for asthenozoospermia]. Zhonghua Nan Ke Xue. 2010;16(5): 420–2.

72. Zhou X, Liu F, Zhai S. Effect of L-carnitine and/or L-acetyl-carnitine in nutrition treatment for male infertility: a systematic review. Asia Pac J Clin Nutr. 2007;16 Suppl 1:383–90. Epub 2007/03/30.

73. Cavallini G, Magli MC, Crippa A, Ferraretti AP, Gianaroli L. Reduction in sperm aneuploidy levels in severe oligoasthenoteratospermic patients after medical therapy: a preliminary report. Asian J Androl. 2012;14(4):591–8. Epub 2012/05/01.

74. Watson AA. Seminal vitamin B12 and sterility. Lancet. 1962;2(7257):644. Epub 1962/09/29.

75. Crha I, Kralikova M, Melounova J, Ventruba P, Zakova J, Beharka R, et al. Seminal plasma homocysteine, folate and cobalamin in men with obstructive and non-obstructive azoospermia. J Assist Reprod Genet. 2010;27(9–10):533–8. Epub 2010/08/03.

76. Boxmeer JC, Smit M, Weber RF, Lindemans J, Romijn JC, Eijkemans MJ, et al. Seminal plasma cobalamin significantly correlates with sperm concentration in men undergoing IVF or ICSI procedures. J Androl. 2007;28(4):521–7. Epub 2007/02/09.

77. Kumamoto Y, Maruta H, Ishigami J, Kamidono S, Orikasa S, Kimura M, et al. [Clinical efficacy of mecobalamin in the treatment of oligozoospermia–results of double-blind comparative clinical study]. Hinyokika Kiyo. 1988;34(6):1109–32.

78. Isoyama R, Baba Y, Harada H, Kawai S, Shimizu Y, Fujii M, et al. [Clinical experience of methylcobalamin (CH3-B12)/clomiphene citrate combined treatment in male infertility]. Hinyokika Kiyo. 1986;32(8):1177–83.

79. Moriyama H, Nakamura K, Sanda N, Fujiwara E, Seko S, Yamazaki A, et al. [Studies on the usefulness of a long-term, high-dose treatment of methylcobalamin in patients with oligozoospermia]. Hinyokika Kiyo. 1987;33(1):151–6.

80. Isoyama R, Kawai S, Shimizu Y, Harada H, Takihara H, Baba Y, et al. [Clinical experience with methylcobalamin (CH3-B12) for male infertility]. Hinyokika Kiyo. 1984;30(4):581–6.

81. Balercia G, Buldreghini E, Vignini A, Tiano L, Paggi F, Amoroso S, et al. Coenzyme Q10 treatment in infertile men with idiopathic asthenozoospermia: a placebo-controlled, double-blind randomized trial. Fertil Steril. 2009;91(5):1785–92. Epub 2008/04/09.

82. Mancini A, Balercia G. Coenzyme Q(10) in male infertility: physiopathology and therapy. Biofactors. 2011;37(5):374–80. Epub 2011/10/13.

83. Safarinejad MR. Efficacy of coenzyme Q10 on semen parameters, sperm function and reproductive hormones in infertile men. J Urol. 2009;182(1): 237–48. Epub 2009/05/19.

84. Nadjarzadeh A, Sadeghi MR, Amirjannati N, Vafa MR, Motevalian SA, Gohari MR, et al. Coenzyme Q10 improves seminal oxidative defense but does not affect on semen parameters in idiopathic oligoasthenoteratozoospermia: a randomized double-blind, placebo controlled trial. J Endocrinol Invest. 2011;34(8):e224–8. Epub 2011/03/15.

85. Nadjarzadeh A, Shidfar F, Amirjannati N, Vafa MR, Motevalian SA, Gohari MR, et al. Effect of coenzyme Q10 supplementation on antioxidant enzymes activity and oxidative stress of seminal plasma: a double-blind randomised clinical trial. Andrologia. 2014;46(2):177–83. Epub 2013/01/08.

86. Joshi R, Adhikari S, Patro BS, Chattopadhyay S, Mukherjee T. Free radical scavenging behavior of folic acid: evidence for possible antioxidant activity. Free Radic Biol Med. 2001;30(12):1390–9. Epub 2001/06/08.

87. Ebisch IM, Thomas CM, Peters WH, Braat DD, Steegers-Theunissen RP. The importance of folate, zinc and antioxidants in the pathogenesis and prevention of subfertility. Hum Reprod Update. 2007;13(2):163–74. Epub 2006/11/14.

88. De Sanctis V, Candini G, Giovannini M, Raiola G, Katz M. Abnormal seminal parameters in patients with thalassemia intermedia and low serum folate levels. Pediatr Endocrinol Rev. 2011;8 Suppl 2:310–3. Epub 2011/06/28.

89. Wong WY, Merkus HM, Thomas CM, Menkveld R, Zielhuis GA, Steegers-Theunissen RP. Effects of folic acid and zinc sulfate on male factor subfertility: a double-blind, randomized, placebo-controlled trial. Fertil Steril. 2002;77(3):491–8. Epub 2002/03/02.

90. Ebisch IM, van Heerde WL, Thomas CM, van der Put N, Wong WY, Steegers-Theunissen RP. C677T methylenetetrahydrofolate reductase polymorphism interferes with the effects of folic acid and zinc sulfate on sperm concentration. Fertil Steril. 2003;80(5):1190–4. Epub 2003/11/11.

91. Ebisch IM, Pierik FH, Jong FH DE, Thomas CM, Steegers-Theunissen RP. Does folic acid and zinc sulphate intervention affect endocrine parameters and sperm characteristics in men? Int J Androl. 2006;29(2):339–45. Epub 2006/03/15.

92. Landau B, Singer R, Klein T, Segenreich E. Folic acid levels in blood and seminal plasma of normo- and oligospermic patients prior and following folic

acid treatment. Experientia. 1978;34(10):1301–2. Epub 1978/10/15.

93. Irvine DS. Glutathione as a treatment for male infertility. Rev Reprod. 1996;1(1):6–12. Epub 1996/01/01.

94. Pompella A, Visvikis A, Paolicchi A, De Tata V, Casini AF. The changing faces of glutathione, a cellular protagonist. Biochem Pharmacol. 2003;66(8):1499–503. Epub 2003/10/14.

95. Atig F, Raffa M, Habib BA, Kerkeni A, Saad A, Ajina M. Impact of seminal trace element and glutathione levels on semen quality of Tunisian infertile men. BMC Urol. 2012;12:6. Epub 2012/03/21.

96. Yun JI, Gong SP, Song YH, Lee ST. Effects of combined antioxidant supplementation on human sperm motility and morphology during sperm manipulation in vitro. Fertil Steril. 2013;100(2):373–8. Epub 2013/05/09.

97. Ansari MS, Rakha BA, Andrabi SM, Ullah N, Iqbal R, Holt WV, et al. Glutathione-supplemented triscitric acid extender improves the post-thaw quality and in vivo fertility of buffalo (Bubalus bubalis) bull spermatozoa. Reprod Biol. 2012;12(3):271–6. Epub 2012/11/17.

98. Lenzi A, Lombardo F, Gandini L, Culasso F, Dondero F. Glutathione therapy for male infertility. Arch Androl. 1992;29(1):65–8. Epub 1992/07/01.

99. Lenzi A, Culasso F, Gandini L, Lombardo F, Dondero F. Placebo-controlled, double-blind, crossover trial of glutathione therapy in male infertility. Hum Reprod. 1993;8(10):1657–62. Epub 1993/10/01.

100. Kodama H, Yamaguchi R, Fukuda J, Kasai H, Tanaka T. Increased oxidative deoxyribonucleic acid damage in the spermatozoa of infertile male patients. Fertil Steril. 1997;68(3):519–24. Epub 1997/10/07.

101. Witschi A, Reddy S, Stofer B, Lauterburg BH. The systemic availability of oral glutathione. Eur J Clin Pharmacol. 1992;43(6):667–9. Epub 1992/01/01.

102. Rao AV, Ray MR, Rao LG. Lycopene. Adv Food Nutr Res. 2006;51:99–164. Epub 2006/10/03.

103. Gupta NP, Kumar R. Lycopene therapy in idiopathic male infertility—a preliminary report. Int Urol Nephrol. 2002;34(3):369–72. Epub 2003/08/06.

104. Oborna I, Malickova K, Fingerova H, Brezinova J, Horka P, Novotny J, et al. A randomized controlled trial of lycopene treatment on soluble receptor for advanced glycation end products in seminal and blood plasma of normospermic men. Am J Reprod Immunol. 2011;66(3):179–84. Epub 2011/02/01.

105. Filipcikova R, Oborna I, Brezinova J, Novotny J, Wojewodka G, De Sanctis JB, et al. Lycopene improves the distorted ratio between AA/DHA in the seminal plasma of infertile males and increases the likelihood of successful pregnancy. Biomed Pap Med Fac Univ Palacky Olomouc Czech Repub. 2013. Epub 2013/03/01.

106. Zembron-Lacny A, Slowinska-Lisowska M, Szygula Z, Witkowski K, Szyszka K. The comparison of antioxidant and hematological properties of N-acetylcysteine and alpha-lipoic acid in physically active males. Physiol Res. 2009;58(6):855–61. Epub 2008/12/20.

107. Ciftci H, Verit A, Savas M, Yeni E, Erel O. Effects of N-acetylcysteine on semen parameters and oxidative/antioxidant status. Urology. 2009;74(1):73–6. Epub 2009/05/12.

108. Safarinejad MR, Safarinejad S. Efficacy of selenium and/or N-acetyl-cysteine for improving semen parameters in infertile men: a double-blind, placebo controlled, randomized study. J Urol. 2009; 181(2):741–51. Epub 2008/12/19.

109. Sharlip I. Rational use of dapoxetine for the treatment of premature ejaculation. Neuropsychopharmacology. 2008;33(11):2785; author reply 6-8. Epub 2008/09/13.

110. Safarinejad MR, Taghva A, Shekarchi B, Safarinejad S. Safety and efficacy of sildenafil citrate in the treatment of Parkinson-emergent erectile dysfunction: a double-blind, placebo-controlled, randomized study. Int J Impot Res. 2010;22(5):325–35. Epub 2010/09/24.

111. Comhaire FH, Christophe AB, Zalata AA, Dhooge WS, Mahmoud AM, Depuydt CE. The effects of combined conventional treatment, oral antioxidants and essential fatty acids on sperm biology in subfertile men. Prostaglandins Leukot Essent Fatty Acids. 2000;63(3):159–65. Epub 2000/09/19.

112. Zhao Y, Zhao H, Zhai X, Dai J, Jiang X, Wang G, et al. Effects of Zn deficiency, antioxidants, and low-dose radiation on diabetic oxidative damage and cell death in the testis. Toxicol Mech Methods. 2013;23(1):42–7. Epub 2012/09/21.

113. Oeda T, Henkel R, Ohmori H, Schill WB. Scavenging effect of N-acetyl-L-cysteine against reactive oxygen species in human semen: a possible therapeutic modality for male factor infertility? Andrologia. 1997;29(3):125–31. Epub 1997/05/01.

114. Peters-Golden M, Canetti C, Mancuso P, Coffey MJ. Leukotrienes: underappreciated mediators of innate immune responses. J Immunol. 2005;174(2):589–94. Epub 2005/01/07.

115. Micic S, Hadzi-Djokic J, Dotlic R, Tulic C. Pentoxifyllin treatment of oligoasthenospermic men. Acta Eur Fertil. 1988;19(3):135–7. Epub 1988/05/01.

116. Wang C, Chan CW, Wong KK, Yeung KK. Comparison of the effectiveness of placebo, clomiphene citrate, mesterolone, pentoxifylline, and testosterone rebound therapy for the treatment of idiopathic oligospermia. Fertil Steril. 1983;40(3):358–65. Epub 1983/09/01.

117. Mangoli V, Mangoli R, Dandekar S, Suri K, Desai S. Selection of viable spermatozoa from testicular biopsies: a comparative study between pentoxifylline and hypoosmotic swelling test. Fertil Steril. 2011;95(2):631–4. Epub 2010/11/16.

118. Numabe T, Oikawa T, Kikuchi T, Horuchi T. Pentoxifylline improves in vitro fertilization and subsequent development of bovine oocytes. Theriogenology. 2001;56(2):225–33. Epub 2001/08/02.

119. Gradil CM, Ball BA. The use of pentoxifylline to improve motility of cryopreserved equine spermatozoa. Theriogenology. 2000;54(7):1041–7. Epub 2000/12/29.

120. Kalthur G, Salian SR, Keyvanifard F, Sreedharan S, Thomas JS, Kumar P, et al. Supplementation of biotin to sperm preparation medium increases the motility and longevity in cryopreserved human spermatozoa. J Assist Reprod Genet. 2012;29(7):631–5. Epub 2012/04/25.

121. Lukiw WJ, Bazan NG. Docosahexaenoic acid and the aging brain. J Nutr. 2008;138(12):2510–4. Epub 2008/11/22.

122. Roqueta-Rivera M, Stroud CK, Haschek WM, Akare SJ, Segre M, Brush RS, et al. Docosahexaenoic acid supplementation fully restores fertility and spermatogenesis in male delta-6 desaturase-null mice. J Lipid Res. 2010;51(2):360–7. Epub 2009/08/20.

123. Maccarrone M, Barboni B, Paradisi A, Bernabo N, Gasperi V, Pistilli MG, et al. Characterization of the endocannabinoid system in boar spermatozoa and implications for sperm capacitation and acrosome reaction. J Cell Sci. 2005;118(Pt 19):4393–404. Epub 2005/09/08.

124. Safarinejad MR, Hosseini SY, Dadkhah F, Asgari MA. Relationship of omega-3 and omega-6 fatty acids with semen characteristics, and anti-oxidant status of seminal plasma: a comparison between fertile and infertile men. Clin Nutr. 2010;29(1):100–5. Epub 2009/08/12.

125. Arab K, Rossary A, Flourie F, Tourneur Y, Steghens JP. Docosahexaenoic acid enhances the antioxidant response of human fibroblasts by upregulating gamma-glutamyl-cysteinyl ligase and glutathione reductase. Br J Nutr. 2006;95(1):18–26. Epub 2006/01/31.

126. Safarinejad MR. Effect of omega-3 polyunsaturated fatty acid supplementation on semen profile and enzymatic anti-oxidant capacity of seminal plasma in infertile men with idiopathic oligoasthenoteratospermia: a double-blind, placebo-controlled, randomised study. Andrologia. 2011;43(1):38–47. Epub 2011/01/12.

127. Conquer JA, Martin JB, Tummon I, Watson L, Tekpetey F. Effect of DHA supplementation on DHA status and sperm motility in asthenozoospermic males. Lipids. 2000;35(2):149–54. Epub 2000/04/11.

128. Brown KM, Arthur JR. Selenium, selenoproteins and human health: a review. Public Health Nutr. 2001;4(2B):593–9. Epub 2001/10/31.

129. Watanabe T, Endo A. Effects of selenium deficiency on sperm morphology and spermatocyte chromosomes in mice. Mutat Res. 1991;262(2):93–9. Epub 1991/02/01.

130. Noack-Fuller G, De Beer C, Seibert H. Cadmium, lead, selenium, and zinc in semen of occupationally unexposed men. Andrologia. 1993;25(1):7–12. Epub 1993/01/01.

131. Scott R, MacPherson A, Yates RW, Hussain B, Dixon J. The effect of oral selenium supplementation on human sperm motility. Br J Urol. 1998;82(1):76–80. Epub 1998/08/12.

132. Keskes-Ammar L, Feki-Chakroun N, Rebai T, Sahnoun Z, Ghozzi H, Hammami S, et al. Sperm oxidative stress and the effect of an oral vitamin E and selenium supplement on semen quality in infertile men. Arch Androl. 2003;49(2):83–94. Epub 2003/03/08.

133. Vezina D, Mauffette F, Roberts KD, Bleau G. Selenium-vitamin E supplementation in infertile men. Effects on semen parameters and micronutrient levels and distribution. Biol Trace Elem Res. 1996;53(1–3):65–83. Epub 1996/01/01.

134. Moslemi MK, Tavanbakhsh S. Selenium-vitamin E supplementation in infertile men: effects on semen parameters and pregnancy rate. Int J Gen Med. 2011;4:99–104. Epub 2011/03/16.

135. Iwanier K, Zachara BA. Selenium supplementation enhances the element concentration in blood and seminal fluid but does not change the spermatozoal quality characteristics in subfertile men. J Androl. 1995;16(5):441–7. Epub 1995/09/01.

136. Yazama F, Furuta K, Fujimoto M, Sonoda T, Shigetomi H, Horiuchi T, et al. Abnormal spermatogenesis in mice unable to synthesize ascorbic acid. Anat Sci Int. 2006;81(2):115–25. Epub 2006/06/28.

137. Kefer JC, Agarwal A, Sabanegh E. Role of antioxidants in the treatment of male infertility. Int J Urol. 2009;16(5):449–57. Epub 2009/04/23.

138. Dawson EB, Harris WA, Rankin WE, Charpentier LA, McGanity WJ. Effect of ascorbic acid on male fertility. Ann N Y Acad Sci. 1987;498:312–23. Epub 1987/01/01.

139. Dawson EB, Harris WA, Powell LC. Relationship between ascorbic acid and male fertility. World Rev Nutr Diet. 1990;62:1–26. Epub 1990/01/01.

140. Greco E, Iacobelli M, Rienzi L, Ubaldi F, Ferrero S, Tesarik J. Reduction of the incidence of sperm DNA fragmentation by oral antioxidant treatment. J Androl. 2005;26(3):349–53. Epub 2005/05/04.

141. Vani K, Kurakula M, Syed R, Alharbi K. Clinical relevance of vitamin C among lead-exposed infertile men. Genet Test Mol Biomarkers. 2012;16(9):1001–6. Epub 2012/06/27.

142. Al-Damegh MA. Rat testicular impairment induced by electromagnetic radiation from a conventional cellular telephone and the protective effects of the antioxidants vitamins C and E. Clinics (Sao Paulo). 2012;67(7):785–92. Epub 2012/08/16.

143. Rolf C, Cooper TG, Yeung CH, Nieschlag E. Antioxidant treatment of patients with asthenozoospermia or moderate oligoasthenozoospermia with high-dose vitamin C and vitamin E: a randomized, placebo-controlled, double-blind study. Hum Reprod. 1999;14(4):1028–33. Epub 1999/04/30.

144. Palamanda JR, Kehrer JP. Involvement of vitamin E and protein thiols in the inhibition of microsomal lipid peroxidation by glutathione. Lipids. 1993;28(5):427–31. Epub 1993/05/01.

145. Kessopoulou E, Powers HJ, Sharma KK, Pearson MJ, Russell JM, Cooke ID, et al. A double-blind randomized placebo cross-over controlled trial using the antioxidant vitamin E to treat reactive oxygen species associated male infertility. Fertil Steril. 1995;64(4):825–31. Epub 1995/10/01.

146. Suleiman SA, Ali ME, Zaki ZM, el-Malik EM, Nasr MA. Lipid peroxidation and human sperm motility: protective role of vitamin E. J Androl. 1996;17(5):530–7. Epub 1996/09/01.

147. Diafouka F, Gbassi GK. Deficiency of alpha-tocopherol in seminal fluid as a probable factor in low fertility in Cote d'Ivoire. Afr J Reprod Health. 2009;13(3):123–5. Epub 2010/08/10.

148. Vigueras-Villasenor RM, Ojeda I, Gutierrez-Perez O, Chavez-Saldana M, Cuevas O, Maria DS, et al. Protective effect of alpha-tocopherol on damage to rat testes by experimental cryptorchidism. Int J Exp Pathol. 2011;92(2):131–9. Epub 2011/02/15.

149. Akiyama M. [In vivo scavenging effect of ethylcysteine on reactive oxygen species in human semen]. Nihon Hinyokika Gakkai Zasshi. 1999;90(3):421–8. Epub 1999/06/01.

150. Croxford TP, McCormick NH, Kelleher SL. Moderate zinc deficiency reduces testicular Zip6 and Zip10 abundance and impairs spermatogenesis in mice. J Nutr. 2011;141(3):359–65. Epub 2011/01/21.

151. Paradiso Galatioto G, Gravina GL, Angelozzi G, Sacchetti A, Innominato PF, Pace G, et al. May antioxidant therapy improve sperm parameters of men with persistent oligospermia after retrograde embolization for varicocele? World J Urol. 2008;26(1): 97–102. Epub 2007/11/06.

152. Tremellen K, Miari G, Froiland D, Thompson J. A randomised control trial examining the effect of an antioxidant (Menevit) on pregnancy outcome during IVF-ICSI treatment. Aust N Z J Obstet Gynaecol. 2007;47(3):216–21. Epub 2007/06/07.

153. Busetto GM, Koverech A, Messano M, Antonini G, De Berardinis E, Gentile V. Prospective open-label study on the efficacy and tolerability of a combination of nutritional supplements in primary infertile patients with idiopathic astenoteratozoospermia. Arch Ital Urol Androl. 2012;84(3):137–40. Epub 2012/12/06.

154. Pawlowicz P, Stachowiak G, Bielak A, Wilczynski J. [Administration of natural anthocyanins derived from chokeberry (aronia melanocarpa) extract in the treatment of oligospermia in males with enhanced autoantibodies to oxidized low density lipoproteins (oLAB). The impact on fructose levels]. Ginekol Pol. 2001;72(12):983–8. Epub 2002/03/09. Zastosowanie naturalnych antocyjanow pochodzacych z ekstraktu aronii czarnoowocowej (aronia melanocarpa) w leczeniu oligospermii u mezczyzn z podwyzszonymi poziomami przeciwcial anty-O-LDL (OLAB). Wplyw na poziom fruktozy w nasieniu.

155. Comhaire FH, El Garem Y, Mahmoud A, Eertmans F, Schoonjans F. Combined conventional/antioxidant "Astaxanthin" treatment for male infertility: a double blind, randomized trial. Asian J Androl. 2005;7(3):257–62. Epub 2005/08/20.

156. Zavaczki Z, Szollosi J, Kiss SA, Koloszar S, Fejes I, Kovacs L, et al. Magnesium-orotate supplementation for idiopathic infertile male patients: a randomized, placebo-controlled clinical pilot study. Magnes Res. 2003;16(2):131–6. Epub 2003/08/02.

157. Anagnostis P, Karras S, Goulis DG. Vitamin D in human reproduction: a narrative review. Int J Clin Pract. 2013;67(3):225–35. Epub 2013/01/09.

158. Yang B, Sun H, Wan Y, Wang H, Qin W, Yang L, et al. Associations between testosterone, bone mineral density, vitamin D and semen quality in fertile and infertile Chinese men. Int J Androl. 2012;35(6):783–92. Epub 2012/06/21.

159. Ashour AE, Abdel-Hamied HE, Korashy HM, Al-Shabanah OA, Abd-Allah AR. Alpha-lipoic acid rebalances redox and immune-testicular milieu in septic rats. Chem Biol Interact. 2011;189(3): 198–205. Epub 2011/01/05.

160. Mohasseb M, Ebied S, Yehia MA, Hussein N. Testicular oxidative damage and role of combined antioxidant supplementation in experimental diabetic rats. J Physiol Biochem. 2011;67(2):185–94. Epub 2010/12/25.

161. Palan P, Naz R. Changes in various antioxidant levels in human seminal plasma related to immuno-infertility. Arch Androl. 1996;36(2):139–43. Epub 1996/03/01.

162. Colone M, Marelli G, Unfer V, Bozzuto G, Molinari A, Stringaro A. Inositol activity in oligoasthenoteratospermia—an in vitro study. Eur Rev Med Pharmacol Sci. 2010;14(10):891–6. Epub 2011/01/13.

163. Ibrahim SF, Osman K, Das S, Othman AM, Majid NA, Rahman MP. A study of the antioxidant effect of alpha lipoic acids on sperm quality. Clinics (Sao Paulo). 2008;63(4):545–50. Epub 2008/08/23.

The Effect of Alcohol Consumption on Male Infertility

6

Edson Borges Jr. and Fábio Firmbach Pasqualotto

Introduction

Substance abuse, particularly of alcohol, is one of the fastest growing health problems in the world. It has been reported that alcoholic beverages is consumed by nearly 90 % of the population in England, which is equivalent to 36 million people (adults aged 16 years or over) [1]. Drinking alcohol is widely socially accepted and associated with relaxation and pleasure, and some people drink alcohol without experiencing harmful effects. However, a growing number of people experience physical, social, and psychological harmful effects of alcohol.

Alcohol consumption has health and social consequences via intoxication (drunkenness), alcohol dependence, and other biochemical effects of alcohol. In addition to chronic diseases that may affect drinkers after many years of heavy use, alcohol contributes to traumatic outcomes that kill or disable at a relatively young age, resulting in the loss of many years of life due to death or disability.

E. Borges Jr., MD, PhD (✉)
Clinical Department, Fertility—Centro de
Fertilização Assistida, Av. Brigadeiro Luiz Antônio,
São Paulo, São Paulo 4545, Brazil
e-mail: edson@fertility.com.br

F.F. Pasqualotto, MD, PhD
Departamento de Urologia, Universidade de Caxias
do Sul e Conception - Centro de Reprodução
Assistida, Caxias do Sul, Rio Grande do Sul, Brazil

There is increasing evidence that besides volume of alcohol, the pattern of the drinking is relevant for the health outcomes. Overall there is a causal relationship between alcohol consumption and more than 60 types of disease and injury. Alcohol is estimated to cause esophageal cancer, liver cancer, cirrhosis of the liver, homicide, epileptic seizures, and motor vehicle accidents worldwide. In addition, a possible association between alcohol consumption and male and female infertility has been suggested.

Infertility affects 10–15 % of couples attempting to conceive [2, 3] during their reproductive lifespan. A male factor is identifiable in 40–60 % of couples and is the sole etiology in at least 20 % of all couples seeking infertility treatments [4, 5]. Despite extensive research, it is still not well known which maternal and especially paternal lifestyle and sociodemographic factors are predictors of a couple's fecundity. Few risk factors for male infertility are known as smoking and alcohol intake [6, 7] but with conflicting results [8, 9]. The inconsistency in the literature seems to be due to (1) the small sample size of most of the studies, (2) differences in the population selected (healthy volunteers or patients suspected to be infertile), and (3) the frequent association between smoking and alcohol consumption reported by several investigators.

A negative effect of chronic alcoholism on male fertility has been previously described. Increased impotence has been reported in subjects suffering from chronic alcoholism, as compared with the case of nondrinkers [10, 11].

S.S. du Plessis et al. (eds.), *Male Infertility: A Complete Guide to Lifestyle and Environmental Factors*,
DOI 10.1007/978-1-4939-1040-3_6, © Springer Science+Business Media New York 2014

Additionally, testicular atrophy, gynecomastia, and loss of sexual interest are often associated with alcoholism in men. In the following chapter different aspects of the effect of alcohol consumption on male infertility will be discussed.

Prevalence of Alcohol Consumption on the World Population

Alcohol is possibly the oldest psychoactive substance used in the world. The World Health Organization (WHO) estimates that there are about two billion people worldwide who consume alcoholic beverages and 76.3 million with diagnosable alcohol use disorders. From a public health perspective, the global burden related to alcohol consumption, both in terms of morbidity and mortality, is considerable in most parts of the world.

Although it is also the most prevalent psychoactive substance in the world, the majority of the world adult population abstains. Globally, 46 % of all men and 73 % of all women abstain from alcohol, and most of these persons have not consumed any alcoholic beverage during their entire lives.

Among those who are current abstainers, some have never consumed alcohol for religious, cultural, or other reasons, and some have consumed alcohol but not in the past year. This latter group includes people who have been harmful drinkers or alcohol dependent in the past and who have stopped because of experiencing the harmful effects of alcohol.

Among those who currently consume alcohol, there is a wide spectrum of alcohol consumption, from the majority who are moderate drinkers through to a smaller number of people who regularly consume a liter of spirits per day or more and who will typically be severely alcohol dependent. However, it is important to note that most of the alcohol consumed by the population is drunk by a minority of heavy drinkers.

The rates of abstainers vary considerably across countries. The overwhelming majority of people in a belt stretching from Northern Africa, over the Eastern Mediterranean, South Central Asia, and Southeast Asia to the islands of Indonesia abstain for reasons often attributable to religion and culture. In other parts of the world such as Europe, less than 20 % of the population abstains on average. In fact it has been reported that alcohol is consumed by nearly 90 % of the United Kingdom population over the age of 16.

According to the WHO Global Status Report on Alcohol, the proportion of last year abstainers among the total adult population reported across countries ranged from a low of 2.5 % in Luxembourg to a high of 99.5 % in Egypt. In relation to lifetime abstainers (have never tried alcohol) among the total adult population, the rates range from 9.4 % in Latvia to 98.4 % in the Comoros.

Given the role of alcohol in different societies, these differences may be quite easily explained. The one consistency that appears to transcend cultures is the difference in abstention rates between males and females. A higher proportion of women abstain from alcohol than men. A second common finding is the role of religion in shaping drinking habits. For instance, countries with Islam as the official religion almost always have higher rates of abstinence. However, in each case, one must keep in mind that patterns of abstinence, like drinking patterns, may vary within specific subpopulations and across different regions of a particular country. This is especially true for multicultural and multiethnic societies, in which different groups may represent quite diverse traditions with respect to alcohol.

Effect of Alcohol Consumption on Male Infertility (Results)

Overview of Alcohol Consumption Effect on Male Infertility

In adults, a possible effect of alcohol exposure during spermatozoa production on semen parameters has been assessed in a limited number of studies with conflicting results: some indicate a detrimental effect [12], but others point towards no or even a protective effect of moderate amounts of alcohol [13]. Whether maternal alcohol consumption during pregnancy is associated with poor semen quality in the male offspring is still to be elucidated. In fact, moderate prenatal exposure to alcohol was associated with lower sperm concentrations, and sons exposed to ≥4.5 drinks per week in utero had approximately one-third lower sperm concentration than sons exposed to 1 drink per week [14].

An ethanol-induced oxidative stress is not restricted to the liver, where ethanol is actively oxidized, but can affect various extrahepatic tissues as shown by experimental data obtained in the rat during acute or chronic ethanol intoxication. Most of these data concern the central nervous system, the heart, and the testes.

That alcohol abuse may lead to testicular lipid peroxidation is suggested by the fact that ethanol is a known testicular toxin and its chronic use leads to both endocrine and reproductive failure. Because testicular membranes are rich in polyenoic fatty acids that are prone to undergo peroxidative decomposition, it is reasonable to consider that lipid peroxidation may contribute to the membrane injury and gonadal dysfunction that occurs as a result of alcohol abuse and/or chronic use. Consistent with such a mechanism for putative alcohol-associated testicular toxicity are the observed reductions in the testicular content of polyenoic fatty acids and glutathione (GSH) content of the testes of alcohol-fed animals as compared to isocalorically fed controls [15].

The increased conversion of xanthine dehydrogenase into xanthine oxidase as well as the activation of peroxisomal acyl-CoA oxidase linked to ethanol administration could contribute to the oxidative stress [16]. Chronic ethanol administration elicits in the testes an enhancement in mitochondrial lipid peroxidation and a decrease in the GSH level, which appear to be correlated to the gross testicular atrophy observed [17]. It is well known that peroxidation injury can be attenuated when it occurs in association with dietary vitamin A supplementation. Thus, it is of interest to note that vitamin A, acting as an antioxidant, stabilizes testicular membranes by reducing lipid peroxidation and prevents the alcohol-induced atrophy that occurs in animals not receiving vitamin-A-enriched diets. Vitamin A supplementation

attenuates the changes in lipid peroxidation, GSH, and testicular morphology [17].

Taken together, these observations suggest that the enhanced peroxidation of testicular lipids that occurs following ethanol exposure may be an important factor in the pathogenesis of alcohol-associated gonadal injury.

Alcohol's Effect on Semen Parameters and Spermatozoa

Dunphy and colleagues [18] evaluated the relationship between male alcohol intake and fertility in 258 couples attending an infertility clinic. No association between the amount of alcohol and sperm parameters was observed in this study. In addition, there was no significant difference in the alcohol intake between normal and abnormal female groups. In addition, there was no significant association between the amount of alcohol consumed per week and the fertility outcome. Data from the Ontario Farm Family Health Study were analyzed to determine whether alcohol use among men and women impact upon fecundability [19]. In this retrospective study, the alcohol use among women and men was not associated with fecundability. A multicenter prospective study evaluated whether the amount and the timing of female and male alcohol use during in vitro fertilization program affected the reproductive outcome. The risk of not achieving a live birth increased by 2.28–8.32 times, depending on the time period, in men who drank one additional drink per day [20].

From a cohort of pregnant women established in 1984–1987, 347 young adult sons were selected for a follow-up study conducted in 2005–2006 [14]. The results of this study showed that the sperm concentration decreased with increasing prenatal alcohol exposure. The adjusted mean sperm concentration among sons of mothers drinking nearly 4.5 drinks per week during pregnancy was 40 million per mL, which was approximately 32 % lower compared with the sons of mother exposed to 1 drink per week. The semen volume and the total sperm count were also associated with the mothers' prenatal alcohol exposure; sons prenatally exposed to 1.0–1.5 drinks per week had the highest values.

Experimental and clinical studies suggest that alcohol consumption may alter both testosterone secretion and spermatogenesis. In fact, it is well known that alcohol consumption produces significant spermatozoon morphological changes which include breakage of the sperm head, distention of the midsection, and tail curling [21]. In addition, seminiferous tubules in alcohol users mostly contain degenerated spermatids with a consequent azoospermia [21]. These effects may be due to alteration of the endocrine system controlling the hypothalamic–pituitary–gonadal (HPG) axis function and/or to a direct effect on testis and/or male accessory glands [21, 22]. In particular, experimental evidence suggests that ethanol is a Leydig cell toxin [22] although dose-dependent effects of alcohol on human spermatogenesis are not well known. A recent case report showed that an azoospermic patient recovered normal sperm parameters 3 months after alcohol consumption discontinuation [23], which has raised the interest for this topic. The present article briefly reviews the main preclinical and clinical evidences on this topic.

Animal Evidence

C57B1 mice have been used to evaluate the effects of ethanol on the testicular function and its reversal following alcohol withdrawal [22]. This interesting and comprehensive study showed that an ethanol-containing diet alters testicular function and that this effect is partially reversible upon discontinuation of alcohol consumption.

In another experimental study [24] male mice were evaluated showing an increased percentage of morphological abnormal spermatozoa. There was a significant effect of paternal alcohol exposure on implantation rate, but no effects on pre- or postnatal mortality or fetal weight were observed. Dhawan and Sharma [25] reported that ethanol resulted in a decreased libido (evaluated by mating behavior) and decreased sperm number [26]. These detrimental effects on sexual/reproductive function were counteracted by the administration of a tri-substituted benzoflavone moiety isolated from Passiflora incarnata Linneaus. Talebi and

colleagues [26] evaluated the effect of ethanol consumption on sperm parameters and chromatin integrity of spermatozoa aspirated from the epididymal cauda of rats allowed to drink ad libitum ethanol compared to control rats. The results showed that progressive and nonprogressive motility were significantly lower in ethanol-consuming rats compared with control animals, whereas the percentage of aniline blue-reacted spermatozoa were similar in both groups. However, the percentages of spermatozoa positive to chromomycin A3, toluidine blue, or acridine orange were significantly higher in ethanol drinking rats compared with controls.

Clinical Evidence

Chronic and persistent alcohol use is known to induce sexual dysfunction, which leads to marked distress and interpersonal difficulty [12, 13, 20, 24]. This, in turn, is known to worsen the alcohol abuse. Sexual dysfunction in the alcoholic may be due to the depressant effect of alcohol itself, alcohol-related disease, or due to a multitude of psychological forces related to the alcohol use. The spectrum of sexual dysfunction encompasses all of the following aspects:

1. Decreased sexual desire—persistent or recurrent deficiency or absence of desire for sexual activity giving rise to marked distress and interpersonal difficulty
2. Sexual aversion disorder—persistent or recurrent aversion and avoidance of all genital sexual contact leading to marked distress and interpersonal difficulty
3. Difficulty in erection—recurrent or persistent, partial or complete failure to attain or maintain an erection until the completion of the sex act
4. Difficulty in achieving orgasm—persistent or recurrent delay in or absence of orgasm, following a normal sexual excitement phase
5. Premature ejaculation—persistent or recurrent ejaculation with minimal sexual stimulation, before, on, or shortly after penetration and before the person wishes it, which causes marked distress

Alcohol has been shown to have a deleterious effect at all levels of the male reproductive system.

It interferes with the HPT axis regulation resulting in an impairment of luteinizing hormone (LH) and follicle-stimulating hormone (FSH) secretion [27, 28]. Moreover, a progressive testicular damage and the consequent decrease of sex hormones lead to a loss of secondary sexual characteristics and the onset of erectile dysfunction and infertility [12, 29].

A significant seminal fluid volume and sperm concentration decrease has been reported in men with alcohol dependence syndrome [30]. Hormonal serum levels, measured in only five of them, showed low testosterone levels and normal LH, FSH, and prolactin values. Thus, hypotestosteronemia may explain the observed reduction of the seminal plasma volume. In addition, a higher percentage of morphologically abnormal spermatozoa were observed in these men compared with controls, but no correlation has been found with the amount or the duration of alcohol consumption. The lack of a compensatory increase of LH and FSH concentrations suggests that alcohol has an inhibitory effect on the central component of the HPT axis [31]. Indeed, alcohol may alter gonadotropin-releasing hormone receptor function at the pituitary levels or the interaction of these receptors with gonadotropin-releasing hormone, resulting in a diminished LH release. In addition, alcohol seems to interfere negatively with the LH biological activity. Furthermore, the increased b-endorphin levels observed after acute or chronic alcohol consumption may contribute to testicular damage. Additionally, sperm parameter abnormalities have been reported to be significantly associated with elevated serum LH, FSH, and 17b-estradiol levels and significantly decreased serum testosterone levels, thus suggesting the presence of a primary testiculopathy in men drinking ethanol [32]. Goverde and colleagues [33] did not find any statistically significant difference for seminal fluid volume, sperm concentration, and percentage of motile spermatozoa in daily drinkers and subfertile patients. On the other hand, a significantly lower percentage of morphologically normal spermatozoa in daily drinkers compared with subfertile patients was reported [33]. Semen volume, sperm count, motility, and the percentage of morphologically normal spermatozoa were reported to be significantly decreased in 66 non-smoking and drug-free alcoholics who consumed a minimum of 180 mL of alcohol per day for a minimum of 5 days per week for one year. The morphological abnormality was mainly relative to the sperm head [34]. Gaur and colleagues [35] reported that only 12 out of 100 alcoholics had normozoospermia compared with 37 % of nonalcoholic control men.

Kuller and colleagues [22] evaluated testicular and liver pathology and related the findings with the estimated alcohol consumption among men who had died suddenly from a variety of causes. Out of the men studied, 14 % had a moderate-to-severe decrease in spermatogenesis, but only nine of these men had also severe or very severe fatty infiltration of the liver. These findings suggest that testicular spermatogenesis seem to be more sensitive to alcohol than liver tissue. A subsequent prospective autopsy study further explored the relationship between alcohol consumption, spermatogenesis, and morphometric analysis of the human testis [28].

The mean testicular weight of heavy drinkers was slightly but significantly lower compared with that of controls. Compared to men with normal spermatogenesis, testicular weight was slightly lower in heavy drinkers with spermatogenic arrest and significantly lower in heavy-drinking men with Sertoli cell-only syndrome. Spermatogenic arrest was not correlated with fatty liver or cirrhosis of the liver, whereas four of the five men with Sertoli cell-only syndrome exhibited a fatty liver.

Possible Mechanisms Through Which the Alcohol Affects Male Reproduction

An ethanol-induced oxidative stress is not restricted to the liver, where ethanol is actively oxidized, but can affect various extrahepatic tissues as shown by experimental data obtained in the rat during acute or chronic ethanol intoxication. Most of these data concern the central nervous system, the heart, and the testes [15].

That alcohol abuse may lead to testicular lipid peroxidation is suggested by the fact that ethanol is a known testicular toxin and its chronic use leads to both endocrine and reproductive failure. Because testicular membranes are rich in polyenoic fatty acids that are prone to undergo peroxidative decomposition, it is reasonable to consider that lipid peroxidation may contribute to the membrane injury and gonadal dysfunction that occurs as a result of alcohol abuse and/or chronic use. Consistent with such a mechanism for putative alcohol-associated testicular toxicity are the observed reductions in the testicular content of polyenoic fatty acids and GSH content of the testes of alcohol-fed animals as compared to isocalorically fed controls [36].

The increased conversion of xanthine dehydrogenase into xanthine oxidase as well as the activation of peroxisomal acyl-CoA oxidase linked to ethanol administration could contribute to the oxidative stress. Chronic ethanol administration elicits in the testes an enhancement in mitochondrial lipid peroxidation and a decrease in the CGS level, which appear to be correlated to the gross testicular atrophy observed. It is well known that peroxidation injury can be attenuated when it occurs in association with dietary vitamin A supplementation. Thus, it is of interest to note that vitamin A, acting as an antioxidant, stabilizes testicular membranes by reducing lipid peroxidation and prevents the alcohol-induced atrophy that occurs in animals not receiving vitamin-A-enriched diets. Vitamin A supplementation attenuates the changes in lipid peroxidation, GSH, and testicular morphology [37]. Taken together, these observations suggest that the enhanced peroxidation of testicular lipids that occurs following ethanol exposure may be an important factor in the pathogenesis of alcohol-associated gonadal injury (Fig. 6.1).

A significant negative association was observed between daily alcohol consumption and polycyclic aromatic hydrocarbon-DNA adducts in spermatozoa [38]. Horak and colleagues analyzed the levels of bulky DNA adducts in spermatozoa and did not find any correlation between alcohol and sperm DNA adducts.

Individual Variability to Alcohol Consumption: Role of Genetic Background and Other Factors

The glutathione S-transferase (GST) M1 genotype may be associated with a greater susceptibility to develop, via direct mechanism at testicular level, alcohol-induced spermatogenesis disorders [39]. The homozygous deletion of the GST M1 gene may indicate increased susceptibility to develop irreversible liver damage in response to the toxic effects of ethanol. The association between alcohol-induced alteration of human spermatogenesis and the GST M1 genotype was investigated in an autopsy study comprising 271 subjects [40]. The results of this study showed that among moderate-drinking men, 42 % of the subjects had normal spermatogenesis, whereas 48 % had partial, and 10 % had complete spermatogenic arrest. Among men with normal spermatogenesis, 42.9 % had the GST M1 genotype with a frequency similar to that found in men with partial or complete spermatogenic arrest (44.8 %). Among the heavy-drinking men, 21.2 % of the subjects had normal spermatogenesis, 36.3 % had partial spermatogenic arrest, 38.2 % showed complete spermatogenic arrest, and 4.2 % showed Sertoli cell-only syndrome. Interestingly, 60 % of the heavy drinkers with normal spermatogenesis had the GST M1 genotype when compared with those with disorders of spermatogenesis. The frequency of GST M1 genotype in heavy drinkers with normal spermatogenesis also differed from that of corresponding moderate drinkers, whereas the frequency of GST M1 genotype in heavy drinkers with disorders of spermatogenesis was similar to moderate drinkers with or without disorders of spermatogenesis. The finding that 20 % of heavy drinkers had normal spermatogenesis suggests that the GST M1 genotype exerts a protective effect on alcohol-induced spermatogenesis disorders. Among factors that may potentiate the toxic action of alcohol protein malnutrition, other nutritional deficiencies or imbalances and the associated liver disease are frequently encountered. Due to a low dietary intake or excessive loss of micronutrients, caused by vomiting or diarrhea,

Fig. 6.1 Possible mechanisms through which alcohol affects male reproduction

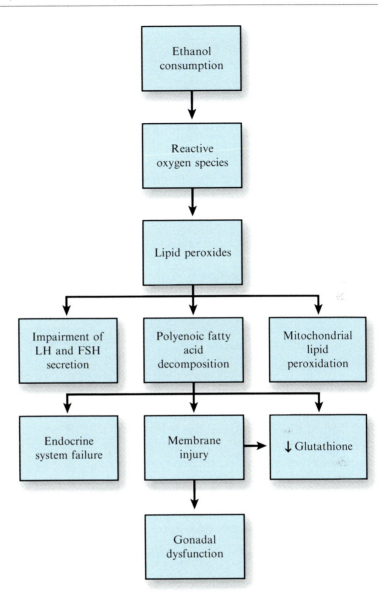

the lack of certain minerals is often present in alcohol users. These include Zn (which plays an important role for the activation of alkaline phosphatase, carbonic anhydrase, and alcohol dehydrogenase), Mg (important in some metabolic processes and for stabilizing DNA, RNA, and ribosomes), and possible states of folate deficiency and hypovitaminosis (A, D, E) in many organs (liver, muscle, heart, testis, and male accessory glands).

In a study performed on a group of alcohol abusers and control group, the patients had significantly low plasma testosterone with low LH and FSH concentrations, associated with oligo-asthenozoospermia and increased oxidative stress. The latter was due to high thiobarbituric acid reactive substances, superoxide dismutase, GST, low glutathione, ascorbic acid, catalase, GSH reductase, and GSH peroxidase.

Discussion and Conclusion

Alcohol-attributable injuries are of a growing concern to the public health community, with alcohol-related injuries such as road traffic accidents, burns, poisonings, falls, and drowning. Sexual disorders have also been reported frequently in chronic alcoholics. Alcohol exposure has been associated with a reduction in seminiferous tubular diameter and germinal epithelium, sperm concentration, percentage of spermatozoa with normal morphology, and sperm motility [30, 41]. In addition, a decrease in testicular and serum levels of testosterone has been reported among ethanol consumers [42, 43].

Alcohol exerts a dose-related toxic effect on testicular function. Spermatogenesis disruption and a primary testicular insufficiency and compensatory increase of FSH and LH secretion have been observed in alcoholics [44, 45].

Drinking alcohol is considered a common social entertainment. A significant association between alcohol and cigarette consumption has been reported by several researchers [46–49]. According to Rubes et al. [46], alcohol consumption cannot be separated from smoking because most smokers consumed moderate to high amounts of alcohol, whereas most nonsmokers were also nondrinkers. In addition, based on previous reports suggesting that moderate drinking does not affect male gametes' quality [19, 50], most of the investigators do not separate, for statistical analysis, those men who have the two habits from those who have only one [46, 47]. Nevertheless, the synergic or additive effects of these substances on the male reproductive physiology cannot be discarded.

In fact, a reduction in sperm concentration and in the percentage of spermatozoa with normal morphology has been detected in chronic alcoholics and in smokers. The above modifications suggest a synergistic or additive effect of both toxic habits on male reproductive function.

It is evident from the findings of different studies that chronic alcohol consumption has a detrimental effect on male reproductive function, which, in turn, will make people who are addicted to alcohol impotent and sterile. However, until relatively recently, alcohol consumption was not discussed. Because of insufficient knowledge and limited research data, health care providers often overlook substance abuse and misuse among adults. Other factors responsible for the lack of attention to substance abuse include the current disapproval of and shame about use and misuse of substances, along with a reluctance to seek professional help for what many consider a private matter.

In conclusion, male patients should be specifically warned of the negative effect of chronic alcohol consumption on their reproductive competence and be advised to refrain from chronic alcohol consumption if they want to procreate and lead a normal sexual life [32].

References

1. Fuller E, editor. Drug use, smoking and drinking among young people in England in 2007. London, UK: The Health and Social Care Information Centre; 2008.
2. Hull MG, Glazener CM, Kelly NJ, Conway DI, Foster PA, Hinton RA, et al. Population study of causes, treatment, and outcome of infertility. Br Med J (Clin Res Ed). 1985;291:1693–7.
3. Mosher WD, Pratt WF. Fecundity and infertility in the United States: incidence and trends. Fertil Steril. 1991;56:192–3.
4. Wang C, McDonald V, Leung A, Superlano L, Berman N, Hull L, et al. Effect of increased scrotal temperature on sperm production in normal men. Fertil Steril. 1997;68:334–9.
5. Thonneau P, Marchand S, Tallec A, Ferial ML, Ducot B, Lansac J, et al. Incidence and main causes of infertility in a resident population (1,850,000) of three French regions (1988–1989). Hum Reprod. 1991;6:811–6.
6. Hull MG, North K, Taylor H, Farrow A, Ford WC. Delayed conception and active and passive smoking. The Avon Longitudinal Study of Pregnancy and Childhood Study Team. Fertil Steril. 2000; 74:725–33.
7. Hassan MA, Killick SR. Negative lifestyle is associated with a significant reduction in fecundity. Fertil Steril. 2004;81:384–92.
8. Bolumar F, Olsen J, Boldsen J. Smoking reduces fecundity: a European multicenter study on infertility and subfecundity. The European Study Group on Infertility and Subfecundity. Am J Epidemiol. 1996;143:578–87.
9. Jensen TK, Hjollund NH, Henriksen TB, Scheike T, Kolstad H, Giwercman A, et al. Does moderate

alcohol consumption affect fertility? Follow up study among couples planning first pregnancy. BMJ. 1998;317:505–10.

10. Oldereid NB, Rui H, Purvis K. Lifestyles of men in barren couples and their relationships to sperm quality. Eur J Obstet Gynecol Reprod Biol. 1992;43: 51–7.

11. Marshburn PB, Sloan CS, Hammond MG. Semen quality and association with coffee drinking, cigarette smoking, and ethanol consumption. Fertil Steril. 1989;52:162–5.

12. La Vignera S, Condorelli RA, Balercia G, Vicari E, Calogero AE. Does alcohol have any effect on male reproductive function? A review of literature. Asian J Androl. 2013;15:221–5.

13. Marinelli D, Gaspari L, Pedotti P, Taioli E. Mini-review of studies on the effect of smoking and drinking habits on semen parameters. Int J Hyg Environ Health. 2004;207:185–92.

14. Ramlau-Hansen CH, Toft G, Jensen MS, Strandberg-Larsen K, Hansen ML, Olsen J. Maternal alcohol consumption during pregnancy and semen quality in the male offspring: two decades of follow-up. Hum Reprod. 2010;25:2340–5.

15. Rosenblum ER, Gavaler JS, Van Thiel DH. Lipid peroxidation: a mechanism for alcohol-induced testicular injury. Free Radic Biol Med. 1989;7:569–77.

16. Faut M, Rodriguez de Castro C, Bietto FM, Castro JA, Castro GD. Metabolism of ethanol to acetaldehyde and increased susceptibility to oxidative stress could play a role in the ovarian tissue cell injury promoted by alcohol drinking. Toxicol Ind Health. 2009;25:525–38.

17. Rosenblum E, Gavaler JS, Van Thiel DH. Lipid peroxidation: a mechanism for ethanol-associated testicular injury in rats. Endocrinology. 1985;116:311–8.

18. Dunphy BC, Barratt CL, Cooke ID. Male alcohol consumption and fecundity in couples attending an infertility clinic. Andrologia. 1991;23:219–21.

19. Curtis KM, Savitz DA, Arbuckle TE. Effects of cigarette smoking, caffeine consumption, and alcohol intake on fecundability. Am J Epidemiol. 1997;146:32–41.

20. Klonoff-Cohen H, Lam-Kruglick P, Gonzalez C. Effects of maternal and paternal alcohol consumption on the success rates of in vitro fertilization and gamete intrafallopian transfer. Fertil Steril. 2003;79: 330–9.

21. Hadi HA, Hill JA, Castillo RA. Alcohol and reproductive function: a review. Obstet Gynecol Surv. 1987;42:69–74.

22. Kuller LH, May SJ, Perper JA. The relationship between alcohol, liver disease, and testicular pathology. Am J Epidemiol. 1978;108:192–9.

23. Sermondade N, Elloumi H, Berthaut I, Mathieu E, Delarouziere V, Ravel C, et al. Progressive alcohol-induced sperm alterations leading to spermatogenic arrest, which was reversed after alcohol withdrawal. Reprod Biomed Online. 2010;20:324–7.

24. Abel EL, Moore C. Effects of paternal alcohol consumption in mice. Alcohol Clin Exp Res. 1987; 11:533–5.

25. Dhawan K, Sharma A. Prevention of chronic alcohol and nicotine-induced azospermia, sterility and decreased libido, by a novel tri-substituted benzoflavone moiety from Passiflora incarnata Linneaus in healthy male rats. Life Sci. 2002;71:3059–69.

26. Talebi AR, Sarcheshmeh AA, Khalili MA, Tabibnejad N. Effects of ethanol consumption on chromatin condensation and DNA integrity of epididymal spermatozoa in rat. Alcohol. 2011;45:403–9.

27. Emanuele MA, Emanuele NV. Alcohol's effects on male reproduction. Alcohol Health Res World. 1998;22:195–201.

28. Pajarinen JT, Karhunen PJ. Spermatogenic arrest and 'Sertoli cell-only' syndrome–common alcohol-induced disorders of the human testis. Int J Androl. 1994;17:292–9.

29. Beckman LJ. Reported effects of alcohol on the sexual feelings and behavior of women alcoholics and nonalcoholics. J Stud Alcohol. 1979;40:272–82.

30. Kucheria K, Saxena R, Mohan D. Semen analysis in alcohol dependence syndrome. Andrologia. 1985;17: 558–63.

31. Salonen I, Pakarinen P, Huhtaniemi I. Effect of chronic ethanol diet on expression of gonadotropin genes in the male rat. J Pharmacol Exp Ther. 1992; 260:463–7.

32. Muthusami KR, Chinnaswamy P. Effect of chronic alcoholism on male fertility hormones and semen quality. Fertil Steril. 2005;84:919–24.

33. Goverde HJ, Dekker HS, Janssen HJ, Bastiaans BA, Rolland R, Zielhuis GA. Semen quality and frequency of smoking and alcohol consumption–an explorative study. Int J Fertil Menopausal Stud. 1995;40:135–8.

34. Guo H, Zhang HG, Xue BG, Sha YW, Liu Y, Liu RZ. [Effects of cigarette, alcohol consumption and sauna on sperm morphology]. Zhonghua Nan Ke Xue. 2006;12:215–7, 221.

35. Gaur DS, Talekar MS, Pathak VP. Alcohol intake and cigarette smoking: impact of two major lifestyle factors on male fertility. Indian J Pathol Microbiol. 2010;53:35–40.

36. Nordmann R, Ribiere C, Rouach H. Ethanol-induced lipid peroxidation and oxidative stress in extrahepatic tissues. Alcohol Alcohol. 1990;25:231–7.

37. Nordmann R. Alcohol and antioxidant systems. Alcohol Alcohol. 1994;29:513–22.

38. Gaspari L, Chang SS, Santella RM, Garte S, Pedotti P, Taioli E. Polycyclic aromatic hydrocarbon-DNA adducts in human sperm as a marker of DNA damage and infertility. Mutat Res. 2003;535:155–60.

39. Horak S, Polanska J, Widlak P. Bulky DNA adducts in human sperm: relationship with fertility, semen quality, smoking, and environmental factors. Mutat Res. 2003;537:53–65.

40. Pajarinen J, Savolainen V, Perola M, Penttila A, Karhunen PJ. Glutathione S-transferase-M1 'null' genotype and alcohol-induced disorders of human spermatogenesis. Int J Androl. 1996;19:155–63.

41. Vine MF, Tse CK, Hu P, Truong KY. Cigarette smoking and semen quality. Fertil Steril. 1996;65:835–42.

42. Bannister P, Losowsky MS. Ethanol and hypogonadism. Alcohol Alcohol. 1987;22:213–7.
43. Adler RA. Clinical review 33: clinically important effects of alcohol on endocrine function. J Clin Endocrinol Metab. 1992;74:957–60.
44. Lindholm J, Fabricius-Bjerre N, Bahnsen M, Boiesen P, Bangstrup L, Pedersen ML, et al. Pituitary-testicular function in patients with chronic alcoholism. Eur J Clin Invest. 1978;8:269–72.
45. Villalta J, Ballesca JL, Nicolas JM, Martinez de Osaba MJ, Antunez E, Pimentel C. Testicular function in asymptomatic chronic alcoholics: relation to ethanol intake. Alcohol Clin Exp Res. 1997;21:128–33.
46. Rubes J, Lowe X, Moore II D, Perreault S, Slott V, Evenson D, et al. Smoking cigarettes is associated with increased sperm disomy in teenage men. Fertil Steril. 1998;70:715–23.
47. Wong WY, Thomas CM, Merkus HM, Zielhuis GA, Doesburg WH, Steegers-Theunissen RP. Cigarette smoking and the risk of male factor subfertility: minor association between cotinine in seminal plasma and semen morphology. Fertil Steril. 2000;74:930–5.
48. Kunzle R, Mueller MD, Hanggi W, Birkhauser MH, Drescher H, Bersinger NA. Semen quality of male smokers and nonsmokers in infertile couples. Fertil Steril. 2003;79:287–91.
49. Martini AC, Molina RI, Estofan D, Senestrari D, Fiol de Cuneo M, Ruiz RD. Effects of alcohol and cigarette consumption on human seminal quality. Fertil Steril. 2004;82:374–7.
50. Chia SE, Lim ST, Tay SK, Lim ST. Factors associated with male infertility: a case-control study of 218 infertile and 240 fertile men. BJOG. 2000;107:55–61.

Drugs: Recreational and Performance Enhancing Substance Abuse

7

Fanuel Lampiao, Taryn Lockey, Collins E. Jana,
David Moon Lee, and Stefan S. du Plessis

Introduction

Infertility can be a shocking diagnosis, and in some regions fertility is regarded as an integral aspect of certain traditional and societal roles; however, near to 15 % of couples are categorized as infertile [1]. The clinical definition of infertility is a couple's inability to achieve a pregnancy after 1 year of unprotected, regular, and well-timed intercourse [2]. There are two types of infertility: primary infertility describes couples that have never achieved parenthood and secondary infertility

F. Lampiao, PhD (✉) • C.E. Jana, MSc
Department of Basic Medical Sciences, College
of Medicine, University of Malawi, Mahatma Gandhi
Campus, Blantyre, Malawi
e-mail: flampiao@medcol.mw

T. Lockey, BSc, BSc (Hons)
Division of Medical Physiology, Department
of Biomedical Sciences, Faculty of Medicine
and Health Sciences, Stellenbosch University,
Tygerberg, Western Cape, South Africa
e-mail: tlockey@live.co.za

D.M. Lee, BA
Center for Reproductive Medicine, Cleveland Clinic
Foundation/Glickman Urological and Kidney Institute,
10681 Carnegie Avenue, Cleveland, OH 44106, USA
e-mail: davidlee89@gmail.com

S.S. du Plessis, BSc (Hons), MSc, MBA,
PhD (Stell) (✉)
Division of Medical Physiology, Department
of Biomedical Sciences, Faculty of Medicine and
Health Sciences, Stellenbosch University, Tygerberg,
Western Cape, South Africa
e-mail: ssdp@sun.ac.za

describes couples with a history of parenthood [3]. Thirty percent of infertile couples are infertile due solely to a male factor, and that statistic rises to 50 % when couples that are experiencing difficulty achieving pregnancy due to a combination of male and female factors are included [4–6].

Abuse of drugs and misuse of prescription medications or household substances seems to be on the rise [7, 8]. According to the World Health Organization, marijuana, opioids, methamphetamine and 3, 4-methylenedioxymethamphetamine (MDMA), and cocaine are the most commonly used recreational drugs in the world. Although creatine and steroid use is not as prevalent as recreational drug use, it has garnered much public attention recently as professional athletes come under more criticism and scrutiny regarding their use. Additionally, as with recreational drug users, the predominant users of creatine and anabolic steroids are young males in their reproductive years [9].

People abuse these drugs for several reasons, which include to gain social acceptance, to relieve boredom, to rebel, to experiment, and to improve their performance [8]. For instance, androgens are now widely used by professional and recreational athletes, weight lifters and bodybuilders, and non-athletes wishing to enhance their appearance [7]. There is an accumulating body of evidence in the literature suggesting that drug abuse negatively affects the reproductive system [10, 11]. Use of steroids in men decreases levels of luteinizing hormone and follicle stimulating hormone (FSH), which lead to decreased endogenous testosterone production, decreased

S.S. du Plessis et al. (eds.), *Male Infertility: A Complete Guide to Lifestyle and Environmental Factors*,
DOI 10.1007/978-1-4939-1040-3_7, © Springer Science+Business Media New York 2014

spermatogenesis, and testicular atrophy. These effects have been shown to lead to infertility [12].

A clinical evaluation for the presence of a male factor influencing a couple's fertility is indicated if there is a failure to conceive after at least 12 months of unprotected, regular, and well-timed intercourse for couples below the age of 35 [13]. Many cases of male infertility do not present with any obvious signs: intercourse, erections, and ejaculation occur without difficulty, and ejaculate appears normal upon visual inspection [5].

In this chapter, we aim to describe the drug, highlight key facts about typical usage, and describe the endocrine and overall fertility effects of each drug. Finally, we will discuss some treatment options for recreational drug and steroid-induced male infertility.

Causes of Male Infertility

Pathological causes of male infertility can be broadly classified as pre-testicular, testicular, and post-testicular. Some pre-testicular causes of infertility are hypo- and hypergonadotropic hypogonadism, Kallman Syndrome and medications or genetic abnormalities that affect the hypothalamic-pituitary-gonadal (HPG) axis. Common testicular causes of infertility are varicocele, cryptorchidism, testicular injury, testicular cancer, and congenital abnormalities. Examples of post-testicular causes of infertility are congenital bilateral absence of the vas deferens (CBVAD), erectile dysfunction, Young's syndrome, nerve injury, and abnormal coital practices [14].

Drug and substance abuse has emerged as a factor of interest of male infertility because these drugs often affect male reproduction via a trifecta of pre-, post-, and direct testicular influences. This chapter will discuss how the commonly used drugs and substances such as marijuana, opioids, methamphetamine and ecstasy, cocaine and creatine and steroids contribute to male infertility (Fig. 7.1).

Marijuana

Marijuana is the common name for the Cannabis plant. There is controversy over the number of cannabis species, with more recent morphological

and genetic data suggesting three distinct species (Cannabis sativa, Cannabis indica, and Cannabis ruderalis) instead of the traditional view of a solitary cannabis species. Marijuana use predates recorded history, and was used for a myriad of purposes. Marijuana seeds were used as fuel and food, fibers in the stalks were used to make rope and clothing, and the flower was used for a variety of pharmaceutical purposes [15]. Marijuana is now known to be a psychostimulant that affects ones' perception of reality by causing mild hallucinations and euphoria [16]. Although it is illegal throughout most of the world, marijuana still remains the most widely used recreational drug in the world [17]. It is able to exert both stimulatory and depressant effects through various receptors—perhaps due, in part, to the wide variety of constituent compounds [18].

Marijuana contains over 420 compounds, but the class of compound predominantly responsible for the psychological and medical effects are called cannabinoids. The most studied of these cannabinoids are delta-9-tetrahydrocannabinol (THC), cannabinol (CBN), and cannabidiol (CBD). Although THC is thought to be responsible for the majority of the psychoactive effects, there is a complex interplay between the various cannabinoid and terpenoid components of marijuana that is yet to be elucidated [19]. THC is also thought to be responsible for exerting most of marijuana's negative effects on male fertility; however, this may be due to the overwhelming number of studies focusing on THC and infertility and the relative absence of studies focusing on other compounds in marijuana and infertility [16].

THC is a lipid soluble compound and can form a reserve within adipose tissue [20]. Due to its lipid solubility, THC was thought to reach its areas of action by diffusion across lipid membranes; however, this hypothesis was rejected after cannabinoid receptors were identified in humans [21]. Only a small quantity of THC is needed to elicit its effects as it can bind directly to lipoproteins [16].

How Is Marijuana Used?

Marijuana is used as both a recreational and medical drug; however, due to its illegal status in

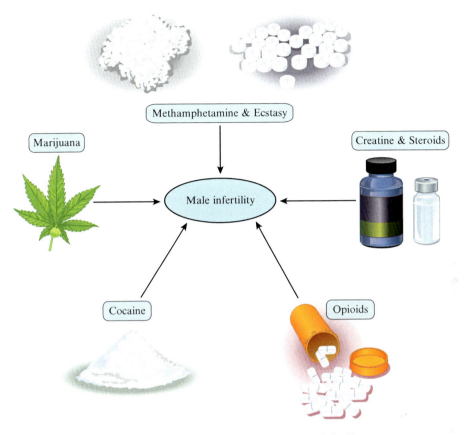

Fig. 7.1 Recreational and performance enhancing substance abuse that causes infertility

most countries it is most commonly used as a recreational drug [22]. Marijuana is still most commonly found in three forms, and these forms are often called by their Indian names: bhang, or 'grass' in the USA, includes flowers, stems, leaves, and seeds of the cannabis plant; ganja is the seedless unfertilized flowers of the female plant; and charas, commonly referred to by its Arabic name 'hashish', is a collection of cannabis resin and trichomes from the cannabis flowers [23]. These preparations can be smoked using a pipe or marijuana cigarette, vaporization, or the historically preferred method of ingestion via marijuana tea, tincture, or food preparations [19, 23].

Endocrine Effects of Marijuana

THC, CBN, and CBD are similar enough to endogenous human cannabinoids, called endocannabinoids, to interact with the endocannabinoid system (ECS) [24] and behave as ligands to the CB1 and CB2 cannabinoid receptors. CB1 receptors are found in the hypothalamus, pituitary, testes, prostate, vas deferens, and spermatozoa, while CB2 receptors have been localized in the hypothalamus and Sertoli cells, with some evidence of their presence in spermatozoa [25–27].

Marijuana has been shown to inhibit the release of the reproductive hormones, growth hormone, and thyroid hormone [28] from the anterior pituitary, which is regulated by the hypothalamus [29–31]. Marijuana also exerts an inhibitory effect on gonadotropin releasing hormone (GnRH), which is responsible for initiating the release of the FSH and luteinising hormone (LH) [29]. It is postulated that this effect might be due to an accumulation of catecholamines in the brain, which can downregulate the release of GnRH [30]. It is generally accepted that both acute and chronic use of marijuana also depresses testosterone levels [31–33]; however, there is conflicting evidence showing no significant changes in LH, FSH, or testosterone levels for chronic users [34].

The presence of CB1 receptors in the pituitary gland of the brain and Leydig cells of the testes indicate that cannabinoids exert a direct effect on the production of these hormones [31], and the presence of both CB1 and CB2 receptors in the GnRH secreting cells of the hypothalamus suggest that the ECS also plays an indirect role in regulating HPG axis activity.

Effects of Marijuana on the Testes, Spermatozoa, and Fertility

Evidence suggests that cannabinoids decrease the weight of the prostate, epididymis, and testes through breakdown of seminiferous tubules; however, these changes have not been measured in humans [30, 35]. The role of CB2 receptors in male reproduction is yet unclear; however, it seems that they do play an important role in male reproduction as they help regulate the survival of Sertoli cells via their protective role against the endogenous cannabinoid N-arachidonoylethanolamine (AEA) [36].

CB1 receptors have been localized in testes and germ cells through all stages of sperm development [35, 37]. Both isoforms of THC are able to bind directly to the head and midpiece of the sperm via the CB1 receptor [38], which helps explain reduction in sperm motility, concentration, and viability [38–41]. Furthermore, the CB1 receptor has been shown to play an important role in regulating capacitation and the acrosome reaction through its binding with the ligand AEA [36, 42, 43], which has been found at significantly lower levels in the seminal plasma of infertile men compared to fertile men and further supports the importance of CB1 in male infertility [44].

Although much is still unclear, the evidence supports marijuana having a negative effect on male reproductive capacity. This is of particular concern because marijuana is the most widely used recreational drug in the world, especially amongst men of reproductive age.

Opioids

Opioids are a class of analgesic medications that are prescribed for treating acute or chronic pain, or relieving coughs or diarrhea, and they are derived from the poppy plant [45]. Some common examples of opioid pain medications include morphine, hydrocodone, and oxycodone [46]. Heroin, which is synthesized from morphine, is an illegal, rapidly acting addictive opioid. Opioids are the third most commonly abused category of drug in the world [46].

How Are Opioids Used?

In modern medicine, opioids are most commonly used for their analgesic properties; however, recreational users consume high doses in order to induce euphoria and other euphoric feelings. Opioids may be ingested, injected, insufflated, used as a suppository or smoked. Accordingly, these drugs are available in pill, liquid, powder, and resin forms [45].

The acute use of opioids can cause an increase in growth hormone, thyroid stimulating hormone (TSH), and prolactin as well as a decrease in LH, testosterone, estradiol, and oxytocin in humans [47]. All of these changes were seen from direct opioid action at the hypothalamic, pituitary, and gonadal levels in humans [47, 48]. It is thought that the decrease in LH caused by opioid inhibition at the hypothalamus consequently leads to a decrease in testosterone levels [49, 50]; however, an alternative explanation is opioid-induced hypersensitivity to testosterone, which inhibits the release of LH [51]. Evidence of the latter explanation is that innocuous doses of testosterone have been shown to be significantly inhibitory of LH release after morphine administration [52].

Effects of Opioids on Testes, Sperm, and Fertility

Opioids affect the function of the testes indirectly through changes in LH and testosterone levels.

A direct mode of influence is suggested due to altered testicular function from reduced testicular interstitial fluid (TIF) volume [53]; however, it is still unclear whether such a mode of influence exists. Spermatozoa are affected both indirectly via altered reproductive hormone pulses and directly via opioid receptors located on the spermatozoa themselves [48, 51–55]. Evidence about the effects of opioids on sperm motility, concentration, and viability is inconsistent. Studies contradict each other in regard to the degree and even the presence of changes in the aforementioned sperm parameters; however, it is generally agreed that there is a significant reduction in number of pregnancies when males are exposed to opioids in animal models [48, 56, 57]. Also, men on prolonged opioid treatments also experienced erectile dysfunction, difficulty with ejaculation, and decreased sex drive [58]. Therefore, despite lack of consensus about the effects of opioids on actual sperm parameters, it is obvious that opioids reduce the likelihood of male reproductive success.

Methamphetamine and MDMA

Methamphetamine and MDMA belong to the drug class amphetamine, which is the second most widely abused type of drug in the world [Word Drug Report]. Methamphetamine in its crystalline form is commonly called crystal meth, ice, Tina, or glass [59]. It is classified as a psychostimulant and causes a heightened sense of alertness and awareness as well as hallucinations [30]. MDMA causes a euphoric high as well as a burst of energy and feelings of elation, empathy, and excitement [60]. MDMA is also known as ecstasy, E, X, and molly [61, 62]. Methamphetamine and MDMA cause the release of both dopamine and serotonin, which are responsible for some of the more pleasurable effects and habit formation [63].

How Are Methamphetamine and MDMA Used?

Unlike MDMA, which is typically only found in tablet form, methamphetamine can be inhaled,

insufflated, or injected (with the addition of water) in its powder form and is typically smoked in its pure crystalline form [61, 64].

Although once used therapeutically, both methamphetamine and MDMA are no longer commonly used in a clinical setting. Today, both drugs are used recreationally as central nervous system stimulants and mild hallucinogens, and MDMA is also used recreationally as an empathogen [61, 64].

Endocrine Effects of Methamphetamine and MDMA

Methamphetamine's effect on reproductive hormones and the HPG axis has not been well studied and little is known [65]; however, a biphasic effect on testosterone levels, which first decrease and then increase, has been reported [66].

Both chronic and acute MDMA use has been shown to significantly affect the HPG axis. Exposure to MDMA decreased GnRH mRNA, LH, and testosterone levels in adult male rats due to MDMA's interruption of the HPG axis at the hypothalamus, most likely specifically on the GnRH neurosecretory system [67].

Effects of Methamphetamine and MDMA on Spermatozoa, Testes, and Fertility

Although it is unknown exactly how or if methamphetamine affects spermatozoa and the testes in humans, it has been shown to affect gametogenesis in male mice and rats. Spermatozoa were found in lower concentrations, with poorer motility and with poorer morphology after acute and subacute exposures as well as significantly increased apoptosis of germ cells in the seminiferous tubules. These changes were accompanied by a decrease in signs of copulation and number of live births [66, 68–70].

MDMA has been shown to decrease the concentration, motility, and DNA integrity of spermatozoa in rats [67, 68]. MDMA disrupts the redox cycle and causes the production of reactive oxygen species. The resultant oxidative stress can damage the DNA in the spermatozoa [71]. Other effects of chronic MDMA use that have been observed include tubular degeneration and interstitial oedema, which may contribute to the other adverse sperm parameters [72].

Cocaine

Cocaine (benzoylmethylecgonine) is the fourth most widely used type of drug in the world [World Drug Report], and cocaine abuse has adverse affects on the cardiovascular, cerebrovascular, pulmonary, and reproductive functions [73]. Cocaine is extracted from the leaves of the coca plant and is commonly known as coke, blow, and crack. It is highly addictive due to its blockage of dopamine reuptake [74].

How Is Cocaine Used?

The coca leaf must be processed into a paste from which freebase cocaine is extracted; then the freebase cocaine is further purified and processed into a crystalline salt, cocaine hydrochloride [75]. Cocaine hydrochloride is the powder form of cocaine that can be insufflated, inhaled, injected, ingested, and absorbed through the gums or as a rectal suppository; however, cocaine hydrochloride can be reduced back into a less pure version of freebase cocaine called crack cocaine. The vaporization temperature of freebase cocaine is 98 °C, much lower than that of cocaine hydrochloride. Because freebase cocaine remains relatively stable at this low vaporization temperature, the predominant method of abuse of freebase cocaine is by inhaling the vapor [76].

Endocrine Effects of Cocaine

Despite the brain having the highest affinity to cocaine amongst selected rat organs, it seems that cocaine's effect on male reproduction via hormonal changes is limited. Multiple studies have found changes in LH and prolactin levels amongst male cocaine users [77, 78]. Interestingly, the fluctuations in testosterone levels seen in animal studies were not seen in humans, and there was no change in testosterone levels corresponding to depression of LH levels [79]. LH and prolactin levels attenuated after 2 weeks of cocaine abstinence, and levels returned to normal after 4 weeks of cocaine abstinence [77, 78].

Effects of Cocaine on Spermatozoa, Testes, and Fertility

Cocaine has been shown to cause testicular lesions, apoptosis of germ cells, reduced testes weight, and reduced seminiferous tubule diameter in rats possibly by direct action since cocaine specific binding sites in rat testes have been identified [80], however, the specific mechanism by which cocaine causes testicular damage is unknown. Although these effects have not been assessed in humans, various changes in semen parameters also support cocaine having detrimental effects on male fertility. Yelian et al. and Hurd et al. observed decreases in human sperm motility when exposed to high concentrations of cocaine [80, 81], although Yelian et al. found that this decrease did not persist or affect the ability of the cocaine exposed human sperm to fertilize hamster oocytes. Bracken and McSharry (1990) found a correlation between prior cocaine use and decreases in sperm motility, concentration, and morphology, which persisted after accounting for other common risk factors for these three semen parameters [82]. It is therefore not surprising to learn that chronic cocaine exposure significantly reduced pregnancy rates in rats. An additional consideration that should be taken when evaluating the male cocaine user is that cocaine specific binding sites have been identified in human spermatozoa which are able to carry cocaine into the ovum. This toxic exposure may affect fetal development and has been shown to cause altered behavior in the offspring of cocaine exposed male rats [83].

Creatine and Steroids

Creatine (α-methyl guanidine-acetic acid) supplements are widely used by athletes as an ergogenic agent [84]. Creatine (Cr) has been shown to enhance muscle mass and performance, stop disease-induced muscle atrophy, improve rehabilitation, and support cellular energetics [85]. Cr, a nonprotein nitrogen, is a compound containing nitrogen but is not itself a protein. It is endogenously synthesized in the liver, kidneys, and to a lesser extent in the pancreas [86–88]. The remaining Cr found in the body is obtained exogenously from a diet of plant and animal origin. Studies have shown that about 95 % of the body's Cr is stored in skeletal muscle whereas the remaining 5 % is shared by the brain, liver, kidney, and testes [89]. In the human body, Cr is mainly found in two forms, the phosphorylated form (phosphocreatine), which constitutes about 60 % of total creatine, and the non-phosphorylated (free) form [89, 90]. Creatine found in skeletal muscle has a different distribution: 67 % is stored in a phosphorylated form, and the remainder is in its free form [89].

Steroids are a synthetic form of testosterone. Since the isolation and characterization of testosterone in 1935, modifications to this molecule have led to synthesis of various derivatives called anabolic-androgenic steroids (AAS) or anabolic steroids [91]. Previously, the use of steroids was only common among professional athletes and body builders, but it has become widely popular among recreational athletes. There are an estimated three million AAS users in the USA alone, of which two thirds are noncompetitive body builders and non-athletes [91].

How Are Creatine and Steroids Used?

Creatine is primarily used as a dietary supplement. Various studies on Cr have shown that its use is associated with positive therapeutic effects in different clinical applications [87]. Studies have also shown that using Cr as a sport supplement enhances muscular force and power and decreases fatigue in longer bout activities. Furthermore, Cr supplementation has been shown to increase muscle mass [87].

The use of AAS has been shown to improve athlete performance, but AAS use has also been associated with adverse health effects. It has been reported that oral administration of steroids produces more adverse effects than steroids administered parenterally; however, most athletes and body builders use anabolic steroids both orally and parenterally, with doses which are up to 40 times more than normal. Therefore, the rate of recurrence of side effects may vary depending on type of drug, dosage, and duration of use among individuals [92, 93].

Endocrine Effects of Creatine and Steroids

Since Cr supplementation has been shown to increase lean muscle mass, total work performed, muscular power, and fat-free mass [87, 94], it has been speculated that Cr stimulates hypertrophy through the endocrine system [94]. To investigate this hypothesis, some studies on the effects of short-term Cr supplementation on anabolic hormones have been conducted; however, contradictory results have been reported from these investigations [95].

Studies conducted on individuals administered Cr (25 g/day for 7 days) or placebo to assess levels of testosterone and cortisol soon after exercise showed that Cr had no effect on endocrine status [95]; however, studies evaluating acute and short-term Cr exposure found that acute oral administration of a 20 g Cr bolus raised growth hormone levels (83 %) [96], whereas short-term Cr administration (20 g/day for 5 days) did not induce any changes in cortisol and growth hormone levels after a session of heavy resistance exercise [97].

Androgens are responsible for the development of secondary sexual characteristics during puberty, as well as creation and maintenance of adult sexual function and fertility. Androgens are tissue specific and this is demonstrated by the conversion of testosterone to other metabolites including dihydrotestosterone (DHT) and estradiol [11]. Since the skeletal muscle lacks 5α-reductase activity, testosterone and DHT emerge to be the only key hormones for androgen action. Aromatization of testosterone to estradiol is important for differentiation of the brain, bone mass secretion, as well as fusion of the epiphyses at the end of puberty [11]. By using supraphysiological doses of steroids, anabolic effects may be induced via a different mechanism free of the androgen receptor [11].

Gynecomastia is a well-known and irreversible side effect of anabolic steroid use caused by elevated circulating estrogen levels. The estrogens are produced from peripheral aromatization of anabolic steroids, and when their concentration in males is elevated in circulation, breast growth is stimulated [92, 98].

Effects of Creatine and Steroids on Testes, Spermatozoa, and Fertility

Studies have shown that creatine kinase (CK) plays an important enzymatic role in the generation, transport, as well as energy utilization in spermatozoa by catalyzing the reversible phosphorylation of Cr to form phosphocreatine [99]. It is now known that there are two forms of CK isoenzymes in human spermatozoa: CK-B and CK-Mi [100].

The proportion of CK-Mi to total CK is a measure of normal sperm development. Huszar et al. (1992) used this proportion to stratify a group of couples seeking IVF into two groups, and they found that the CK proportion was predictive of male fertilizing potential. They also found that the CK proportion can be used to detect some idiopathic male infertility [101]. Huszar et al. (2005) reported that CK activity was higher in spermatozoa of oligozoospermic men when compared to CK activity in spermatozoa of normozoospermic men and that there was no relationship between sperm CK activity and motility or morphology [102]. Additionally, spermatozoa containing elevated levels of total CK

content were regarded as not being mature and also poor in various functions [103].

Testosterone has strong genitotropic effects, so it is no surprise that anabolic steroids, which are testosterone derivatives, affect the reproductive system as well. The use of anabolic steroids causes an elevated level of testosterone [11], which puts negative feedback on the hypothalamic-pituitary axis resulting in inhibition of FSH and luteinizing hormone (LH) production [98]. Prolonged use of high doses of anabolic steroids results in decreased levels of testosterone, LH, and FSH and can lead to hypogonadotrophic hypogonadism [92]. Generally, it has been reported that suspension of anabolic steroid use restores gonadal functions within a number of months [92, 98].

Possible Treatment of Male Infertility

Some infertility problems can be treated in a way that permits natural conception. Treatable causes of male infertility include: blockage of sperm transport (for example, vasectomy); hormonal problems; some sexual problems (for example, problems with getting and keeping an erection) and some reversible conditions (for example, use of anabolic steroids) [9]. Most of the drugs that contribute to male infertility discussed in this chapter do so by disrupting the production hormones required for the normal process of spermatogenesis such as FSH, LH, and testosterone [29, 32, 33]. Consequently, discontinuation of use of these drugs would lead to production of normal spermatozoa that are capable of fertilizing the egg; however, this amelioration has not been studied in all of the aforementioned drugs. Studies have shown that for marijuana use and anabolic steroid use, abstaining from drug use can attenuate and even reverse the negative reproductive effects for males [92, 98], but opioids, methamphetamine, MDMA, and cocaine also exert a direct influence on testicular function. Reproductive damage caused by these drugs may not respond to cessation of drug use. A possible method of treating infertility caused due to drug abuse is by hormone replacement therapy, however, hormone replacement therapy has not been studied as a treatment for infertility caused by recreational drug or anabolic steroid use. More potential treatments may be discovered as further elucidation of the mechanism of damage for these drugs occurs. Unfortunately, there is a paucity in the literature concerning the amelioration of this sort of drug-induced damage, and treatment options are quite limited. Patient education about negative reproductive effects caused by these drugs may be effective in halting the progression or even prevention of an infertility outcome.

Conclusion

Marijuana, opioids, methamphetamine, MDMA, cocaine, and anabolic steroids have a negative effect on male reproductive capacity through both direct and indirect modes of influence. With the majority of drug users being males in their reproductive years and as a decline in semen parameters have been observed over the past 50 years, assessing drug use during patient history is especially pertinent today, despite limited treatment options.

References

1. Dyer S, Mokoena N, Maritz J, van der Spuy Z. Motives for parenthood among couples attending a level 3 infertility clinic in the public health sector in South Africa. Hum Reprod. 2008;23(2):352–7.
2. Isidori A, Latini M, Romanelli F. Treatment of male infertility. Contraception. 2005;72:314–8.
3. Walsh TJ, Wu AK, Croughan MS, Turek PJ. Differences in the clinical characteristics of primarily and secondarily infertile men with varicocele. Fertil Steril. 2009;91:826–30.
4. Poland ML, Moghissi KS, Giblin PT, Ager JW, Oslon JM. Variation of semen measures within normal men. Fertil Steril. 1985;44:396–400.
5. Baker HW. Medical treatment for idiopathic male infertility: is it curative or palliative? Baillieres Clin Obstet Gynaecol. 1997;11:673–89.
6. Thonneau P, Marchand S, Tallec A, Ferial ML, Ducot B, Lansac J, Spira A. Incidence and main causes of infertility in a resident population (1,850,000) of three French regions (1988–1989). Hum Reprod. 1991;6(6):811–6.

7. Bagatell CJ, Bremmer WJ. Androgens in men—uses and abuses. Drug Ther. 1996;334:707–14.
8. Maravelias C, Dona A, Stefanidou M, Spiliopoulou C. Adverse effects of anabolic steroids in athletes. A constant threat. Toxicol Lett. 2005;158:167–75.
9. Metzl JD, Small E, Levine SR, Gershel JC. Creatine use among young athletes. Pediatrics. 2001;108(2): 421–5.
10. Boyadjiev NP, Georgieva KN, Massaldjieva RI, Gueorguiev SI. Reversible hypogonadism and azoospermia as a result of anabolic-androgenic steroid use in a bodybuilder with personality disorder. A case report. J Sport Med Phys Fitness. 2000;40:271–4.
11. Dohle GR, Smit M, Weber RF. Androgens and male fertility. World J Urol. 2003;21:341–5.
12. Eklof AC, Thurelius AM, Garle M, Rane A, Sjoqvist F. The anti-doping hot-line, a means to capture the abuse of doping agents in the Swedish society and a new service function in clinical pharmacology. Eur J Clin Pharmacol. 2003;59:571–7.
13. Practice Committee of American Society of Reproductive Medicine. Diagnostic evaluation of the infertile male: a committee opinion. Fertil Steril. 2012;98(2):294–301.
14. Wiser HJ, Sandlow J, Köhler TS. Causes of male infertility. Male Infertil. 2012;Part 1: 3–14.
15. Russo EB. History of cannabis and its preparations in saga, science, and sobriquet. Chem Biodivers. 2007;4(8):1614–48.
16. Maykut MO. Health consequences of acute and chronic marijuana use. Prog Neuropsychopharmacol Biol Psychiatry. 1985;9(3):209–38.
17. Di Marzo V. A brief history of cannabinoid and endocannabinoid pharmacology as inspired by the work of British Scientist. Trends Pharmacol Sci. 2006;27(3):134–40.
18. Rossato M, Pagano C, Vettor R. The cannabinoid system and male reproductive function. J Neuro Endocrinol. 2008;20(1):90–3.
19. Turner CE, Elsohly MA, Boeren EG. Constituents of Cannabis sativa L. XVII A review of the natural constituents. J Nat Prod. 1980;43(2):169–234.
20. Fronczak CM, Kim ED, Bargawi AB. The insults of illicit drug use on male fertility. J Androl. 2012; 33(4):515–28.
21. Pacher P, Bátkai S, Kunos G. The endocannabinoid system as an emerging target of pharmacotherapy. Pharmacol Rev. 2006;58(3):389–462.
22. Iversen LL. Pharmacology. Medical uses of marijuana? Nature. 1993;365(6441):12–3.
23. Dalterio S, Bartke A, Burstein S. Cannabinoids inhibit testosterone secretion by mouse testes in vitro. Science. 1977;196(4297):1472–3.
24. Rossato M, Pagano C, Vettor R. The cannabinoid system and male reproductive functions. J Neuroendocrinol. 2008;20 Suppl 1:90–3.
25. Maccarrone M, Wenger T. Effects of cannabinoids on hypothalamic and reproductive function. Handb Exp Pharmacol. 2005;168:555–71.

26. Abood ME. Molecular biology of cannabinoid receptors. Cannabinoids. 2005;168:81–115.
27. Grimaldi P, Orlando P, Di Siena S, et al. The endocannabinoid system and pivotal role of the CB2 receptor in mouse spermatogenesis. Proc Natl Acad Sci U S A. 2009;106(27):11131–6.
28. Wang H, Dey SK, Maccarrone M. Jekyll. Two faces of cannabinoid signaling in male and female fertility. Endocr Rev. 2006;27(5):427–48.
29. Brown TT, Dobs AS. Endocrine effects of marijuana. J Clin Pharmacol. 2002;42(11):90S–6.
30. Braude MC. Marijuana effects on the endocrine and reproductive systems. Discussion and recommendations. NIDA Res Monogr. 1984;44:124–9.
31. Cone EJ, Johnson RE, Moore JD, Roache JD. Acute effects of smoking marijuana on hormones, subjective effects and performance in male human subjects. Pharmacol Biochem Behav. 1986;24(6):1749–54.
32. Kolodny RC, Lassin P, Toro G, Masters WH, Cohen S. Depression of plasma testosterone with acute marijuana administration. In: Braude MC, Szara S, editors. The pharmacology of Marijuana. New York: Raven Press; 1976. p. 217–25.
33. Battista N, Meccariello R, Cobellis G, Fasano S, Di Tommaso M, Pirazzi V, Konje JC, Pierantoni R, Maccarrone M. The role of endocannabinoids in gonadal function and fertility along the evolutionary axis. Mol Cell Endocrinol. 2012;355(1):1–14.
34. Block RI, Farinpour R, Schlechte JA. Effects of chronic marijuana use on testosterone, luteinizing hormone, follicle stimulating hormone, prolactin and cortisol in men and women. Drug Alcohol Depend. 1991;28(2):121–8.
35. Chianese R, Cobellis G, Pierantoni R, Fasano S, Meccariello R. Non mammalian vertebrate models and the endocannabinoid system; relationships with gonadotropin-releasing hormone. Mol Cell Endocrinol. 2007;286:1–22.
36. Maccarrone M. CB2 receptors in reproduction. Br J Pharmacol. 2008;153:189–98.
37. Gye MC, Kang HH, Kang HJ. Expression of cannabinoid receptor 1 in mouse testes. Arch Androl. 2005;51:247–55.
38. Gerard CM, Mollereau C, Vassart G, Parmentier M. Molecular cloning of a human cannabinoid receptor which is also expressed in testes. Biochem J. 1991;279:129–34.
39. Rossato M, Ion Popa F, Ferigo M, Clari G, Foresta C. Human sperm express cannabinoid receptor cb1, the activation of which inhibits motility, acrosome reaction, and mitochondrial function. J Clin Endocrinol Metab. 2005;90(2):984–91.
40. Banerjee A, Singh A, Srivastava P, Turner H, Krishna A. Effects of chronic bhang (cannabis) administration on the reproductive system of male mice. Birth Defects Res B Dev Reprod Toxicol. 2011;92(3):195–205.
41. Kolodny RC, Masters WH, Kolodner RM, Toro G. Depression of plasma testosterone levels after chronic intensive marijuana use. N Engl J Med. 1974;290(16):872–4.

42. Schuel H, Burkman LJ, Lippes J, Crickard K, Mahony MC, Giuffrida A, Picone RP, Makriyannis A. Evidence that anandamide-signaling regulates human sperm functions required for fertilization. Mol Reprod Dev. 2002;63(3):376–87.
43. Fasano S, Meccariello R, Cobellis G, et al. The endocannabinoid system: an ancient signaling involved in the control of male fertility. Ann N Y Acad Sci. 2009;1163:112–24.
44. Lewis SE, Rapino C, Di Tommaso M, et al. Differences in the endocannabinoid system of sperm from fertile and infertile men. PLoS One. 2012; 7(10):e47704.
45. Melzack R. The tragedy of needless pain. Sci Am. 1990;262:27–33.
46. Manchikanti L, Fellows B, Ailinani H, Pampati V. Therapeutic use, abuse, and nonmedical use of opioids: a ten year perspective. Pain Physician. 2010;13(5):401–35.
47. Vuong C, Van Uum SH, O'Dell LE, Lutfy K, Friedman TC. The effects of opioids and opioid analogs on animal and human endocrine systems. Endocr Rev. 2010;31(1):98–132.
48. Agirregoitia E, Valdivia A, Carracedo A, Casis L, Gil J, Subiran N, Ochoa C, Irazusta J. Expression and localization of delta-, kappa-, and mu-opioid receptors in human spermatozoa and implications for sperm motility. J Clin Endocrinol Metab. 2006;91(12):4969–75.
49. Mauras N, Vedhuis JD, Rogol AD. Role of endogenous opiates in pubertal maturation: opposing actions of naltroxone in prepubertal and late pubertal boys. J Clin Endocrinol Metab. 1986;62:1256–63.
50. Petraglia F, Bernasconi S, Lughetti L, Loche S, Romanini F, Facchinetti F, Marcellini C, Genazzani AR. Naloxone-induced luteinizing hormone secretion in normal, precocious and delayed puberty. J Clin Endocrinol Metab. 1986;63:1112–6.
51. Kalra PS, Sahu A, Kalra SP. Opiate-induced hypersensitivity to testosterone feedback: pituitary involvement. Endocrinology. 1988;122(3):997–1003.
52. Mimi Giri JMK. Opiodergic modulation of in vitro pulsatile gonadotropin-releasing hormone release from the isolated medial basal hypothalamus of the male guinea pig. Endocrinology. 1994;135(5): 2137–43.
53. Mirin SM, Meyer RE, Mendelson JH, Ellingboe J. Opiate use and sexual function. Am J Psychiatry. 1980;137(8):909–15.
54. Safarinejad MR, Asgari SA, Farshi A, Ghaedi G, Kolahi AA, Iravani S, Khoshdel AR. The effects of opiate consumption on serum reproductive hormone levels, sperm parameters, seminal plasma antioxidant capacity and sperm DNA integrity. Reprod Toxicol. 2013;36:18–23.
55. Bowe JE, Li XF, Kinsey-Jones JS, Paterson S, Brain SD, Lightman SL, O'Byrne KT. Calcitonin gene-related peptide-induced suppression of luteinizing hormone pulses in the rat: the role of endogenous opioid peptides. J Physiol. 2005;566(Pt 3):921–8.

56. Ciceroa TJ, Davis LA, LaReginac MC, Meyer ER, Schlegel MS. Chronic opiate exposure in the male rat adversely affects fertility. Pharmacol Biochem Behav. 2002;72:157–63.
57. Ragni G, De Lauretis L, Gambaro V, Di Pietro R, Bestetti O, Recalcati F, Papetti C. Semen evaluation in heroin and methadone addicts. Acta Eur Fertil. 1985;16(4):245–9.
58. Subirán N, Candenas L, Pinto FM, Cejudo-Roman A, Agirregoitia E, Irazusta J. Autocrine regulation of human sperm motility by the met-enkephalin opioid peptide. Fertil Steril. 2012;98(3):617–25.
59. Plüddemann A, Myers BJ, Parry CD. Surge in treatment admissions related to methamphetamine use in Cape Town, South Africa: implications for public health. Drug Alcohol Rev. 2008;27(2):185–9.
60. Rogers G, Elston J, Garside R, Roome C, Taylor R, Younger P, Zawada A, Somerville M. The harmful health effects of recreational ecstasy: a systematic review of observational evidence. Health Technol Assess. 2009;13(6):1–338.
61. Methylenedioxymethamphetamine (MDMA, ecstasy). Drugs and Human Performance Fact Sheets. National Highway Traffic Safety Administration. 2014. http://www.nhtsa.gov/people/injury/research/job185drugs/methylenedioxymethamphetamine.htm. Accessed 14 Nov 2013.
62. Csomor M. There's something (potentially dangerous) about molly. CNN Health. 2012. http://www.cnn.com/2012/08/16/health/molly-mdma-drug. Accessed 14 Nov 2013.
63. Graham DL, Herring NR, Schaefer TL, Vorhees CV, Williams MT. Glucose and corticosterone changes in developing and adult rats following exposure to (+/−)-3,4-methylendioxymethamphetamine or 5-methoxydiisopropyltryptamine. Neurotoxicol Teratol. 2010;32(2):152–7.
64. Golub M, Costa L, Crofton K, et al. NTP-CERHR Expert Panel report on the reproductive and developmental toxicity of amphetamine and methamphetamine. Birth Defects Res B Dev Reprod Toxicol. 2005;74(6):471–584.
65. Kobesissy FH, Jeung JA, Warren MW, Geier JE, Gold MS. Changes in leptin, ghrelin, growth hormone and neuropeptide-Y after an acute model of MDMA and methamphetamine exposure in rats. Addict Biol. 2008;13(1):15–25.
66. Yamamoto Y, Yamamoto K, Hayase T. Effect of methamphetamine on male mice fertility. J Obstet Gynaecol Res. 1999;25(5):353–8.
67. Dickerson SM, Walker DM, Reveron ME, Duvauchelle CL, Gore AC. The recreational drug ecstasy disrupts the hypothalamic-pituitary-gonadal reproductive axis in adult male rats. Neuroendocrinology. 2008;88(2):95–102.
68. Nudmamud-Thanoi S, Thanoi S. Methamphetamine induces abnormal sperm morphology, low sperm concentration and apoptosis in the testis of male rats. Andrologia. 2011;43(4):278–82.

69. Yamamoto Y, Yamamoto K, Hayase T, Abiru H, Shiota K, Mori C. Methamphetamine induces apoptosis in seminiferous tubules in male mice testis. Toxicol Appl Pharmacol. 2002;178:155–60.
70. Saito TR, Aoki S, Saito M, et al. Effects of methamphetamine on copulatory behavior in male rats. Jikken Dobutsu. 1991;40(4):447–52.
71. Barenys M, Macia N, Camps L, de Lapuente J, Gomez-Catalan J, Gonzalez-Linares J, Borras M, Rodamilans M, Llobet JM. Chronic exposure to MDMA (ecstasy) increases DNA damage in sperm and alters testes histopathology in male rats. Toxicol Lett. 2009;191(1):40–6.
72. Mangelsdorf I, Buschmann J, Orthen B. Some aspects relating to the evaluation of the effects of chemicals on male fertility. Toxicol Pharmacol. 2003;37:356–69.
73. Mendelson JH, Mello NK. Cocaine and other commonly abused drugs. In: Fauci AS, Braunwald E, Kasper DL, Hauser SL, Longo DL, Jameson JL, Loscalzo J, editors. Harrison's principles of internal medicine, vol. 17. New York: The McGraw-Hill; 2008. p. 2733–6.
74. Leshner AI. Molecular mechanisms of cocaine addiction. N Engl J Med. 1996;335(2):128–9.
75. Casale JF, Klein RFX. Illicit production of cocaine. Forensic Sci Rev. 1993;5:95–107.
76. Gorelick DA. The pharmacology of cocaine, amphetamines, and other stimulants. In: Ries RK, Fiellin DA, Miller SC, Saitz R, editors. Principles of addiction medicine. Philadelphia, PA: Lippincott Williams & Wilkins; 2009. p. 133–58.
77. Mendelson JH, Sholar MB, Mutschler NH, et al. Effects of intravenous cocaine and cigarette smoking on luteinizing hormone, testosterone, and prolactin in men. J Pharmacol Exp Ther. 2003; 307(1):339–48.
78. Gawin FH, Kleber HD. Neuroendocrine findings in a chronic cocaine abusers: a preliminary report. Br J Psychiatry. 1985;147:569–73.
79. Festa ED, Jenab S, Chin J, et al. Frequency of cocaine administration affects behavioral and endocrine responses in male and female Fischer rats. Cell Mol Biol (Noisy-le-Grand). 2003;49(8): 1275–80.
80. Yelian FD, Sacco AG, Ginsburg KA, Doerr PA, Armant DR. The effect of in vitro cocaine exposure on human sperm motility, intracellular calcium and oocyte penetration. Fertil Steril. 1994;61:915–21.
81. Hurd WW, Kelly MS, Ohl DA, Gauvin JM, Smith AJ, Cummins CA. The effect of cocaine on sperm motility characteristics and bovine cervical mucus characteristics. Fertil Steril. 1992;57:178–82.
82. Bracken MB, Eskenazi B, Sachse K, McSharry JE, Hellenbrand K, Leo-Summers L. Association of cocaine use with sperm concentration, motility and morphology. Fertil Steril. 1990;53:315–22.
83. Mesa JL, González-Gross MM, Gutiérrez Sáinz A, Castillo Garzón MJ. Oral creatine supplementation

and skeletal muscle metabolism in physical exercise. Sports Med. 2002;32(14):903–44.

84. Salomons GS, editor. Creatine and creatine kinase in health and disease. 1st ed. New York: Springer; 2007.

85. Brunzel NA. Renal function: nonprotein nitrogen compounds, function tests, and renal disease. In: Scardiglia J, Brown M, McCullough K, Davis K, editors. Clinical chemistry. New York, NY: McGraw-Hill; 2003. p 373–99.

86. Persky AM, Brazeau GA. Clinical pharmacology of the dietary supplement creatine monohydrate. Pharmacol Rev. 2001;53(2):161–76.

87. Walker JB. Creatine: biosynthesis, regulation, and function. Adv Enzymol Relat Areas Mol Biol. 1979;50:177–242.

88. Balsom PD, Soderlund K, Ekblom B. Creatine in humans with special reference to creatine supplementation. Sports Med. 1994;18:268–80.

89. Brosnan JT, Brosnan ME. The metabolic burden of creatine synthesis. Amino Acids. 2011;40(5):1325–31.

90. de Souza GL, Hallak J. Anabolic steroids and male infertility: a comprehensive review. BJU Int. 2011;108(11):1860–5.

91. Kuipers H. Anabolic steroids: side effects. In: Fahey TD, editor. Encyclopedia of sports, medicine and science. Internet Society for Sport Science; 1998. http://www.sportsci.org/encyc/anabstereff/anab-stereff.html. Accessed 14 Nov 2013.

92. Rogol AD, Yesalis CE. Clinical review 31: anabolic-androgenic steroids and athletes: what are the issues? J Clin Endocrinol Metab. 1992;74(3):465–9.

93. Rawson ES. Effects of creatine supplementation and resistance training on muscle strength and weightlifting performance. J Strength Cond Res. 2003;17(4):822–31.

94. Volek JS, Bush JA. Response of testosterone and cortisol concentrations to high-intensity resistance exercise following creatine supplementation. J Strength Cond Res. 1997;11(3):182–7.

95. Schedel JM, Tanaka H, Kiyonaga A, Shindo M, Schutz Y. Acute creatine loading enhances human growth hormone secretion. J Sports Med Phys Fitness. 2000;40(4):336–42.

96. Op't Ejinde B, Hespel P. Short-term creatine supplementation does not alter the hormonal response to resistance training. Med Sci Sports Exerc. 2001; 33(3):449–53.

97. Wu FCW. Endocrine aspects of anabolic steroids. Clin Chem. 1997;43(7):1289–92.

98. Wallimann TH. Creatine kinase in non-muscle tissues and cells. Mol Cell Biochem. 1994;133(134): 193–220.

99. Wallimann T, Moser H, Zurbriggen B, Wegmann G, Eppenberger H. Creatine kinase isoenzymes in spermatozoa. J Muscle Res Cell Motil. 1986;7(1): 25–34.

100. Huszar GC, Vigue L. Correlation between sperm creatine phosphokinase activity and sperm concentrations in normospermic and oligospermic men. Gamete Res. 1988;19(1):67–75.

101. Huszar GVL, Morshedi M. Sperm creatine phosphokinase M-isoform ratios and fertilizing potential of men: a blinded study of 84 couples treated with in vitro fertilization. Fertil Steril. 1992; 57(4):882–8.

102. Huszar GVL, Oehninger S. Creatine kinase immunocytochemistry of human sperm-hemizona complexes: selective binding of sperm with mature creatine kinase-staining pattern. Fertil Steril. 1994;61(1):136–42.

103. Liu PY, Handelsman DJ. The present and future state of hormonal treatment for male infertility. Hum Reprod Update. 2003;9:9–23.

Testicular Heat Stress and Sperm Quality

8

Damayanthi Durairajanayagam, Rakesh K. Sharma, Stefan S. du Plessis, and Ashok Agarwal

Introduction

In the male, exposure to heat has a deleterious effect on fertility and is considered a significant risk factor for male infertility [1]. Testicular temperatures should ideally be hypothermic compared to the core body temperature of 36.9 °C. This is essential for maintaining normal spermatogenesis and ideal sperm characteristics. A crucial feature that contributes towards this is the anatomical position of the human testes, which is located outside the body. Homeothermic animals have the ability to maintain a stable core body temperature despite fluctuating environmental temperatures. This is achieved by regulating heat production and loss by means of adjusting the body's metabolism.

In most homeothermic birds and mammals, including humans, testicular function depends on temperature. Temperatures that either fall below or above the physiological range required for optimal testicular function could potentially disrupt spermatogenesis. Certain land mammals (such as elephants and rhinoceroses) and aquatic mammals (such as whales and dolphins) have intra-abdominal testes throughout their lifespan. The abdomen is metabolically active and it therefore generates a lot of heat. However, spermatogenesis functions optimally in these mammals despite the proximity of their testes to the abdomen.

Humans, on the other hand, have intra-scrotal testes that develop within the abdomen and, towards the end of the gestation period, begins its descent through the inguinal canals into the scrotum. In humans, normal testicular function is temperature dependent and the extra-abdominal testes are maintained at temperatures below that of core body temperature [2]. Under normal healthy environmental conditions, testicular thermoregulation maintains scrotal hypothermy to ensure optimal testicular function [1].

Testicular Thermoregulation

The normal physiological temperature of the human testis ranges between 32 and 35 °C [3]. Thermoregulation in the testis occurs via two mechanisms: the physiological properties of the scrotum and the counter-current mechanism.

The scrotum is a loose sac-like structure that houses each testicle. The main function of the scrotum in most mammals is to prevent heat from reaching at the testis by means of adjusting to heat stress [4]. The scrotum has features that allow free dissipation of heat through passive

D. Durairajanayagam, PhD • R.K. Sharma, PhD
• A. Agarwal, PhD (✉)
Center for Reproductive Medicine, Cleveland Clinic,
Cleveland, OH, USA
e-mail: agarwaa@ccf.org

S.S. du Plessis, BSc (Hons), MSc, MBA, PhD (Stell)
Division of Medical Physiology, Department of
Biomedical Sciences, Faculty of Medicine and Health
Sciences, Stellenbosch University,
Tygerberg, Western Cape, South Africa

S.S. du Plessis et al. (eds.), *Male Infertility: A Complete Guide to Lifestyle and Environmental Factors*,
DOI 10.1007/978-1-4939-1040-3_8, © Springer Science+Business Media New York 2014

convection and radiation. These include a large total skin surface area that changes according to the surrounding temperature, a large number of sweat glands, minimal subcutaneous fat, and sparse hair. When external temperatures rise and cause the scrotal temperature to increase beyond a threshold value, cutaneous receptors on the scrotal skin are activated, initiating secretions of the scrotal sweat glands and active heat loss occurs through the evaporation of sweat [4, 5]. Vasodilation of the scrotal vessels, the very thin scrotal skin and the near-absence of surface hair further contribute to heat dissipation.

The spermatic cord is made up of the testicular artery, veins, cremaster muscle, and vas deferens. The testicular artery is greatly coiled while the veins have thin walls and poor muscularization. The bulk of the spermatic cord is composed of numerous testicular veins that anastomose and drain into the convoluted pampiniform plexus [6]. The testicular arterial and venous blood vessels are intimately associated with each other, facilitating the transfer of heat between the inflowing arterial blood to the outflowing venous blood in the spermatic cord. Thus, the arterial blood arriving at the testis is effectively cooled while the venous blood disperses this heat through the scrotal skin [7]. In a normal individual, this counter-current heat exchange regulates the temperature of the arterial blood supply to the testis and epididymis at 2–4 °C below rectal temperature [7].

Thermoregulation of the testis is further aided by two muscles: the cremasteric and dartos muscles. The cremaster muscle is skeletal-type muscle that is associated with the spermatic cord and testis. A reflex contraction of the cremasteric muscle can be produced by gently stroking the skin on the medial side of the thigh (cremasteric reflex). The dartos muscle is a layer of smooth muscle fibers that surround the testis subcutaneously. When the ambient temperature falls, both the cremaster and the dartos muscles contract involuntarily, raising the testes and bringing them closer to the warmer body. The scrotal skin wrinkles with the contraction of these muscles, reducing the exposed surface area to avoid further heat

loss. Conversely, when ambient temperatures increase, the dartos and cremasteric muscles relax causing the testes to lower away from the body and the scrotal skin to become looser around the testes, aiding heat loss.

Mechanism of Heat Stress: Testicular and Germ Cell Changes

Germ cells have high mitotic activity, which makes them more susceptible to heat stress [8]. The type of germ cells that is most sensitive to heat is the pachytene and diplotene spermatocytes and early round spermatids in both the rat [9, 10] and in humans [11]. In fact, the spermatogenic process, particularly the differentiation and maturation of spermatocytes and spermatids, is temperature dependent and occurs ideally at a temperature of at least 1–2 °C below core body temperature [1, 10]. As such, raising the scrotal temperature causes testicular germinal epithelial atrophy and spermatogenic arrest [12], leading to lower sperm counts. The supportive role of Sertoli [13] and Leydig [14] cells towards germ cell development are also impacted by heat stress. Levels of a biochemical marker of spermatogenesis, inhibin B [15], decrease along with sperm concentration when scrotal temperatures are high [16]. Irreversible testicular weight loss follows shortly after heat exposure [17]. Histopathological changes in the testis following heat exposure include degeneration of the mitochondria, dilatation of the smooth endoplasmic reticulum, and wider intercellular spaces in both Sertoli and spermatid cells [18].

The fundamental mechanism by which loss of germ cells occurs in response to heat stress is due to apoptosis [9, 19]. The intensity of heat stress and duration of heat exposure influence germ cell apoptosis. For example, 2 days after a single exposure to heat (43 °C for 15 min), late pachytene and early spermatids degenerate [20]. However, shorter heat exposure of the rat testes (43 °C for 10 min) does not result in apoptotic germ cells whereas a longer heat exposure (43 °C for 30 min) intensifies germ cell apoptosis [21].

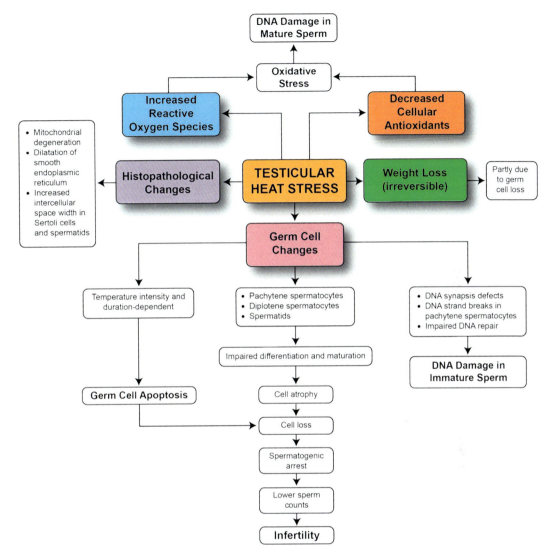

Fig. 8.1 Schematic highlighting various mechanisms by which testicular heat stress causes germ cell apoptosis, DNA damage in mature and immature sperm and male infertility

Similarly, higher heat exposure (45 °C for 15 min) causes generalized, nonspecific damage to many different germ cell types in adult rats.

Besides apoptosis, heat stress also causes defects in DNA synapsis and DNA strand breaks in pachytene spermatocytes and induces DNA damage in mature spermatozoa [20]. Sperm DNA damage that occurs in the heat-stressed testis is likely due to excessive generation of reactive oxygen species (which causes the sperm cell to be in a state of oxidative stress) as well impaired DNA repair in the germ cells [20, 22]. In experimentally cryptorchid rats, heat stress (due to increased scrotal temperatures) increases generation of reactive oxygen species leading to oxidative stress [23, 24]. Moreover, in adult rats, the effects of scrotal hyperthermia (43 °C for 30 min once daily for 6 consecutive days) include decreased levels of glutathione, superoxide dismutase, and glutathione peroxidase and increased lipid peroxidation in the testes [18]. Further, gene expression for DNA repair and cellular antioxidants are suppressed during testicular heat stress [25] (Fig. 8.1).

In summary, heat-induced changes due to increased scrotal temperatures in the testes lead to apoptosis of germ cells and sperm DNA damage, which subsequently suppresses spermatogenesis [18, 20].

Impact of Failed Thermoregulation on Semen Parameters

Semen analysis is carried out as a routine laboratory assessment of the infertile male. Fundamental sperm parameters evaluated during a standard semen analysis include sperm concentration, motility, and morphology [26]. The total count and concentration of sperm reflect semen quality and the male reproductive potential whereas sperm concentration and motility are best able to predict fertility [27]. Repeated testicular exposure to elevated levels of heat could lead to chronic thermo-dysregulation, which in time could lead to significant changes in sperm characteristics [1, 28].

Mean scrotal temperature is higher in infertile men than in fertile ones [29], and the higher the scrotal temperature, the more sperm quality is altered [29]. Men (mean age 31.8 years) who were infertile for at least 2 years (without female factor infertility) were found to have lower sperm count, percentage of motile sperm and testicular volume in both testes and higher mean scrotal temperatures compared to fertile men [29]. However, testicular hyperthermia causes modification of sperm characteristics in both the fertile and infertile male [29]. Physiological increases in scrotal temperature are associated with substantially reduced sperm concentration that results in poor semen quality [30]. An increase of 1 °C above baseline values suppresses spermatogenesis by 14 %, decreasing sperm production [31].

Elevated testicular and epididymal temperatures decrease the synthesis of sperm membrane coating protein, resulting in higher amounts of morphologically abnormal sperm [31]. Within 6–8 months of exposure to elevated temperatures, the mean value of sperm with abnormal morphology was found to double [31]. Sperm motility is also suppressed in the hyperthermic testis [32]. Exposure to high temperature causes deterioration in sperm morphology and impairs motility as well as sperm production, all of which have a deleterious effect on male fertility [33, 34].

Pathological Failure of Thermoregulation

Increased testicular temperatures due to either endogenous or exogenous stimuli decrease sperm concentration, motility, and the number of morphologically normal sperm [11, 35]. Pathophysiological abnormalities such as varicocele and cryptorchidism cause testicular hyperthermia, which could lead to male infertility [36]. Thus, any disruption (either acute or chronic) to the thermoregulation of the testis would have severe adverse effects on the spermatogenic process.

Febrile Episodes

When the hypothalamic thermoregulation of the core body temperature is compromised with the onset of fever, thermoregulation at the level of the testes is also impacted. In a case study of a fertile patient with influenza who was febrile (39.9 °C) for 1 day, semen samples analyzed 18–66 days post fever showed underlying effects on sperm chromatin structure and a temporary release of abnormal sperm [37]. In another study, the incidence of fever was reported to have a significant effect on spermatogenesis, and the more days of fever (between 1 and 11 days); the more increasingly adverse were its effects on sperm concentration, percentage of normal and immotile sperm [11]. Certain stages of spermatogenesis were found to be more predisposed to the effects of higher temperatures caused by a fever than others: sperm concentration was affected when fever occurred during meiosis (33–56 days before ejaculation) and spermiogenesis (post-meiotic phase, 9–32 days before ejaculation) while sperm morphology and motility were affected when fever occurred during spermiogenesis [11].

Varicocele

Varicocele is the most common and treatable cause of male infertility and it affects 15 % of the male population. It is implicated in 40 % of men with primary infertility and in 80 % of men with secondary infertility [38, 39]. A varicocele is the abnormal tortuosity and dilatation of the testicular veins in the pampiniform plexus causing retrograde blood flow in the internal spermatic veins and venous stasis. Consequently, the cooling of the testicular arterial blood via the counter current heat exchange becomes ineffective and testicular temperature increases towards that of the core body [40]. Increased scrotal temperature found in infertile men is most commonly caused by varicocele [29, 41]. Both Mieusset et al. [29] and Goldstein and Eid [42] reported that infertile men with varicocele have higher mean scrotal temperatures on (1) the affected testis compared to the unaffected side and (2) both testes compared to that in fertile men. Intra-testicular temperatures in the affected testis were 2.43–2.72 °C higher than that of a normal testis [42]. The underlying mechanism of varicocele-related infertility is not clear but is attributable to factors such as increased scrotal temperature, oxidative stress, and hormonal imbalance [43]. Varicocele patients have increased apoptosis (programmed cell death) [44], and the increase in scrotal temperature (but not varicocele grade) is associated with oxidative stress-induced apoptosis [43]. Chan et al. [45] found that heat shock proteins 70 and 90 were significantly upregulated in varicocele patients. Heat shock proteins are produced in response to various stress inducers including heat, and their increased expression suggest that they play a role in the mechanism of varicocele-related infertility [45].

Cryptorchidism

Cryptorchidism is among the most common congenital defects in newborns and occurs in 2–4 % of full-term male births [46]. About 50 % of these cases resolve spontaneously within the first year of birth and those that do not resolve naturally require surgical intervention. Failure of the testis to descend leads to infertility and increased risk of testicular cancer. The severity of infertility in human cryptorchidism depends on the position of the testis, whether one or both of the testis is maldescended, how soon it is surgically corrected and perhaps the underlying pathology [47]. In its supra-scrotal position, the testis is hyperthermic. This causes heat-induced loss of spermatogonial differentiation and apoptosis of all germ cells (including germ stem cells) as well as an indirect effect of increased oxidative stress and abnormal energy metabolism [23, 48, 49]. In addition, the changes in Sertoli cell junctions and abnormal levels of Leydig cell hormones noted in the cryptorchid testis are linked to hyperthermia [50, 51]. Furthermore, despite sperm appearing to be morphologically normal [52], heat stress produced in conditions of cryptorchidism and varicocele induces sperm DNA fragmentation [52, 53].

Assessing Testicular Temperature

Testicular and intra-scrotal temperatures can be measured either directly or indirectly and in the form of either a single or continuous measurement (Table 8.1). Intra-scrotal skin surface temperatures reflect the temperature of the underlying testis as the testis and epididymis constitute the largest thermal mass in the hemiscrotum [36, 54]. Testicular temperature may range between 31 and 36 °C depending on the method used for the measurement of temperature and the presence of any underlying pathology [55]. Accuracy and reproducibility of the temperature are important as temperature differences in a normal (euthermic) and pathologic (hyperthermic) testis may be as small as 0.6–1.4 °C [36]. Even these small increases can hamper spermatogenesis and epididymal maturation [36].

Single or Discontinuous Measurements

In this method evolved by Zorgniotti and MacLeod [36], the subject disrobes from the waist below and lays supine for about 6 min (to equilibrate to an ambient room temperature of about 21–23 °C) [32, 36]. A mercury thermometer is pre-warmed by placing the bulb of the thermometer in contact with

Table 8.1 Methods of measuring scrotal (testicular) temperature in humans

Method	Description	Advantage	Disadvantage	Reference(s)
Single measurement or discontinuous method				
Mercury thermometer	1. Pre-warmed bulb positioned directly over the most prominent part of the anterior testis	1. Simple and inexpensive	1. Clinical thermometer unsuitable as its mercury column is constricted	[32, 36, 54, 55]
	2. Thermometer bulb held longitudinally against the scrotum	2. Provides accurate measurements	2. Applicable only when subject is unclothed	
	3. Loose scrotal skin drawn around the thermometer bulb using the thumb and index finger	3. Gives repeatable and standardized values	3. Reproducible only under static conditions (e.g., lying down for several minutes)	
Skin surface thermocouples	1. Attached to the scrotal skin overlying the anterior testis using an adhesive	1. Small dimensions	1. May be displaced from the site of contact with the testis beneath	[55, 65]
	2. Electrode cables secured at trouser waistband	2. Light weigh	2. Minor movements of the scrotum could alter the readings	
		3. Assessment done in a clothed state		
Thermal resistor (thermistor) needles	1. Placed within the scrotum or testis	1. Direct measurement	1. Invasive procedure	[4, 54, 55, 108]
			2. Depth of thermistor placement could contribute to differences in reading (temperature in the peripheral testis is lower than the mediastinum testis)	
			3. Use of anesthesia and evaporation of the antiseptic solution applied during scrotal skin preparation would alter the temperature	
			4. Extremes of ambient temperature, scrotal skin inflammation, and intrascrotal disease would affect the temperature	

Infrared thermometry	1. Measures heat emitted from the scrotal skin	1. Easy way to measure temperature in different body positions	1. For better accuracy, these thermometers needs to be calibrated using a black body prior to use	[55, 109, 110]
	2. A pistol-type, non-contact, digital infrared thermometer with an accuracy of ±0.1 °C was preferred	2. Permits repeated measurement on the same area	2. Variations in skin's thermal radiation or emissivity could affect readings	
	3. Replicate readings taken at the skin over the most prominent part of the testis		3. Only the surface temperature is measured and not deep scrotal temperature	
			4. Lacks sensitivity to record small differences in temperature	
Thermography	1. Measured heat emitted from the scrotal skin		1. Does not provide the required accuracy for research as the comparison with the grey scale can introduce inaccuracies	[55]
			2. Provides relative differences but not absolute numbers	
			3. Unable to obtain a preferred sensitivity of ±0.1 °C	
Liquid crystal thermometry	1. Measured using temperature-sensitive crystals		1. Unable to obtain a preferred sensitivity of ±0.1 °C	[55, 109]
Continuous measurement method				
Thermoport thermocouples or thermoprobes	1. Attached to skin on the anterior face of the each scrotum using transparent tape	1. Allows for a dynamic recording of temperature		[56–58]
	2. Connected to a portable data recorder attached to a belt	2. Representative of testicular temperature during normal daily activities		
Thermistor	1. Thermistor attached to underwear			[54, 55]
	2. Connected to a light-weight data logger			

a light source or immersing it in warm water, allowing the mercury column in the thermometer to expand to a temperature that is slightly higher than the estimated temperature of the testis (i.e., around 37 °C). The thermometer is then quickly positioned directly over the most prominent part of the anterior testis and the bulb is held longitudinally against the scrotum. The loose scrotal skin is drawn around the thermometer bulb using the thumb and index finger (to include the immersion mark, if present). The mercury column will begin to drop until it reaches equilibrium (usually about 8 s). The reading at that point plus 0.1 °C represents the intra-scrotal temperature [36]. The process is then repeated in the contralateral testis. This method was modified from the "invagination method" by Brindley [32] and allows for repeatable and consistent values to be obtained for use in a clinical evaluation of, for example, a varicocele [56].

Continuous Measurements

During continuous measurement, two cutaneous thermocouples (thermoprobes) are attached to the skin on the anterior face of the each scrotum using transparent tape, and these are connected to a small portable data recorder attached to a belt. Temperatures are recorded at 2-min intervals. Measurements recorded in the data recorder are downloaded to a computer through a specific program [57]. The use of a portable data recorder for continuous determination of scrotal temperature allows for a dynamic recording of temperature [58]. However, scrotal skin temperatures have also been measured noninvasively for an entire day using a thermistor attached to underwear that is connected to a light-weight data logger [56].

Risk Factors for Scrotal Hyperthermia

The temperature difference between the body and scrotum can be affected by a variety of external thermogenic factors including body posture or position, clothing, obesity, lifestyle and occupational exposure, and ambient seasonal temperature changes (Fig. 8.2).

Posture

Changes in posture affect testicular temperature. Scrotal temperature is lowest when standing disrobed [36, 59]. Heat dissipation can occur unhindered from the unsupported testis when the body is unclothed and in an upright position. When comparing body positions, scrotal temperature in the supine or seated position is higher than that in the standing position [32, 36, 58, 59]. When walking (upright and moving), scrotal temperatures are 0.3–1 °C lower than those generated when sitting regardless of clothing type [32, 59]. Scrotal temperatures are highest during sleep when the body is supine and movement is minimized [32, 58, 60] compared to other body positions. When comparing sleepwear, scrotal temperatures were the lowest when sleeping in the nude compared to sleeping in pyjamas or underwear [32]. When in a supine position, the testes are resting on the thighs and are in direct contact (conduction) with the relatively higher body temperature. Additional layers of clothing trap air and conserve heat. Using an electric blanket or quilt on top of typical nightclothes while lying down in bed after a hot bath will give a cumulative effect that is likely to lead to genital heat stress. When assessing diurnal variation, Hjollund et al. [56] found that scrotal temperatures, when measured at a 5-min interval for a continuous 24 h, were higher at night by 1.2 °C compared to those during the day.

Sitting

The length of time spent in a seated position, either due to occupational nature, long commutes and sedentary leisure activities, also contributes to testicular heat stress. A predominantly sedentary (sitting) position at work has been shown to increase scrotal temperatures [30, 56, 57]. When sitting, the testes are trapped between the thighs. Moreover, the normal seated position leads to poor ventilation in the groin area, which contributes to an increase in scrotal temperature. The positioning of the legs while sitting (i.e., legs together, apart or crossed) impacts the scrotal temperature in both the disrobed [59] and clothed state [32, 57].

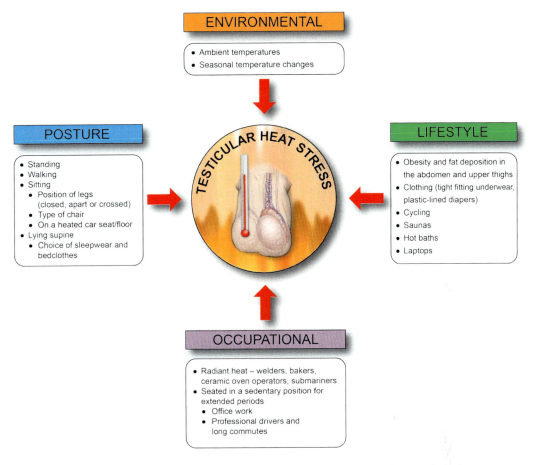

Fig. 8.2 Various lifestyle, occupational, postural, and environmental factors contributing to testicular heat stress

Paraplegic men in wheelchairs who remain seated for extended periods with closed and unmoving legs were found to have higher deep scrotal temperature and poor sperm motility than normal men who were seated freely for 20 min or more (without the position of their thighs being specified, i.e., kept close together or apart) [32]. However, when compared in a supine position, there was no significant difference in scrotal temperatures between the paraplegic and normal men [32].

The insulating effect of the seated posture is compounded by being sedentary but counteracted by physical activity. The average scrotal temperature in healthy volunteers while sitting on a conventional chair for a period longer than 35 min is 36.4 °C compared to 34.5 °C during walking [61]. Increased limb movement during physical activity increases perigenital air circulation, and this allows for better dissipation of heat, which then results in lower scrotal temperatures, compared to when being seated in a sedentary manner.

In a study comparing the increase in scrotal temperatures while seated on different types of chairs, Koskelo et al. [62] reported a 3 °C increase in scrotal temperature upon 20 min of sitting on a conventional cushioned office chair. However, they found no difference in temperature when subjects sat in a saddle chair. This is probably due to the open hip and knee angles, which allow for adequate scrotal ventilation [62]. Similarly, sitting with crossed legs causes a bigger increase in scrotal temperature than sitting with the legs apart (at an angle of about 70°) [63]. After remaining in a seated position with crossed legs for 15 min, the thermogenic effect caused by this position further persisted for a minimum of 5 min, even after standing up [63].

When sitting on surfaces with a higher temperature, the increase in scrotal temperature attributed to the seated posture is further compounded by the warmth exuding from the seated surface. In a Korean study, Song and Seo [64] investigated the effects of sitting directly on a heated floor on scrotal temperature among 6 healthy male volunteers in a controlled environmental chamber. They concluded that the floor surface temperature and the rate of metabolism while in a sedentary posture affect scrotal temperature and recommended that surface temperature of a heated floor be maintained within 23–33 °C to avoid impairment of spermatogenesis [64].

Clothing

Irrespective of the body position, wearing clothing has an insulating effect that increases scrotal temperature. In the standing and supine positions, clothing increases scrotal temperatures by 1.5–2 °C compared to the naked state [63, 65]. In men at rest who are lightly clothed, the layer of air trapped in the space between the skin and clothes is on average 3.5 °C higher than that of ambient air (at a temperature of between 21 and 32 °C) [66]. The reduction in air exchange when in a clothed state contributes to the increase in scrotal skin temperature [63]. Clothing that permits better air flow would mean that scrotal heat could be more easily dissipated, keeping temperatures closer to physiological levels. Kompanje [27] suggested that Scottish kilt-wearing possibly produced a more ideal physiological scrotal environment, especially since nearly 70 % of men chose to not wear anything underneath their kilt. In the Asian region, men often wear only a sarong when at leisure, which similarly helps in dispersing body and environmental heat to keep lower testicular temperatures.

Tight Underwear, Boxers, Jockey Shorts
It is still debated whether the type of underwear has a significant impact on testicular temperature and hence, male fertility. Studies have reported that the regular use of tight underwear over a period of time leads to a reduction in sperm motility [67, 68]. Another study found that men who wear tight underwear have decreased sperm count and sperm motility compared to those who wear loose underwear [69]. Conversely, in a study involving 97 men presenting for primary infertility (aged between 25 and 52 years), scrotal temperatures did not differ between men who wore boxer shorts and those who wore brief style underwear [12]. The authors further reasoned that brief style underwear gives a supportive effect that pushes the testes closer to the body while the boxer shorts lacks this effect. However, any additional layer of clothing that is worn over the underwear (e.g., trousers) would result in the same supportive effect on the testes [12].

Diapers
The use of disposable plastic-lined diapers is more common these days than cotton, reusable diapers. Even cotton diapers are usually used in combination with a plastic lining as a protective covering to prevent leakages. The use of plastic material reduces the skin's breathability, which would lead to a warm and moist perigenital area, thereby contributing to higher scrotal temperature. Partsch et al. [70] studied 14 neonates (term aged 0–4 weeks) and pre-term with a gestational age of 28–36 weeks (postnatal age 14–85 days), 22 infants (aged 1–12 months), and 12 toddlers (age 13–55 months) and reported that young boys wearing disposable plastic-lined nappies have increased scrotal temperatures compared to those wearing reusable cotton diapers (without protective pants). However, in another study, Grove et al. [71] found no differences in the scrotal temperature profiles of approximately 70 young boys (aged 3–25 months) wearing disposable diapers with a plastic lining compared to those wearing reusable cotton diapers covered with plastic pants. Only when the cotton diapers were used without any plastic covering were scrotal temperatures lower than those in the boys using disposable diapers [70, 71]. That being said, as cotton diapers are almost always used along with the plastic pants, it would seem that practically speaking, both the classic and modern diaper choices did not differ significantly on their effect on scrotal temperature. As to whether

diapering preferences (and the higher scrotal temperatures is generates) at a young age could contribute towards a compromised male fertility potential as an adult, Jung and Schuppe [72] reasoned that pachytene spermatocytes and round spermatids (the most temperature-sensitive testicular cells) [10] are not yet present in the age group when most children use diapers. The authors concluded that there was no convincing evidence linking genital heat stress with poor semen quality in their adulthood [72].

Lifestyle

Obesity

Obesity is a common lifestyle-related societal problem of the modern era. Many adults who are in the reproductive age group have a higher than normal body mass index (BMI, normal range: 18.0–24.9). In fact, the rate of obesity is higher in infertile men than in men with normal semen parameters [73]. A BMI ≥ 25 is associated with an average 25 % reduction in sperm count and motility [74]. Obesity is often associated with decreased physical activity and prolonged periods of sitting or being sedentary, which have been found to increase testicular temperatures and consequently suppress sperm production [75]. Obese males are more likely to have increased fat deposition in the abdomen and upper thighs and larger waist and hip circumferences. Additionally, scrotal lipomatosis (deposition of fat around the spermatic cord) in obese men could inhibit spermatogenesis by several means, i.e., (1) provide insulation that could disrupt the radiation of testicular heat, (2) compress blood vessels, leading to testicular congestion (venous stasis) and impaired heat exchange, (3) compress the testicular artery leading to ischemia of the testis, (4) hamper the cord's ability to reposition the testes in response to temperature changes, and (5) disrupt local thermoregulation due to excess fat in the suprapubic region [76, 77]. The compromised efficiency of testicular thermoregulation may well lead to elevated testicular temperatures. However, scrotal lipomatosis could also occur in those who are not obese [76]. In one study,

removal of excess fat in the scrotal and suprapubic region helped improve sperm count, motility, and morphology in nearly 65 % of infertile patients, and nearly 20 % of these patients went on to initiate a pregnancy [77].

Sauna

Saunas are a popular method of relaxation and detoxification or cleansing in many parts of the world. Temperatures in saunas typically range between 80 and 100 °C at the level of the bather's head, with humidity ranging from 40 to 60 g of water/kg dry air [78]. Conventional saunas provide wet heat through warmed, humid air (radiation and convection) as well as warmed surfaces (radiation and conduction), while modern saunas such as infrared saunas provide dry, radiant heat.

Brown-Woodman et al. [79] examined the effect of a single sauna exposure (85 °C for 20 min) on sperm parameters at 10 weeks postexposure compared to 3 weeks preexposure. They found that this one acute testicular heat stress episode was sufficient to cause the sperm count to reduce within a week post-exposure, only to normalize in the fifth-week post-exposure [79]. In a study that continuously (i.e., every 5 s) monitored scrotal temperature during a sauna exposure (87.6 ± 1.3 °C and <15 % humidity), scrotal temperatures were found to reach core body temperature within about 10 min of exposure to the exogenous heat [58]. Saikhun's group assessed the effects of sauna exposure on sperm parameters after a 2-week sauna exposure (at 80–90 °C for 30 min) [35]. They found that sperm movement characteristics had declined but were restored within a week after concluding the sauna exposure. They reported that sperm parameters such as semen volume, sperm count, number of motile and morphologically normal sperm as well as sperm penetration levels had remained unchanged [35]. More recently, Garolla et al. [80] investigated the effects of biweekly Finnish (dry) sauna sessions (89–90 °C for 15 min) for 3 months on ten normozoospermic men. They found that these frequent sauna exposures (that lasted long enough to cover an entire spermatogenic cycle) caused a significant reduction in sperm count and progressive motility (although they were still within normal range) and altered mitochondrial function, DNA protamination, and chromatin condensation in the sperm [80]. However, sperm morphology and viability remained unaffected while heat shock proteins (and their regulating heat shock factors) that confer a protective effect were found to be upregulated after testicular heating [80]. These studies collectively showed that following sauna exposure, the negative impact on spermatogenesis was significant but reversible.

Hot Baths

Other lifestyle habits such as indulging in a relaxing soak in a hot tub, heated whirlpool, or a warm bath could negatively impact male fertility. Shefi et al. [81] studied the effects of wet heat exposure in a group of 11 infertile men (mean age 36.5 years) who practiced whole body immersion in either a hot tub, heated jacuzzi, or warm bath (at temperatures that were higher than that of body temperature) for more than 30 min weekly (mean weekly exposure was 149 min) for longer than 3 months. Comparison of semen parameters in samples analyzed before vs. 3 months after the discontinuation of the wet hyperthermia, showed improvements, mainly in sperm motility [81]. They concluded that in certain infertile men, refraining from these types of heat exposure could perhaps reverse the detrimental effects of hyperthermia on their semen quality.

Cycling

A regular, moderate exercise regimen bestows numerous health benefits. However, certain forms of exercise done in the pursuit of fitness, cycling, for example, may negatively affect male fertility. Scrotal temperatures during cycling may be influenced by the duration and intensity of the exercise as well as posture [82] and clothing. As a physical activity, cycling improves perigenital air circulation, which aids in the dissipation of testicular heat [82]. At the same time, cycling involves extended periods of being in a seated posture on a saddle seat for the majority of the exercise and wearing a body-fitting spandex outfit, which would contribute an insulating effect on scrotal temperatures, especially in professional cyclists [83]. However, in their study, Jung et al. [82] found that 25 healthy volunteers (median BMI of 23.2) who wore cotton wool clothing while performing moderate cycling (median speed of 25.5 km/h, power around 25 W) sitting on the saddle of a stationary cycle for 60 min had mean scrotal temperatures below 35.6 °C. Increases in scrotal temperatures did not differ significantly between the left and right scrotum and with time [82].

Laptop Usage

Sheynkin et al. [84] demonstrated among 29 healthy volunteers that using a laptop in a lap position close to the genital area (i.e., a seated position with approximated thighs) for an hour contributes to a 0.6–0.8 °C increase in scrotal temperatures compared to a 2.1 °C increase in scrotal temperatures in the same sitting position without using a working laptop. This increase in genital heat could be attributed to heat exposure from laptops that have internal operating temperatures of more than 70 °C and to the seated posture for those 60 min. Although this study did not examine changes in semen parameters, the authors suggested that since scrotal heat impairs spermatogenesis, then laptop usage also likely affects these parameters [84].

Occupation

Welders: Radiant Heat

Welders are occupationally exposed to intense radiant heat, toxic metals and their oxides, and toxic welding fumes during welding. Bonde [85] reported that 17 manual metal arc alloyed steel welders (mean age 35.9 years) with moderate exposure to radiant heat (31.1–44.8 °C) and with minimal exposure to welding fume toxicants experienced a reversible decrease in semen quality. The percentage of sperm with normal morphology decreased within 6 weeks of exposure to radiant heat but increased 4 weeks after cessation of exposure [85]. In another study, 17 welders (mean age 43.8 years) with 1–10 years or more of welding exposure possibly had some adverse effects on sperm motility, morphology and physiologic function, although they maintained a normal range of sperm concentration [86].

Bakers: Radiant Heat

Bakers are reported to take longer to initiate a pregnancy than controls, as only 14 % of bakers' partners were pregnant within 3 months (compared to 55 % of controls) and 29 % of bakers' partners were pregnant within 6 months (compared to 74 % of controls) [87]. This suggests that the bakers' occupational exposure to heat may be a contributory factor to subfertility.

Ceramic Oven Operators: Radiant Heat

Figà-Talamanca et al. [88] reported that healthy ceramics oven operators with chronic occupational exposure to high temperatures (37 °C, 8 h/day) had a higher incidence of abnormal sperm parameters compared to controls. These individuals faced difficulty in establishing a pregnancy and had a higher occurrence of not being able to father a child compared to controls [88].

Professional Drivers

Long hours of driving and remaining in a seated position have shown to have detrimental effects on male reproductive function. The negative effect of extended periods of driving on sperm parameters is attributed to an increase in scrotal temperature [57].

Sas and Szollosi [89] investigated the effects of prolonged driving on spermiogenesis in 2,984 patients, of whom 281 were occupational drivers. They found that the incidence of abnormal sperm was higher among the patients who drove professionally and more severe in those with longer occupational driving experience. Similarly, workers involved in the transport occupational group had lower sperm concentrations [90] and a higher risk of abnormal sperm motility [91] compared to other occupational groups. Figà-Talamanca et al. [92] reported that compared to control subjects, taxi drivers in the city of Rome had a higher amount of sperm with abnormal morphology and that this was more apparent in the longer-serving drivers. However, sperm concentration and motility in these drivers ($n = 72$) were comparable to that of the 50 healthy control subjects, who were of similar age and had similar smoking habits. This study also suggested that prolonged driving time could compromise sperm morphology and thereby sperm quality [92]. In a study of 402 fertile couples in France, Thonneau et al. [93] found that compared to other couples, the time to pregnancy was significantly prolonged for those couples in which the male partner remained seated driving in a vehicle for longer than 3 h daily.

In addition to the effect of prolonged sitting on a car seat (which in itself causes about a 2 °C increase in scrotal temperature) [57], the use of a heated car seat for longer than 60 min was shown to cause an increase in scrotal temperature of 0.5–0.6 °C, nearing core body temperature [94]. This additional factor would likely add towards the decline in sperm quality.

Submariners

Velez de la Calle [95] and co-workers looked into the infertility risk factors in a military population from a large military naval base in Brest, France. They found that male mechanics, cooks, and submariners who were occupationally exposed to very hot working conditions while in the submarine (temperatures in the rear end of the submarine close to the motor range between 40 and 60 °C) had sought help for infertility issues.

Ambient Temperature and Seasonality

A 1 °C increase in ambient temperature induces a 0.1 °C increase in scrotal temperature [32]. In a study of semen samples taken from more than 1,000 fertile men from four European cities (Copenhagen, Denmark; Paris, France; Edinburgh, Scotland; and Turku; Finland), Jorgenson's group found a general seasonal variation in sperm concentration (summer values were 70 % of winter values) and total sperm count (summer values were 72 % of winter values), but not for sperm motility or morphology [96]. The difference of approximately 30 % in sperm count from winter (highest) to summer (lowest) could be attributed to differences in lifestyle or environmental exposures among the men [96]. Similarly, in a preliminary study of 4,435 pre-vasectomy patients, Tjoa et al. [97] reported a circannual rhythm (biological rhythmicity approximating 1 year) in human sperm concentration and total sperm count, with a higher sperm count in winter compared to summer. Gyllenborg et al. [98] found that sperm counts among a group of unselected Danish semen donor candidates were lowest in the summer although semen volume and sperm motility remained unchanged. However, Mallidis et al. [99] did not find any effect of season in semen samples provided by normal healthy Australian men.

Mild Scrotal Heating as a Method of Contraception

Scrotal temperatures that are maintained lower than that of the core body temperature would help improve spermatogenesis and the fertility potential of men facing infertility issues. However, fertile men may find that higher scrotal temperatures could work in their favor. Commonly used methods of male contraception include hormonal approach, the use of condoms and vasectomy [100]. However, local application of heat could provide the means for a non-hormonal, noninvasive, reversible method of contraception targeting the testicular level [100]. In a preliminary study, Mieusset and Bujan [101] induced mild testicular heating (assumed as 1–2 °C) by immobilizing the testis close to the inguinal canal daily during waking hours in 9 men aged between 23 and 34 years. These methods did not affect the men's libido or sexual rhythm, and no pregnancies were reported during the study period [101]. Sperm count and motility normalized within 1–1.5 years in all the subjects involved in this study [101]. In another clinical study, Wang et al. [102] reported that hot water baths taken in combination with testosterone suppressed sperm count and motility. Thus, it would seem that mild scrotal heating could potentially serve as an alternate contraceptive method. However, the endocrine parameters involved in regulating spermatogenesis such as the hypothalamic and pituitary hormones may well be affected by the intentional increase in scrotal temperature.

Scrotal Cooling

Several studies have showed that scrotal cooling can improve sperm count, motility, and morphology [103]. Devices that have been used for testicular cooling include a curved rubber collar filled with ice cubes that was taped to both the thighs for 30 min daily for 14 consecutive days [104] and a gel ice pack that solidified upon freezing, which was wrapped in a cloth or towel and inserted in the underwear on the anterior aspect of the scrotum nightly for 2 months—the cooling effect occurred upon the thawing of the ice pack within 3–4 h [105]. Other techniques included a cotton suspensory bandage placed in close contact with the scrotum (worn for 16–22 h from 8 to 20 weeks) that released fluid (water or alcohol) to maintain a damp scrotum [106] and a device attached with a belt to the abdomen and scrotum that released a continuous air stream to achieve scrotal cooling nightly for 12 weeks [107]. In a study to assess the feasibility of a clinical trial, Osman and his group evaluated the use of a nongreasy hydrogel pad, the Babystart® FertilMate™ Scrotum Cooling Patch, in patients with mild, moderate, and severe oligoasthenospermia [103]. The pad contained 0.5 % w/w natural I-menthol and was reported to be more practical and comfortable to use than other cooling devices [103]. When the testes were cooled, spermatogenesis improved and pregnancy occurred leading to the suggestion that hyperthermia played a role in causing or aggravating male infertility [29]. The factors affecting scrotal (testicular) temperatures and their effect on sperm parameters and male infertility are summarized in Table 8.2.

Conclusion

Scrotal hyperthermia is a substantial risk factor for male infertility. Repetitive transient scrotal hyperthermia in the current modern lifestyle is likely to have a negative impact upon spermatogenesis, specifically in men who are of reproductive age and desire to have children. The normal healthy male is equipped with local

Table 8.2 Factors affecting scrotal (testicular) temperatures and their effect on sperm parameters and male fertility

Exogenous factors contributing to heat stress	Effects on scrotal/ testicular temperature	Reference(s)	Impact on sperm parameters and male fertility	Reference(s)
Posture (physical inactivity)				
1. Standing	Lower (vs. sitting or supine)	[32, 36, 58, 59]	No data	–
2. Sitting (regardless of position of legs, i.e., crossed, close together or apart)	Increased (vs. standing or supine)	[32, 36, 57–59]	Reduced motility (legs close together)	[32]
3. Sitting (legs apart)	Lower (when legs apart vs. when legs close together or crossed)	[57, 63]	No data	–
4. Sitting (on different chair types—cushioned and non-cushioned, plywood and wooden, knee-support, saddle chair)	Increased (in conventional office chair—legs narrowly apart) vs. saddle chair—legs wide apart	[62]	No data	–
5. Sitting (on heated floor, car seat)	Increased (vs. conventional floor or car seat)	[64, 94]	No data	–
6. Supine (and during night sleep)	Increased close to core body temperature (vs. standing or sitting)	[16, 30, 32, 56, 58, 60, 61, 107]	No effect on semen parameter	[16]
	Lower (when naked vs. clothed or wearing underwear)			
7. Sitting (sedentary position at work)	Increased (vs. standing or supine)	[30, 56, 57]	Not a risk factor for abnormal semen quality	[30]
	Strong correlation between scrotal temperatures and duration of sedentary work			
Posture (physical activity)				
8. Moderate walking	Lower (vs. sitting)	[16, 30, 32, 56–61, 107]	No data	–
Clothing				
1. Clothed state	Increased (vs. naked or unclothed state)	[32, 57, 63–66]	No data	–
2. Underwear (form-fitting)	Increased (vs. loose-fitting)	[32, 59, 68, 111]	No data	–
	No difference (vs. loose-fitting)	[12, 65]	No data	–

(continued)

Table 8.2 (continued)

Exogenous factors contributing to heat stress	Effects on scrotal/testicular temperature	Reference(s)	Impact on sperm parameters and male fertility	Reference(s)
3. Diapers (disposable)	No difference (vs. reusable cloth diapers with plastic covering)	[71]	No data	–
	Higher (vs. reusable cloth diapers without plastic covering)	[70, 71]	No data	–
Lifestyle				
1. Obesity	Increased	[76, 77]	Suppressed sperm production	[75]
2. Sauna	Increased to core body temperature	[58]	Reduced sperm count within a week	[79]
	Increased to core body temperature	[35]	No change in semen volume, sperm count, morphology. Reduced motility, reversible once exposure is discontinued	[35]
	Increased to core body temperature	[80]	Reduced sperm count (less efficient spermatogenesis but reversible) and lower (but reversible) progressive motility. No change in sperm morphology and viability. Altered DNA protamination and nuclear condensation. Increased expression of genes associated with hypoxia and heat stress (up-regulation of heat shock proteins and their regulating heat shock factors)	[80]
3. Hot baths	Increased	[68, 81]	Reduced sperm motility	[81]
4. Exercise—moderate cycling	Lowered during cycling (maximum value reached is above physiological range)	[72]	Sperm density and morphology unaffected (in professional cyclists during competition year)	[83]
5. Laptop usage in lap position	Increased	[84]	No data	–
Occupational exposure				
1. Welders—radiant heat	No data	–	Adverse effects on sperm count, motility, concentration, and proportion of sperm with normal morphology reduced	[85, 86]
2. Bakers—radiant heat	No data	–	Longer time to pregnancy	[87]
3. Ceramic oven operators—radiant heat	No data	–	Longer time to pregnancy	[88]

8 Testicular Heat Stress and Sperm Quality

4. Professional drivers	No data	–	Lower percentage of sperm with normal morphology, higher risk of lowered sperm motility	[89, 92, 93]
5. Submariners in a nuclear-powered submarine	No data	–	Increased infertility issues	[95]
Temperature variations				
1. Ambient temperature	Increased	[32]	No data	–
	No effect	[63]	No data	–
2. Seasonal changes	No data	–	Circannual rhythm in sperm count	[97, 98]
			Higher sperm count in winter	
	No data	–	No effect	[99]
Exogenous factors contributing to heat stress				
Pathological conditions				
1. Febrile episode	–	–	Reduced sperm concentration, sperm morphology and motility affected if fever occurs during spermiogenesis	[11, 37]
2. Varicocele	Increased	[29, 36, 58, 63]	Induces sperm DNA fragmentation	[52, 53]
3. Cryptorchidism	Increased	[3, 36, 112]	Lower sperm output	[52, 53]
			Induces sperm DNA fragmentation	
Exogenous application or removal of heat				
1. Mild scrotal heating	Increased	[29, 59, 101, 113, 114]	Reduced sperm count and percentage of motile sperm and sperm with normal morphology	[29, 101, 113, 114]
			No pregnancy established during exposure period	
2. Scrotal cooling	Decreased	[29, 104–107, 111]	Improved spermatogenesis	[29, 104–107, 111, 115]
			Improved semen quality	
			Improved sperm density and motility	

thermoregulatory mechanisms to maintain a hypothermic testis. However, posture, clothing, lifestyle factors, occupation, and environmental exposure can cause testicular heat stress. Extended hours of exposure to genital heat stress factors exacerbate their effect on semen quality and sperm parameters. Each of these factors does not occur solitarily, but many of them occur simultaneously at any given time, compounding their effect on testicular temperatures. This is especially pertinent in infertile men who already have a compromised reproductive potential.

Nevertheless, simple but significant measures can be taken by individuals to help alleviate the deleterious impact of heat stress on male fertility. These include interspersing periods of activity or movement (walking, running) between extended time spent sitting or lying down, wearing clothing that does not restrict genital airflow, maintaining a healthy weight, and making lifestyle modifications that will promote scrotal hypothermia (e.g., avoiding sauna or hot baths or using a laptop on the lap). Understandably, the occupational requirements of certain lines of work and seasonal variations, although less easily tackled, should not be a deterrent for achieving scrotal hypothermia.

References

1. Thonneau P, Bujan L, Multigner L, Mieusset R. Occupational heat exposure and male fertility: a review. Hum Reprod. 1998;13(8):2122–5.
2. Morgentaler A, Stahl BC, Yin Y. Testis and temperature: an historical, clinical, and research perspective. J Androl. 1999;20(2):189–95.
3. Mieusset R, Bujan L. Testicular heating and its possible contributions to male infertility: a review. Int J Androl. 1995;18(4):169–84.
4. Waites GM. Thermoregulation of the scrotum and testis: studies in animals and significance for man. Adv Exp Med Biol. 1991;286:9–17.
5. Candas V, Becmeur F, Bothorel B, Hoeft A. Qualitative assessment of thermal and evaporative adjustments of human scrotal skin in response to heat stress. Int J Androl. 1993;16(2):137–42.
6. Schoor RA, Elhanbly SM, Niederberger C. The pathophysiology of varicocele-associated male infertility. Curr Urol Rep. 2001;2(6):432–6.
7. Glad Sorensen H, Lambrechtsen J, Einer-Jensen N. Efficiency of the countercurrent transfer of heat and 133Xenon between the pampiniform plexus and testicular artery of the bull under in-vitro conditions. Int J Androl. 1991;14(3):232–40.

8. Shiraishi K. Heat and oxidative stress in the germ line. In: Agarwal A, Aitken RJ, Alvarez JG, editors. Studies on men's health and fertility (oxidative stress in applied basic research and clinical practice). New York, NY: Springer Science + Business Media; 2012. p. 149–78.
9. Lue YH, Hikim AP, Swerdloff RS, Im P, Taing KS, Bui T, et al. Single exposure to heat induces stage-specific germ cell apoptosis in rats: role of intratesticular testosterone on stage specificity. Endocrinology. 1999;140(4):1709–17.
10. Chowdhury AK, Steinberger E. Early changes in the germinal epithelium of rat testes following exposure to heat. J Reprod Fertil. 1970;22(2):205–12.
11. Carlsen E, Andersson AM, Petersen JH, Skakkebaek NE. History of febrile illness and variation in semen quality. Hum Reprod. 2003;18(10):2089–92.
12. Munkelwitz R, Gilbert BR. Are boxer shorts really better? A critical analysis of the role of underwear type in male subfertility. J Urol. 1998;160(4):1329–33.
13. Cai H, Ren Y, Li XX, Yang JL, Zhang CP, Chen M, et al. Scrotal heat stress causes a transient alteration in tight junctions and induction of TGF-beta expression. Int J Androl. 2011;34(4):352–62.
14. Kanter M, Aktas C. Effects of scrotal hyperthermia on Leydig cells in long-term: a histological, immunohistochemical and ultrastructural study in rats. J Mol Histol. 2009;40(2):123–30.
15. Jensen TK, Andersson AM, Hjollund NH, Scheike T, Kolstad H, Giwercman A, et al. Inhibin B as a serum marker of spermatogenesis: correlation to differences in sperm concentration and follicle-stimulating hormone levels. A study of 349 Danish men. J Clin Endocrinol Metab. 1997;82(12):4059–63.
16. Hjollund NH, Storgaard L, Ernst E, Bonde JP, Olsen J. Impact of diurnal scrotal temperature on semen quality. Reprod Toxicol. 2002;16(3):215–21.
17. Setchell BP, Ploen L, Ritzen EM. Effect of local heating of rat testes after suppression of spermatogenesis by pretreatment with a GnRH agonist and an anti-androgen. Reproduction. 2002;124(1):133–40.
18. Kanter M, Aktas C, Erboga M. Heat stress decreases testicular germ cell proliferation and increases apoptosis in short term: an immunohistochemical and ultrastructural study. Toxicol Ind Health. 2011;29(2):99–113.
19. Lue YH, Lasley BL, Laughlin LS, Swerdloff RS, Hikim AP, Leung A, et al. Mild testicular hyperthermia induces profound transitional spermatogenic suppression through increased germ cell apoptosis in adult cynomolgus monkeys (Macaca fascicularis). J Androl. 2002;23(6):799–805.
20. Paul C, Murray AA, Spears N, Saunders PT. A single, mild, transient scrotal heat stress causes DNA damage, subfertility and impairs formation of blastocysts in mice. Reproduction. 2008;136(1):73–84.
21. Collins P, Lacy D. Studies on the structure and function of the mammalian testis. II Cytological and histochemical observations on the testis of the rat after a single exposure to heat applied for different lengths of time. Proc R Soc Lond B Biol Sci. 1969;172(26):17–38.

22. Paul C, Melton DW, Saunders PT. Do heat stress and deficits in DNA repair pathways have a negative impact on male fertility? Mol Hum Reprod. 2008; 14(1):1–8.
23. Ahotupa M, Huhtaniemi I. Impaired detoxification of reactive oxygen and consequent oxidative stress in experimentally cryptorchid rat testis. Biol Reprod. 1992;46(6):1114–8.
24. Ikeda M, Kodama H, Fukuda J, Shimizu Y, Murata M, Kumagai J, et al. Role of radical oxygen species in rat testicular germ cell apoptosis induced by heat stress. Biol Reprod. 1999;61(2):393–9.
25. Rockett JC, Mapp FL, Garges JB, Luft JC, Mori C, Dix DJ. Effects of hyperthermia on spermatogenesis, apoptosis, gene expression, and fertility in adult male mice. Biol Reprod. 2001;65(1):229–39.
26. World Health Organization (WHO) Department of Reproductive Health and Research. WHO laboratory manual for the examination and processing of human semen. 5th ed. Geneva, Switzerland: WHO; 2010.
27. Kompanje EJO. 'Real men wear kilts'. The anecdotal evidence that wearing a Scottish kilt has influence on reproductive potential: how much is true? Scott Med J. 2013;58(1):e1–5.
28. Mieusset R, Quintana Casares P, Sanchez Partida LG, Sowerbutts SF, Zupp JL, Setchell BP. Effects of heating the testes and epididymides of rams by scrotal insulation on fertility and embryonic mortality in ewes inseminated with frozen semen. J Reprod Fertil. 1992;94(2):337–43.
29. Mieusset R, Bujan L, Mondinat C, Mansat A, Pontonnier F, Grandjean H. Association of scrotal hyperthermia with impaired spermatogenesis in infertile men. Fertil Steril. 1987;48(6):1006–11.
30. Hjollund NH, Bonde JP, Jensen TK, Olsen J. Diurnal scrotal skin temperature and semen quality. The Danish First Pregnancy Planner Study Team. Int J Androl. 2000;23(5):309–18.
31. Wang C, McDonald V, Leung A, Superlano L, Berman N, Hull L, et al. Effect of increased scrotal temperature on sperm production in normal men. Fertil Steril. 1997;68(2):334–9.
32. Brindley GS. Deep scrotal temperature and the effect on it of clothing, air temperature, activity, posture and paraplegia. Br J Urol. 1982;54(1):49–55.
33. Dada R, Gupta NP, Kucheria K. Deterioration of sperm morphology in men exposed to high temperature. J Anat Soc India. 2001;50(2):107.
34. Dada R, Gupta NP, Kucheria K. Spermatogenic arrest in men with testicular hyperthermia. Teratog Carcinog Mutagen. 2003;Suppl 1:235–43.
35. Saikhun J, Kitiyanant Y, Vanadurongwan V, Pavasuthipaisit K. Effects of sauna on sperm movement characteristics of normal men measured by computer-assisted sperm analysis. Int J Androl. 1998;21(6):358–63.
36. Zorgniotti AW, Macleod J. Studies in temperature, human semen quality, and varicocele. Fertil Steril. 1973;24(11):854–63.

37. Evenson DP, Jost LK, Corzett M, Balhorn R. Characteristics of human sperm chromatin structure following an episode of influenza and high fever: a case study. J Androl. 2000;21(5):739–46.
38. Gorelick JI, Goldstein M. Loss of fertility in men with varicocele. Fertil Steril. 1993;59(3):613–6.
39. Brugh III VM, Matschke HM, Lipshultz LI. Male factor infertility. Endocrinol Metab Clin North Am. 2003;32(3):689–707.
40. Setchell BP. The Parkes Lecture. Heat and the testis. J Reprod Fertil. 1998;114(2):179–94.
41. Agger P. Scrotal and testicular temperature: its relation to sperm count before and after operation for varicocele. Fertil Steril. 1971;22(5):286–97.
42. Goldstein M, Eid JF. Elevation of intratesticular and scrotal skin surface temperature in men with varicocele. J Urol. 1989;142(3):743–5.
43. Shiraishi K, Takihara H, Matsuyama H. Elevated scrotal temperature, but not varicocele grade, reflects testicular oxidative stress-mediated apoptosis. World J Urol. 2010;28(3):359–64.
44. Ku JH, Shim HB, Kim SW, Paick JS. The role of apoptosis in the pathogenesis of varicocele. BJU Int. 2005;96(7):1092–6.
45. Chan CC, Sun GH, Shui HA, Wu GJ. Differential spermatozoal protein expression profiles in men with varicocele compared to control subjects: upregulation of heat shock proteins 70 and 90 in varicocele. Urology. 2013;81(6):1379.e1–8.
46. Barthold JS, Gonzalez R. The epidemiology of congenital cryptorchidism, testicular ascent and orchiopexy. J Urol. 2003;170(6 Pt 1):2396–401.
47. Agoulnik AI, Huang Z, Ferguson L. Spermatogenesis in cryptorchidism. Methods Mol Biol. 2012;825:127–47.
48. Peltola V, Huhtaniemi I, Ahotupa M. Abdominal position of the rat testis is associated with high level of lipid peroxidation. Biol Reprod. 1995;53(5):1146–50.
49. Li YC, Hu XQ, Xiao LJ, Hu ZY, Guo J, Zhang KY, et al. An oligonucleotide microarray study on gene expression profile in mouse testis of experimental cryptorchidism. Front Biosci. 2006;11:2465–82.
50. Lee PA, Coughlin MT. Leydig cell function after cryptorchidism: evidence of the beneficial result of early surgery. J Urol. 2002;167(4):1824–7.
51. Liu Y, Li X. Molecular basis of cryptorchidism-induced infertility. Sci China Life Sci. 2010;53(11): 1274–83.
52. Bertolla RP, Cedenho AP, Hassun Filho PA, Lima SB, Ortiz V, Srougi M. Sperm nuclear DNA fragmentation in adolescents with varicocele. Fertil Steril. 2006;85(3):625–8.
53. Banks S, King SA, Irvine DS, Saunders PT. Impact of a mild scrotal heat stress on DNA integrity in murine spermatozoa. Reproduction. 2005;129(4):505–14.
54. Zorgniotti AW. Non-invasive scrotal thermometry. Adv Exp Med Biol. 1991;286:111–4.
55. Zorgniotti AW. Elevated intrascrotal temperature. II: Indirect testis and intrascrotal temperature measurement for clinical and research use. Bull N Y Acad Med. 1982;58(6):541–4.

56. Hjollund NH, Storgaard L, Ernst E, Bonde JP, Olsen J. The relation between daily activities and scrotal temperature. Reprod Toxicol. 2002;16(3):209–14.
57. Bujan L, Daudin M, Charlet JP, Thonneau P, Mieusset R. Increase in scrotal temperature in car drivers. Hum Reprod. 2000;15(6):1355–7.
58. Jockenhovel F, Grawe A, Nieschlag E. A portable digital data recorder for long-term monitoring of scrotal temperatures. Fertil Steril. 1990;54(4):694–700.
59. Rock J, Robinson D. Effect of induced intrascrotal hyperthermia on testicular function in man. Am J Obstet Gynecol. 1965;93(6):793–801.
60. Lerchl A, Keck C, Spiteri-Grech J, Nieschlag E. Diurnal variations in scrotal temperature of normal men and patients with varicocele before and after treatment. Int J Androl. 1993;16(3):195–200.
61. Jung A, Hofstotter JP, Schuppe HC, Schill WB. Relationship between sleeping posture and fluctuations in nocturnal scrotal temperature. Reprod Toxicol. 2003;17(4):433–8.
62. Koskelo R, Zaproudina N, Vuorikari K. High scrotal temperatures and chairs in the pathophysiology of poor semen quality. Pathophysiology. 2005;11(4):221–4.
63. Mieusset R, Bengoudifa B, Bujan L. Effect of posture and clothing on scrotal temperature in fertile men. J Androl. 2007;28(1):170–5.
64. Song GS, Seo JT. Changes in the scrotal temperature of subjects in a sedentary posture over a heated floor. Int J Androl. 2006;29(4):446–57.
65. Zorgniotti A, Reiss H, Toth A, Sealfon A. Effect of clothing on scrotal temperature in normal men and patients with poor semen. Urology. 1982;19(2):176–8.
66. Elebute EA. The relationship of skin temperatures of clothed adults to ambient temperature in a warm environment. Afr J Med Med Sci. 1976;5(2):175–8.
67. Laven JS, Haverkorn MJ, Bots RS. Influence of occupation and living habits on semen quality in men (scrotal insulation and semen quality). Eur J Obstet Gynecol Reprod Biol. 1988;29(2):137–41.
68. Lynch R, Lewis-Jones DI, Machin DG, Desmond AD. Improved seminal characteristics in infertile men after a conservative treatment regimen based on the avoidance of testicular hyperthermia. Fertil Steril. 1986;46(3):476–9.
69. Tiemessen CH, Evers JL, Bots RS. Tight-fitting underwear and sperm quality. Lancet. 1996; 347(9018):1844–5.
70. Partsch CJ, Aukamp M, Sippell WG. Scrotal temperature is increased in disposable plastic lined nappies. Arch Dis Child. 2000;83(4):364–8.
71. Grove GL, Grove MJ, Bates NT, Wagman LM, Leyden JJ. Scrotal temperatures do not differ among young boys wearing disposable or reusable diapers. Skin Res Technol. 2002;8(4):260–70.
72. Jung A, Schuppe HC. Influence of genital heat stress on semen quality in humans. Andrologia. 2007;39(6): 203–15.
73. Hammoud AO, Gibson M, Peterson CM, Meikle AW, Carrell DT. Impact of male obesity on infertility: a critical review of the current literature. Fertil Steril. 2008;90(4):897–904.
74. Kort HI, Massey JB, Elsner CW, Mitchell-Leef D, Shapiro DB, Witt MA, et al. Impact of body mass index values on sperm quantity and quality. J Androl. 2006;27(3):450–2.
75. Ivell R. Lifestyle impact and the biology of the human scrotum. Reprod Biol Endocrinol. 2007;5:15.
76. Shafik A, Olfat S. Lipectomy in the treatment of scrotal lipomatosis. Br J Urol. 1981;53(1):55–61.
77. Shafik A, Olfat S. Scrotal lipomatosis. Br J Urol. 1981;53(1):50–4.
78. Keast ML, Adamo KB. The Finnish sauna bath and its use in patients with cardiovascular disease. J Cardiopulm Rehabil. 2000;20(4):225–30.
79. Brown-Woodman PD, Post EJ, Gass GC, White IG. The effect of a single sauna exposure on spermatozoa. Arch Androl. 1984;12(1):9–15.
80. Garolla A, Torino M, Sartini B, Cosci I, Patassini C, Carraro U, et al. Seminal and molecular evidence that sauna exposure affects human spermatogenesis. Hum Reprod. 2013;28(4):877–85.
81. Shefi S, Tarapore PE, Walsh TJ, Croughan M, Turek PJ. Wet heat exposure: a potentially reversible cause of low semen quality in infertile men. Int Braz J Urol. 2007;33(1):50–6, discussion 56–7.
82. Jung A, Strauss P, Lindner HJ, Schuppe HC. Influence of moderate cycling on scrotal temperature. Int J Androl. 2008;31(4):403–7.
83. Lucia A, Chicharro JL, Perez M, Serratosa L, Bandres F, Legido JC. Reproductive function in male endurance athletes: sperm analysis and hormonal profile. J Appl Physiol. 1996;81(6):2627–36.
84. Sheynkin Y, Jung M, Yoo P, Schulsinger D, Komaroff E. Increase in scrotal temperature in laptop computer users. Hum Reprod. 2005;20(2):452–5.
85. Bonde JP. Semen quality in welders exposed to radiant heat. Br J Ind Med. 1992;49(1):5–10.
86. Kumar S, Zaidi SS, Gautam AK, Dave LM, Saiyed HN. Semen quality and reproductive hormones among welders—a preliminary study. Environ Health Prev Med. 2003;8(2):64–7.
87. Thonneau P, Ducot B, Bujan L, Mieusset R, Spira A. Effect of male occupational heat exposure on time to pregnancy. Int J Androl. 1997;20(5):274–8.
88. Figa-Talamanca I, Dell'Orco V, Pupi A, Dondero F, Gandini L, Lenzi A, et al. Fertility and semen quality of workers exposed to high temperatures in the ceramics industry. Reprod Toxicol. 1992;6(6):517–23.
89. Sas M, Szollosi J. Impaired spermiogenesis as a common finding among professional drivers. Arch Androl. 1979;3(1):57–60.
90. Henderson J, Rennie GC, Baker HW. Association between occupational group and sperm concentration in infertile men. Clin Reprod Fertil. 1986;4(4):275–81.
91. Chia SE, Ong CN, Lee ST, Tsakok FH. Study of the effects of occupation and industry on sperm quality. Ann Acad Med Singapore. 1994;23(5):645–9.
92. Figa-Talamanca I, Cini C, Varricchio GC, Dondero F, Gandini L, Lenzi A, et al. Effects of prolonged autovehicle driving on male reproduction function: a study among taxi drivers. Am J Ind Med. 1996;30(6): 750–8.

93. Thonneau P, Ducot B, Bujan L, Mieusset R, Spira A. Heat exposure as a hazard to male fertility. Lancet. 1996;347(8995):204–5.
94. Jung A, Strauss P, Lindner HJ, Schuppe HC. Influence of heating car seats on scrotal temperature. Fertil Steril. 2008;90(2):335–9.
95. Velez de la Calle JF, Rachou E, le Martelot MT, Ducot B, Multigner L, Thonneau PF. Male infertility risk factors in a French military population. Hum Reprod. 2001;16(3):481–6.
96. Jorgensen N, Andersen AG, Eustache F, Irvine DS, Suominen J, Petersen JH, et al. Regional differences in semen quality in Europe. Hum Reprod. 2001; 16(5):1012–9.
97. Tjoa WS, Smolensky MH, Hsi BP, Steinberger E, Smith KD. Circannual rhythm in human sperm count revealed by serially independent sampling. Fertil Steril. 1982;38(4):454–9.
98. Gyllenborg J, Skakkebaek NE, Nielsen NC, Keiding N, Giwercman A. Secular and seasonal changes in semen quality among young Danish men: a statistical analysis of semen samples from 1927 donor candidates during 1977–1995. Int J Androl. 1999;22(1):28–36.
99. Mallidis C, Howard EJ, Baker HW. Variation of semen quality in normal men. Int J Androl. 1991; 14(2):99–107.
100. Mathew V, Bantwal G. Male contraception. Indian J Endocrinol Metab. 2012;16(6):910–7.
101. Mieusset R, Bujan L. The potential of mild testicular heating as a safe, effective and reversible contraceptive method for men. Int J Androl. 1994;17(4): 186–91.
102. Wang C, Cui YG, Wang XH, Jia Y, Sinha Hikim A, Lue YH, et al. Transient scrotal hyperthermia and levonorgestrel enhance testosterone-induced spermatogenesis suppression in men through increased germ cell apoptosis. J Clin Endocrinol Metab. 2007;92(8):3292–304.
103. Osman MW, Nikolopoulos L, Haoula Z, Kannamannadiar J, Atiomo W. A study of the effect of the FertilMate Scrotum Cooling Patch on male fertility. SCOP trial (scrotal cooling patch)—study protocol for a randomised controlled trial. Trials. 2012;13:47.
104. Robinson D, Rock J, Menkin MF. Control of human spermatogenesis by induced changes of intrascrotal temperature. JAMA. 1968;204(4):290–7.
105. Mulcahy JJ. Scrotal hypothermia and the infertile man. J Urol. 1984;132(3):469–70.
106. Zorgniotti AW, Cohen MS, Sealfon AI. Chronic scrotal hypothermia: results in 90 infertile couples. J Urol. 1986;135(5):944–7.
107. Jung A, Eberl M, Schill WB. Improvement of semen quality by nocturnal scrotal cooling and moderate behavioural change to reduce genital heat stress in men with oligoasthenoteratozoospermia. Reproduction. 2001;121(4):595–603.
108. Zorgniotti AW, Sealfon AI, Toth A. Chronic scrotal hypothermia as a treatment for poor semen quality. Lancet. 1980;1(8174):904–6.
109. Zorgniotti AW, Sealfon AI. Measurement of intrascrotal temperature in normal and subfertile men. J Reprod Fertil. 1988;82(2):563–6.
110. Zorgniotti AW, Toth A, Macleod J. Infrared thermometry for testicular temperature determinations. Fertil Steril. 1979;32(3):347–8.
111. Jung A, Leonhardt F, Schill WB, Schuppe HC. Influence of the type of undertrousers and physical activity on scrotal temperature. Hum Reprod. 2005;20(4):1022–7.
112. Mieusset R, Fouda PJ, Vaysse P, Guitard J, Moscovici J, Juskiewenski S. Increase in testicular temperature in case of cryptorchidism in boys. Fertil Steril. 1993;59(6):1319–21.
113. Shafik A. Testicular suspension as a method of male contraception: technique and results. Adv Contracept Deliv Syst. 1991;7(3–4):269–79.
114. Mieusset R, Grandjean H, Mansat A, Pontonnier F. Inhibiting effect of artificial cryptorchidism on spermatogenesis. Fertil Steril. 1985;43(4):589–94.
115. Jung A, Schill WB, Schuppe HC. Improvement of semen quality by nocturnal scrotal cooling in oligozoospermic men with a history of testicular maldescent. Int J Androl. 2005;28(2):93–8.

Sexual Issues: Role of Sexually Transmitted Infections on Male Factor Fertility

9

William B. Smith II, Landon W. Trost, Yihan Chen, Amanda Rosencrans, and Wayne J.G. Hellstrom

Introduction

A variety of sexually transmitted infections (STIs) of the male genitourinary (GU) tract have been associated with male factor infertility. In both men and women, these infections may result in significant morbidity and make a formidable contribution to worldwide health expenditures. Although the literature on male GU infections is less robust compared to females, approximately 15 % of male factor infertility is postulated to be secondary to GU inflammation and infections, many of which are sexually transmitted [1–4]. As nearly one quarter of male infertility is considered idiopathic in etiology, the possible contribution of GU infections on infertility may be greater than current estimates [5, 6].

Although the true worldwide prevalence is unknown, the most recent World Health Organization (WHO) report on the global inci-dence of STIs estimates that there were approximately 500 million new cases of *C. trachomatis*, *N. gonorrhoeae* (NG), *syphilis*, and *T. vaginalis* in 2008 [7]. Approximately 53 % of these cases were in the male population, with rates 11 % higher than in 2005. In the male andrological population, the prevalence of GU inflammatory and infectious entities is estimated at 7–8 % [2, 8]. Commonly reported STI-related sequelae in this population include chronic urethritis, epididymi-tis, epididymo-orchitis, male accessory gland infection (MAGI), and nonspecific GU inflam-mation. Given their prevalence and potential for morbidity, it is important to understand their association with and possible contribution toward male factor infertility.

Several different mechanisms for STI-induced infertility have been suggested: (a) outflow obstruction of the urethra, vas deferens, ejacula-tory duct, and/or epididymis secondary to fibrosis and stricture formation; (b) damage to spermato-zoa lipid bilayer and DNA via reactive oxygen species (ROS); (c) testicular and/or epididymal damage affecting spermatogenesis; and (d) gen-eration and binding of antisperm antibodies (ASA). See Fig. 9.1 for graphical depiction of the proposed mechanisms of inflammation/infection-associated infertility. It is noteworthy that since infections present with varying symptomatology, clinical definitions, and diagnostic criteria, it is inherently difficult to accurately categorize indi-vidual infectious syndromes, draw direct com-parisons from available literature, and directly elucidate mechanisms of injury [1, 3, 9].

W.B. Smith II, MBA, BA • Y. Chen, BA
A. Rosencrans, MS, BA • W.J.G. Hellstrom, MD,
FACS (✉)
Department of Urology, Tulane University School of Medicine, 1430 Tulane Avenue, SL-42, New Orleans, LA 70112, USA
e-mail: wsmith@tulane.edu; ychen7@tulane.edu; arosencr@tulane.edu; whellst@tulane.edu

L.W. Trost, MD
Department of Urology, Mayo Clinic,
200 First Street SW, Rochester, MN 55905, USA
e-mail: trost.landon@mayo.edu

S.S. du Plessis et al. (eds.), *Male Infertility: A Complete Guide to Lifestyle and Environmental Factors*,
DOI 10.1007/978-1-4939-1040-3_9, © Springer Science+Business Media New York 2014

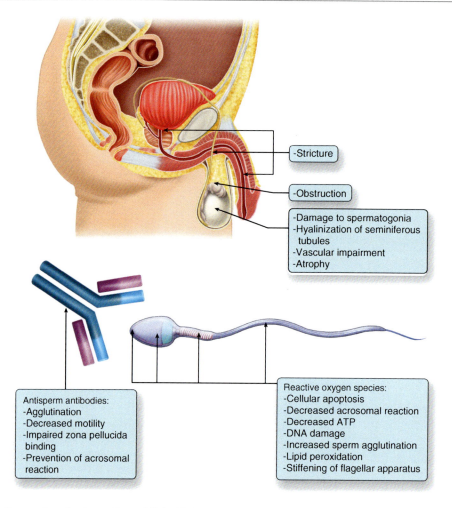

Fig. 9.1 Proposed mechanisms of bacterial/viral-induced male subfertility/infertility

This chapter will address the role of sexually transmitted GU infections in male factor infertility. The impact of inflammation will be discussed first, as it is an underlying component of most STIs. The remainder of the chapter will be devoted to the discussion of individual pathogens and those physiologic sequelae most frequently associated with male factor infertility. See Table 9.1 for the summary of the proposed mechanisms and data on pathologic organisms associated with male factor infertility.

Etiology of Infectious/Inflammatory-Associated Male Factor Infertility

At the developmental level, spermatogonia mature within the seminiferous tubules into spermatocytes, secondary spermatocytes, spermatids, and ultimately spermatozoa. These spermatozoa are then released from the testis and undergo additional maturation in the epididymis [10, 11]. Interruption at any point in this developmental

Table 9.1 Proposed mechanisms and data of pathologic organisms associated with male infertility

Organism/proposed mechanism	Evidence associating with infertility	Organism/proposed mechanism	Evidence associating with infertility
Bacteria		Viruses	
Neisseria gonorrhoea	Among STIs, strongest data on association with infertility	*Cytomegalovirus*	
• Urethral stricture		• NA	Insufficient data
• Ejaculatory duct obstruction			
• Epididymal obstruction		*Epstein-Barr*	
• Vasal obstruction		• NA	Insufficient data
• Epididymo-orchitis			
		Hepatitis B	
		• NA	Insufficient data
Chlamydia trachomatis	Conflicting data		
• Epididymo-orchitis		*Human herpesvirus 6*	
• MAGI		• NA	Insufficient data
• Asthenospermia			
• Caspase-mediated sperm death		*Human immunodeficiency virus*	
		• Present in reproductive tract	Associated with progressive deterioration of semen parameters; CD4 counts may correlate; HAART may also contribute
Ureaplasma urealyticum			
• Attach directly to spermatozoa	Conflicting data; may decrease success with ART	• Asthenospermia	
• Damages paternal DNA		• Reduced ejaculate volume	
		• Oligospermia	
Ureaplasma parvum		*Human papillomavirus*	
• Unknown	Insufficient data	• Asthenospermia	Limited data on association with infertility
Mycoplasma genitalium		*Herpes simplex virus 1/2*	
• Unknown	Limited data on association with infertility	• Present in semen	Limited data on association with infertility
		• Attach to sperm	
Mycoplasma hominis		• Asthenospermia	
• Attach/invade spermatozoa	Conflicting data	• Decreased sperm concentration	
		• Reduce endogenous antioxidants	

ART assisted reproductive techniques, *HAART* highly active antiretroviral therapy, *MAGI* male accessory gland infection, *STI* sexually transmitted infections process, as may occur with inflammation, may lead to abnormal sperm function and resultant subfertility/infertility.

Male GU infections, particularly those in the testis and epididymis, are rarely identified in the absence of inflammation [11]. Inflammatory processes involving the male GU tract recruit leukocytes into the semen with subsequent production of ROS and ASA [11]. Leukocytospermia, defined by the WHO as $>1 \times 10^6$ white blood cells per mL of semen, is a typical consequence of GU inflammation and is seen occasionally in the setting of subclinical GU infection [12–16].

ROS are oxygen-derived free radicals and are therefore highly active oxidizing agents. These include superoxide anions, hydroxyl radicals, hydrogen peroxide, nitric oxide, and peroxide, among others [17]. Leukocytes produce ROS through oxidative bursts [11, 18, 19] and indirectly via cytokine activation of the xanthine oxidase system [20–23]. Although invading pathogens may also produce ROS, leukocytes are the predominant source [11, 24, 25]. ROS production in limited amounts is required for capacitation, hyperactivation, acrosome reaction, and sperm-oocyte fusion [11, 26]. However, when present in excess, oxidative stress increases, which hinders spermatogenesis in the testis and epididymis and results in direct injury to spermatozoa [11, 15, 23, 26–28].

Several potential underlying mechanisms for ROS-induced impairment of spermatogenesis have been proposed. ROS directly damage the lipid membrane via peroxidation, which stiffens the flagellar apparatus. Additionally, consumption of hydrogen atoms by ROS reduces the availability of intracellular adenosine triphosphate (ATP) [11, 25, 29–33]. This process impairs motility and increases agglutination [20, 34]. Oxidative stress also causes transverse DNA mutation, increased rates of apoptosis [35, 36], and decreased acrosomal reactions [37, 38]. Although semen is rich in antioxidants [39], spermatozoa's low cytoplasm content makes them particularly vulnerable to oxidative damage [40]. Indeed, couples in which the male is found to have elevated ROS levels are less likely to conceive than those in which the male is found to

have lower ROS levels [41, 42]. As such, any inflammatory condition has the potential to reduce male fertility.

Urethritis, Epididymitis, Epididymo-Orchitis, and Male Accessory Gland Infection

Urethritis

Urethritis is characterized by dysuria and/or urethral discharge, although it may also be asymptomatic. Urethritis is more often seen in young, sexually active men, with *C. trachomatis* and NG most commonly isolated. *C. trachomatis* is the most frequently reported STI in the United States with 1,412,791 cases identified in 2011, followed by NG with 321,839 [43]. NG infection becomes readily apparent in 90 % of men, with symptoms of urethritis usually developing within 1 week of exposure [44]. Concomitant *C. trachomatis* infection is present in 25–30 % of men with gonococcal urethritis, and chlamydial infection alone accounts for 15–40 % of all nongonococcal urethritis (NGU) cases [45, 46]. In the majority of NGU, no pathogen is detected; however, the CDC estimates that *Mycoplasma genitalium* accounts for 15–25 % of US cases. Less common sexually transmitted causes of male urethritis include *Trichomonas vaginalis* and herpes simplex virus (HSV). Ureaplasma as a causative organism remains controversial, with its role less clearly defined [46].

Currently available data do not definitively demonstrate or disprove a causal link between urethritis and male factor infertility. Isolated, appropriately treated cases of acute urethritis are unlikely to lead to male factor infertility. Ness and colleagues reviewed 17 studies comparing semen in fertile and infertile men and did not consistently find an association between urethritis and alterations in sperm characteristics or fertility status [47]. However, these studies were inconsistent in design and power and did not include healthy controls. Similarly, other authors have reported inconsistent relationships between these two clinical entities [9]. Although urethritis was previously a common etiology for urethral stricture disease (USD), it is now one of the least prevalent causes [48, 49]. Furthermore, to significantly alter semen characteristics or result in azoospermia, USD as an isolated cause would have to be very severe and would be associated with significant urinary symptomatology. Untreated urethritis that progresses to upper genital tract infection, however, may lead to altered semen parameters, and, in severe cases, complete obstruction and azoospermia [50–52].

Epididymitis and Epididymo-orchitis

While treated urethritis alone seems to have little impact on male fertility, cases of epididymo-orchitis or untreated urethritis progressing to epididymo-orchitis are more causally linked [50, 51, 53]. Before the widespread utilization of antibiotics, it is estimated that urethritis progressed to epididymo-orchitis in 10–30 % of cases [47, 54]. Isolated orchitis without epididymitis is uncommon except in the case of mumps orchitis and therefore is not discussed outside of this section.

The incidence of epididymitis in the United States is approximately 600,000 cases annually [55], with greatest prevalence among men aged 15–30 years[46]. Concurrent epididymitis and orchitis occur in approximately 60 % of cases [9, 55–57]. Epididymitis presents as intense scrotal pain, while epididymo-orchitis includes testicular pain and swelling. These conditions are most commonly caused by *C. trachomatis* and NG in men 15–35 years of age [58]. For men outside this age range or those practicing anal intercourse, *E. coli* is the more frequent culprit [55].

Altered semen characteristics including abnormal sperm morphology, decreased motility, and reduced concentration have been observed in 8–33 % of patients after unilateral epididymitis or epididymo-orchitis [9, 47, 57, 59, 60]. In at least 60 % of patients with acute infection, spermatogenesis is significantly reduced [61]. Changes are similar when comparing chronic epididymitis and chronic epididymo-orchitis [1]. Epididymitis frequently leads to impaired sperm motility and number, with occasional development of epididymal obstruction and resultant azoospermia reported [11]. Abnormal sperm function may result without complete occlusion of the epididymis, and infertility may approach 40 % in men with a history of bilateral infection even following resolution of the epididymo-orchitis [47, 54, 59, 62, 63]. Obstruction may also develop in the vas deferens or the ejaculatory duct [64–67]. Seminal alterations can be transient, but affected individuals, particularly those with recurrent and chronic infections, are at risk for developing epididymal obstruction and testicular atrophy. Of interest, patients presenting with unilateral infection who undergo contralateral testicular biopsy demonstrate evidence of gonadal damage and azoospermia in the contralateral testis, suggesting the presence of subclinical bilateral involvement [59].

ASA production may also play a role in the postinfectious development of subfertility. Epididymal and/or testicular inflammation in the context of infection can disrupt the Sertoli cell blood-testis barrier and expose spermatic antigens to the immune response [1, 6, 35, 68, 69]. Resulting ASAs may cause sperm agglutination, reduced motility, and impaired zona pellucida binding and penetration and prevent the acrosome reaction. ASAs can be found in approximately 10 % of infertile men and 2 % of fertile men [70]. The likelihood of infertility is proportional to the amount of antibody binding [71]. The relative contribution of this mechanism to infertility in the context of genital tract infections has not, however, been well defined.

Compared to other GU infections, epididymitis/epididymo-orchitis is most strongly associated with male factor infertility, likely due to a combination of both direct impairment of semen parameters through inflammatory processes and the indirect development of mechanical obstruction [1, 22, 35].

Male Accessory Gland Infection

Studies attempting to define the connection between different forms of MAGI and infertility are inconsistent in their conclusions.

MAGI defined by the WHO includes infection of the seminal vesicles, bulbourethral glands, and prostate [72]. Unfortunately, the literature uses variations in definition, with some analyses incorporating urethritis and/or epididymal disease, further confounding assessments.

Prostatitis is the most common urologic diagnosis in men under 50. In general, the most frequently isolated organisms in prostatitis are gram-negative rods, while NG, *C. trachomatis*, gram-positives, and mycoplasma (controversial) are less often identified [9, 73, 74]. In contrast to bacterial prostatitis, many patients (80 %) have no evidence for infection at the time of presentation. Additionally, the time for sperm contact during ejaculation is limited [22, 75]. Given the low rate of bacterial infections with MAGI and minimal direct interaction with sperm, the relative direct impact of STI on fertility is likely small. However, indirectly MAGI leads to leukocytospermia, elevated ROS production, and suppression of prostatic secretion of citric acid and gamma-glutamyl transpeptidase, which may increase spermatogenic oxidative stress [25]. Additionally, chronic MAGI has been associated with scarring and obstruction of the ejaculatory ducts, leading to ejaculatory duct obstruction [65, 76]. Although EDO is most often partial in nature, it may lead to poor sperm quality and low seminal volume levels [65, 67].

Despite these potential mechanisms, a review by Weidner and colleagues demonstrated no evidence for decreased sperm density, morphology, or motility in patients with chronic prostatitis [9]. Currently, there is no consensus on the role of MAGI on male subfertility/infertility with conflicting data available [77–79].

Genitourinary Pathogens Associated with Infertility

Bacteria

Neisseria gonorrhoeae
The evidence for NG as a cause of male factor infertility is probably the strongest among the STIs; however, the majority of data is observa-

tional in nature, without a direct causal link established.

Observed and hypothesized sequelae of NG infection include urethral strictures, ejaculatory duct obstruction [76], epididymal obstruction, and, less commonly, systemic dissemination. Infection becomes symptomatic typically within 2 weeks, and, if untreated, may lead to epididymo-orchitis. In a WHO comparison of samples from high and low NG prevalence regions in Uganda, 27.9 % of men from the high prevalence sample had evidence of current epididymitis, 6 % of which were bilateral [80–82]. As a corollary, 44 % of those men with epididymitis were childless compared to 19 % of their non-epididymitis counterparts. Prior to widespread antibiotic therapies, NG subsequently led to epididymitis in 17–30 % of cases. Other reports from the 1970s to 1980s era, during which limited antibiotic access was available in Africa, indicate that the majority (65–80 %) of urologic practices involved treatment of USD and infertility [81, 83]. Although less common in the current era, increasing prevalence of drug-resistant NG strains may lead to a resurgence of epididymitis and infertility [84].

Chlamydia trachomatis
Although *C. trachomatis* is primarily located in the penile urethra, it may spread throughout the GU tract, resulting in epididymo-orchitis with or without MAGI [4, 85, 86]. Data on the impact of chlamydial infection on male fertility are inconclusive. In vitro, *C. trachomatis* co-incubation with spermatozoa leads to asthenospermia and premature cell death, likely secondary to a caspase-mediated mechanism triggered by elementary bodies [87]. In an observational analysis of sperm donor samples, Veznik and colleagues found spermatozoa in chlamydia-positive samples to have significantly lower motility rates and significantly increased rates of teratospermia compared to controls. In contrast, other studies have failed to demonstrate any significant difference in sperm count, motility, or morphology [88–91].

Although *C. trachomatis* infection influences a number of factors related to fertility, its overall contribution toward subfertility/infertility remains poorly defined. Given its high prevalence among young sexually active men and its tendency to remain asymptomatic for long periods, additional research is warranted.

Mollicutes

The class *Mollicutes* encompasses eight genera of bacteria, including the ureaplasmas and mycoplasmas [92]. The genital ureaplasmas and mycoplasmas are commonly found in the human GU system, with prevalence associated with increasing sexual exposure [93, 94]. *U. urealyticum* has been associated with NGU [45, 92] and has been observed in 10–40 % of infertile men [61].

Although the true association with infertility remains unknown, the majority of studies have not demonstrated an increased prevalence of *U. urealyticum* in infertile cohorts compared to controls. Two studies which demonstrated an increased rate of infection in infertile patient vs. controls include Xu and colleagues (38.7 % vs. 0.1 %) and Megory and colleagues (40 % vs. 28 %), respectively [61, 95, 96]. In contrast, other studies have failed to identify any differences in *U. urealyticum* rates between infertile and fertile males [97, 98].

Limited research has been undertaken to assess the impact of antibiotic administration on fertility. In reviewing data on 60 infertile patients with asymptomatic *U. urealyticum* or *C. trachomatis* infections and pyospermia, Pajovic and colleagues demonstrated significant improvements in semen characteristics, including seminal volume, pH, sperm concentration, and motility following antibiotic therapy [99].

Although *U. urealyticum* has been shown to attach directly to spermatozoa in vivo, there are conflicting data regarding its impact on fertility [76, 92, 95]. Observed no differences in semen parameters, while others have reported decreased sperm concentration [100–102], lower pH, increased viscosity [101], and reduced motility [97, 102]. Reichart also observed motility varying proportionately with pH and hypothesized that this occurs as a result of mitochondrial energy competition in infected spermatozoa [103].

Beyond the impact on semen analysis parameters, *U. urealyticum* may damage paternal DNA [104]. This is especially problematic with in vitro fertilization (IVF), as it permits normal fertilization while impairing embryonic development. Sperm infected with *U. urealyticum* results in decreased rates of pregnancy with IVF compared to controls [105]. Additional research is required to further assess the impact of *U. urealyticum* on fertility as well as the role and impact of treatment on outcomes.

U. parvum has been reported in 4.2–19.2 % of infertile males. There is currently little evidence, however, that this organism has any effect on male fertility [92, 106].

M. genitalium is a causative agent identified in NGU [107], with a prevalence ranging from 0.9 to 5 % among men presenting to infertility clinics [92, 108]. Gdoura and colleagues have identified an association between the presence of *M. genitalium* DNA and decreased sperm concentration, although there is currently minimal literature available regarding its role and impact of treatment in male factor infertility.

The true prevalence of *M. hominis* is unknown. Estimates range from 0 % of French couples attending a fertility clinic to 10–28 % of infertile men in Africa [92, 109, 110]. In evaluating the pathogenicity of *M. hominis*, Diaz-Garcia et al. observed rapid attachment and invasion of healthy spermatozoa without associated change in sperm viability. These results suggest that short-term infections may be of little consequence [111]. Similarly, an analysis of 234 men infected with *M. hominis* did not detect any changes in sperm parameters compared to controls [112]. In contrast, a more recent study identified an association between *M. hominis* and impaired semen factors, including low sperm concentration ($p=0.007$) and altered morphology ($p=0.03$) [92].

In summary of the currently available literature, with the exception of *U. urealyticum*, none of the above-described ureaplasma/mycoplasma organisms are definitively linked to male factor infertility. Although limited data are available on all ureaplasma/mycoplasma organisms, *M. urealyticum* is of particular concern due to its high prevalence and ability to directly alter sperm DNA. Further research is needed to assess the significance of the Mollicutes as well as the role for their potential treatment.

Viruses

Previous studies have associated viral infections with altered semen parameters and have suggested a deleterious impact on male fertility [113, 114]. Among 241 patients undergoing routine semen analysis at a male infertility clinic, the prevalence of sexually transmissible viral pathogens was 16.2 % [115]: cytomegalovirus (CMV) (8.7 %), human papillomaviruses (HPV) (4.5 %), HSV-1/HSV-2 (3.7 %), human herpesvirus 6 (HHV-6) (3.7 %), and Epstein-Barr virus (EBV) (0.4 %). Although prevalent, CMV, HHV-6, and EBV have not been associated with altered semen parameters [114–117]. Additionally, EBV is rarely found in semen, as it resides in the B-lymphocyte, which occupies only a small proportion of seminal WBCs [116]. Hepatitis B, although not commonly isolated, can be readily transmitted through semen but is not linked to infertility [118]. Human immunodeficiency virus [11], HSV, and HPV have each been associated with male infertility and are reviewed in greater detail below.

Human Immunodeficiency Virus

Among sexually transmitted viruses, HIV is most strongly associated with male factor infertility, particularly in the context of acquired immunodeficiency syndrome (AIDS) and highly active antiretroviral therapy (HAART), although specific mechanisms have not been fully elucidated. In the United States, there are approximately 1.15 million people over age of 13 living with HIV, with an incidence of 50,000 new infections per year [119, 120]. Of those living with HIV, 18 % are unaware of their infection.

Once a male is infected and viral titers rise, HIV is present in the reproductive tract both in infected leukocytes [121] and possibly in spermatozoa as well [122]. Early, asymptomatic HIV infection does not appear to alter semen quality appreciably [8, 114, 123–128]. In a longitudinal cohort study by van Leeuwen and colleagues, 55 men with HIV-1 infection of variable duration in the absence of HAART were followed for 96 weeks, and despite significantly decreased CD4 cell count and increased HIV-1 RNA, no significant changes in semen parameters over time were observed [124].

Although the rate of deterioration appears to be gradual, longer-term HIV infection is associated with progressive reductions in fertility [125, 127]. A number of studies have reported that deterioration in sperm quality is correlated with decreasing CD4 blood count, with lower CD4 levels associated with asthenozoospermia, oligospermia, and reduced ejaculate volume [8, 121, 126–132].

In addition to the direct effects of HIV, HAART is associated with and potentially accelerates the decline of sperm quality in HIV infection, particularly with regard to motility, morphology, and ejaculate volume [118, 127, 132–136]. It is hypothesized that these effects are related, at least in part, to mitochondrial toxicity observed with the nucleoside analogs or through inhibition of apoptosis with protease inhibitors. However, the exact mechanisms for reduced fertility in the context of higher viral loads, lower CD4 counts, and HAART remain poorly described and require additional evaluation.

Herpes Simplex Virus

HSV is responsible for genital herpes infection and is present in over 50 million people in the United States [46]. There is currently only a modest amount of data linking HSV to male factor infertility. HSV-1 and HSV-2, in contrast to other serotypes, are present in the semen and directly attached to sperm [115, 137–139]. el Borai and colleagues identified HSV DNA in 24 % (37/153) of semen samples from men attending an infertility clinic [113, 138]. Interestingly, none of the men who had previously fathered children had any evidence of HSV

DNA in their semen. In another study describing 80 men attending a maternity center for reproductive counseling, HSV was detected in 46 % of semen samples and was associated with reduced sperm count and motility [139]. Among infertile patients undergoing semen analysis, those with HSV+DNA samples have significantly reduced sperm concentration, count, motility, and neutral alpha-glucosidase and citrate concentrations. These results suggest HSV may impact semen quality not only through damaging spermatozoa but also via impairing epididymal and prostatic function; however, the direct impact of HSV on fertility remains unclear and requires additional investigation [115, 116, 139, 140].

Human Papillomavirus

There are over 100 subtypes of HPV, with varying specificity for different body sites. HPV 16 and 18 are the most commonly isolated strains worldwide and may be immunized against with the currently available HPV vaccination. Despite available preventative measures, anogenital HPV infection in the United States was estimated at 5.5 million cases per year in 2010 [43]. Data linking HPV to male infertility are limited, with one study reporting its association with abnormal sperm motility [141]. Given the limited data, the role of HPV in infertility and impact of disease prevention is poorly understood.

Conclusion

Although current data are limited and largely remain observational in nature, GU infections are associated with increased risk for male factor infertility. Among the infectious syndromes, epididymitis, epididymo-orchitis, and obstructive processes appear to be the most causally related. In evaluating individual pathogens, NG is likely the most significant bacteria resulting in subfertility/infertility, while the impact of *C. trachomatis* is less clearly defined. Studies evaluating the impact of the Mollicutes are ongoing, with *U. urealyticum* being the most heavily investigated

due to its prevalence and known impact on spermatozoa DNA. Of the sexually transmitted viruses, HIV appears to be the most detrimental to male fertility status, and data on the impact of HAART are mixed. HSV and HPV are not as widely studied, but their impact is not likely as significant. The current data regarding STIs are limited by its observational nature and lack of adequate control groups. Given the prevalence of STIs in the general population, ongoing research is warranted to better define their direct impact on fertility as well as potential benefits with treatment.

References

1. Haidl G, Allam JP, Schuppe HC. Chronic epididymitis: impact on semen parameters and therapeutic options. Andrologia. 2008;40(2):92–6.
2. Comhaire F. Towards more objectivity in the management of male infertility. The need for a standardized approach. Int J Androl. 1987;10:1.
3. Dohle G, Colpi G, Hargreave T, Papp G, Jungwirth A, Weidner W. EAU guidelines on male infertility. Eur Urol. 2005;48(5):703–11.
4. Pellati D, Mylonakis I, Bertoloni G, Fiore C, Andrisani A, Ambrosini G, et al. Genital tract infections and infertility. Eur J Obstet Gynecol Reprod Biol. 2008;140(1):3–11.
5. Nagler HM, Martinis FG. Varicocele. In: Lipshultz LI, Howards SS, editors. Infertility in the male. St. Louis: Mosby Year Book, Inc.; 1997. p. 336–59.
6. Sabanegh Jr ES, Agarwal A. Sexual issues: role for sexually transmitted infections on male-factor fertility. In: Wein AJ, Kavoussi LR, Partin AW, Peters CA, editors. Campbell-Walsh urology. 10th ed. Philadelphia, PA: Elsevier Inc.; 2010. p. 616–47.
7. WHO. Global incidence and prevalence of selected curable sexually transmitted infections—2008. Geneva, Switzerland: World Health Organization (WHO); 2012. p. 2012.
8. Rusz A, Pilatz A, Wagenlehner F, Linn T, Diemer T, Schuppe HC, et al. Influence of urogenital infections and inflammation on semen quality and male fertility. World J Urol. 2011;30(1):23–30.
9. Weidner W, Krause W, Ludwig M. Relevance of male accessory gland infection for subsequent fertility with special focus on prostatitis. Hum Reprod Update. 1999;5(5):421–32.
10. Russell L. Movement of spermatocytes from the basal to the adluminal compartment of the rat testis. Am J Anat. 1977;148(3):313–28. Epub 1977/03/01.
11. Sarkar O, Bahrainwala J, Chandrasekaran S, Kothari S, Mathur PP, Agarwal A. Impact of inflammation

on male fertility. Front Biosci (Elite Ed). 2011; 3:89–95.

12. Zorn B, Sesek-Briski A, Osredkar J, Meden-Vrtovec H. Semen polymorphonuclear neutrophil leukocyte elastase as a diagnostic and prognostic marker of genital tract inflammation—a review. Clin Chem Lab Med. 2003;41(1):2–12.

13. WHO. WHO laboratory manual for the examination of human semen and sperm-cervical mucus interaction. 4th ed. Cambridge: Cambridge University Press; 2003.

14. Branigan EF, Muller CH. Efficacy of treatment and recurrence rate of leukocytospermia in infertile men with prostatitis. Fertil Steril. 1994;62(3):580–4.

15. Armstrong JS, Rajasekaran M, Chamulitrat W, Gatti P, Hellstrom WJ, Sikka SC. Characterization of reactive oxygen species induced effects on human spermatozoa movement and energy metabolism. Free Radic Biol Med. 1999;26(7–8):869–80.

16. Trum JW, Mol BW, Pannekoek Y, Spanjaard L, Wertheim P, Bleker OP, et al. Value of detecting leukocytospermia in the diagnosis of genital tract infection in subfertile men. Fertil Steril. 1998;70(2):315–9.

17. Sikka SC. Relative impact of oxidative stress on male reproductive function. Curr Med Chem. 2001;8(7):851–62.

18. Fraczek M, Kurpisz M. Inflammatory mediators exert toxic effects of oxidative stress on human spermatozoa. J Androl. 2007;28(2):325–33.

19. Blake DR, Allen RE, Lunec J. Free radicals in biological systems—a review orientated to inflammatory processes. Br Med Bull. 1987;43(2):371–85.

20. Sanocka D, Jedrzejczak P, Szumała-Kaekol A, Fraczek M, Kurpisz M. Male genital tract inflammation: the role of selected interleukins in regulation of pro-oxidant and antioxidant enzymatic substances in seminal plasma. J Androl. 2003;24(3):448–55.

21. Whittington K, Ford WC. Relative contribution of leukocytes and of spermatozoa to reactive oxygen species production in human sperm suspensions. Int J Androl. 1999;22(4):229–35.

22. Wolff H. The biologic significance of white blood cells in semen. Fertil Steril. 1995;63(6):1143–57.

23. Rajasekaran M, Hellstrom WJ, Naz RK, Sikka SC. Oxidative stress and interleukins in seminal plasma during leukocytospermia. Fertil Steril. 1995;64(1):166–71.

24. Hong JE, Santucci LA, Tian X, Silverman DJ. Superoxide dismutase-dependent, catalase-sensitive peroxides in human endothelial cells infected by Rickettsia rickettsii. Infect Immun. 1998;66(4):1293–8.

25. Potts JM, Pasqualotto FF. Seminal oxidative stress in patients with chronic prostatitis. Andrologia. 2003;35(5):304–8.

26. Aitken RJ. The Amoroso lecture. The human spermatozoon—a cell in crisis? J Reprod Fertil. 1999;115(1):1–7.

27. Aitken RJ, Clarkson JS. Cellular basis of defective sperm function and its association with the genesis of reactive oxygen species by human spermatozoa. J Reprod Fertil. 1987;81(2):459–69.

28. Agarwal A, Saleh RA. Role of oxidants in male infertility: rationale, significance, and treatment. Urol Clin North Am. 2002;29(4):817–27.

29. Twigg JP, Irvine DS, Aitken RJ. Oxidative damage to DNA in human spermatozoa does not preclude pronucleus formation at intracytoplasmic sperm injection. Hum Reprod. 1998;13(7):1864–71.

30. de Lamirande E, Gagnon C. Reactive oxygen species and human spermatozoa. I. Effects on the motility of intact spermatozoa and on sperm axonemes. J Androl. 1992;13(5):368–78.

31. de Lamirande E, Gagnon C. Reactive oxygen species and human spermatozoa. II. Depletion of adenosine triphosphate plays an important role in the inhibition of sperm motility. J Androl. 1992; 13(5):379–86.

32. Walrand S, Valeix S, Rodriguez C, Ligot P, Chassagne J, Vasson M-P. Flow cytometry study of polymorphonuclear neutrophil oxidative burst: a comparison of three fluorescent probes. Clin Chim Acta. 2003;331(1–2):103–10.

33. Aitken RJ. Free radicals, lipid peroxidation and sperm function. Reprod Fertil Dev. 1995;7(4): 659–68.

34. Tremellen K. Oxidative stress and male infertility—a clinical perspective. Hum Reprod Update. 2008;14(3):243–58.

35. Comhaire FH, Mahmoud AM, Depuydt CE, Zalata AA, Christophe AB. Mechanisms and effects of male genital tract infection on sperm quality and fertilizing potential: the andrologist's viewpoint. Hum Reprod Update. 1999;5(5):393–8.

36. Vaithinathan S, Saradha B, Mathur PP. Methoxychlor induces apoptosis via mitochondria- and FasL-mediated pathways in adult rat testis. Chem Biol Interact. 2010;185(2):110–8.

37. Depuydt C, Zalata A, Christophe A, Mahmoud A, Comhaire F. Mechanisms of sperm deficiency in male accessory gland infection. Andrologia. 1998;30 Suppl 1:29–33.

38. Zalata AA, Christophe AB, Depuydt CE, Schoonjans F, Comhaire FH. White blood cells cause oxidative damage to the fatty acid composition of phospholipids of human spermatozoa. Int J Androl. 1998; 21(3):154–62.

39. Agarwal A, Makker K, Sharma R. Clinical relevance of oxidative stress in male factor infertility: an update. Am J Reprod Immunol. 2008;59(1):2–11.

40. Drevius LO. Bull spermatozoa as osmometers. J Reprod Fertil. 1972;28(1):29–39.

41. Aitken RJ, Irvine DS, Wu FC. Prospective analysis of sperm-oocyte fusion and reactive oxygen species generation as criteria for the diagnosis of infertility. Am J Obstet Gynecol. 1991;164(2):542–51.

42. Irvine DS. Epidemiology and aetiology of male infertility. Hum Reprod. 1998;13 Suppl 1:33–44.

43. Centers for Disease Control and Prevention (CDC). Sexually transmitted disease surveillance 2011.

Atlanta, GA: U.S. Department of Health and Human Services; 2012.

44. Sherrard J, Barlow D. Gonorrhoea in men: clinical and diagnostic aspects. Genitourin Med. 1996;72(6):422–6.

45. Bradshaw CS, Tabrizi SN, Read TRH, Garland SM, Hopkins CA, Moss LM, et al. Etiologies of nongonococcal urethritis: bacteria, viruses, and the association with orogenital exposure. J Infect Dis. 2006;193(3):336–45.

46. CDC. Sexually transmitted diseases treatment guidelines 2010. Center for Disease Control (CDC): Division of STD Prevention. 2010. p. 1–116.

47. Ness RB, Markovic N, Carlson CL, Coughlin MT. Do men become infertile after having sexually transmitted urethritis? An epidemiologic examination. Fertil Steril. 1997;68(2):205–13.

48. Lumen N, Hoebeke P, Willemsen P, De Troyer B, Pieters R, Oosterlinck W. Etiology of urethral stricture disease in the 21st century. J Urol. 2009;182(3):983–7.

49. McMillan A, Pakianathan M, Mao JH, Macintyre CC. Urethral stricture and urethritis in men in Scotland. Genitourin Med. 1994;70(6):403–5.

50. Jequier AM. Obstructive azoospermia: a study of 102 patients. Clin Reprod Fertil. 1985;3(1):21–36. Epub 1985/03/01.

51. De Schryver A, Meheus A. Epidemiology of sexually transmitted diseases: the global picture. Bull World Health Organ. 1990;68(5):639–54. Epub 1990/01/01.

52. Rusz A, Pilatz A, Wagenlehner F, Linn T, Diemer T, Schuppe HC, et al. Influence of urogenital infections and inflammation on semen quality and male fertility. World J Urol. 2012;30(1):23–30. Epub 2011/07/13.

53. Bernitsky L, Roy J. Male infertility and genitourinary infections. Infertility. 1986;9(2):129–44.

54. Pelouze PS. Gonorrhea in the male and female, a book for practitioners. Philadelphia, PA: WB Saunders and Co.; 1941. 483 p.

55. Trojian TH, Lishnak TS, Heiman D. Epididymitis and orchitis: an overview. Am Fam Physician. 2009;79(7):583–7.

56. Ludwig M. Diagnosis and therapy of acute prostatitis, epididymitis and orchitis. Andrologia. 2008; 40(2):76–80.

57. Schuppe HC, Meinhardt A, Allam JP, Bergmann M, Weidner W, Haidl G. Chronic orchitis: a neglected cause of male infertility? Andrologia. 2008;40(2):84–91.

58. Redfern TR, English PJ, Baumber CD, McGhie D. The aetiology and management of acute epididymitis. Br J Surg. 1984;71(9):703–5.

59. Osegbe DN. Testicular function after unilateral bacterial epididymo-orchitis. Eur Urol. 1991;19(3):204–8.

60. Weidner W, Garbe C, Weißbach L, Harbrecht J. Initiale Therapie der akuten eiseitigen Epididymitis mit Ofloxacin. II. Andrologische Befunde [Germany]. Der Urologe Ausgabe A. 1990;29(5):277–80.

61. Keck C, Gerber-Schäfer C, Clad A, Wilhelm C, Breckwoldt M. Seminal tract infections: impact on male fertility and treatment options. Hum Reprod Update. 1998;4(6):891–903.

62. Berger RE, Alexander ER, Monda GD, Ansell J, McCormick G, Holmes KK. Chlamydia trachomatis as a cause of acute 'idiopathic' epididymitis. N Engl J Med. 1978;298(6):301–4.

63. Campbell MF. The surgical pathology of epididymitis. Ann Surg. 1928;88(1):98–111.

64. Pryor JP, Hendry WF. Ejaculatory duct obstruction in subfertile males: analysis of 87 patients. Fertil Steril. 1991;56(4):725–30.

65. Dohle GR. Inflammatory-associated obstructions of the male reproductive tract. Andrologia. 2003;35(5):321–4.

66. Smith JF, Walsh TJ, Turek PJ. Ejaculatory duct obstruction. Urol Clin North Am. 2008;35(2):221–7.

67. Goluboff ET, Stifelman MD, Fisch H. Ejaculatory duct obstruction in the infertile male. Urology. 1995;45(6):925–31.

68. Francavilla F, Santucci R, Barbonetti A, Francavilla S. Naturally-occurring antisperm antibodies in men: interference with fertility and clinical implications. An update. Front Biosci. 2007;12:2890–911.

69. Bronson R, Cooper G, Rosenfeld D. Sperm antibodies: their role in infertility. Fertil Steril. 1984;42(2):171–83.

70. Guzick DS, Overstreet JW, Factor-Litvak P, Brazil CK, Nakajima ST, Coutifaris C, et al. Sperm morphology, motility, and concentration in fertile and infertile men. N Engl J Med. 2001;345(19):1388–93.

71. Chamley LW, Clarke GN. Antisperm antibodies and conception. Semin Immunopathol. 2007;29(2):169–84.

72. Rowe PJ, Comhaire FH. WHO manual for the standardized investigation, diagnosis and management of the infertile male. Cambridge: Cambridge University Press; 2000.

73. Wolff H, Neubert U, Volkenandt M, Zöchling N, Schlüpen EM, Bezold G, et al. Detection of Chlamydia trachomatis in semen by antibody-enzyme immunoassay compared with polymerase chain reaction, antigen-enzyme immunoassay, and urethral cell culture. Fertil Steril. 1994;62(6):1250–4.

74. Kalugdan T, Chan PJ, Seraj IM, King A. Polymerase chain reaction enzyme-linked immunosorbent assay detection of mycoplasma consensus gene in sperm with low oocyte penetration capacity. Fertil Steril. 1996;66(5):793–7.

75. Potts J, Payne RE. Prostatitis: infection, neuromuscular disorder, or pain syndrome? Proper patient classification is key. Cleve Clin J Med. 2007;74 Suppl 3:S63–71.

76. Núñez-Calonge R, Caballero P, Redondo C, Baquero F, Martínez-Ferrer M, Meseguer MA. Ureaplasma urealyticum reduces motility and induces membrane

alterations in human spermatozoa. Hum Reprod. 1998;13(10):2756–61.

77. Purvis K, Christiansen E. Infection in the male reproductive tract. Impact, diagnosis and treatment in relation to male infertility. Int J Androl. 1993;16(1):1–13.

78. Huwe P, Diemer T, Ludwig M, Liu J, Schiefer HG, Weidner W. Influence of different uropathogenic microorganisms on human sperm motility parameters in an in vitro experiment. Andrologia. 1998;30 Suppl 1:55–9.

79. Everaert K, Mahmoud A, Depuydt C, Maeyaert M, Comhaire F. Chronic prostatitis and male accessory gland infection—is there an impact on male infertility (diagnosis and therapy)? Andrologia. 2003;35(5):325–30.

80. Arya OP, Taber SR, editors. Venereal diseases and fertility in rural Uganda. Presented to the Medical Society for the Study of Venereal Diseases; 1975; Malta.

81. WHO. Neisseria gonorrhoeae and gonococcal infections. World Health Organization technical report series. 1978(616). p. 1–142.

82. Arya OP, Bennett FJ. Role of the medical auxiliary in the control of sexually transmitted disease in a developing country. Br J Vener Dis. 1976;52(2): 116–21.

83. Osoba AO. Sexually transmitted diseases in tropical Africa. A review of the present situation. Br J Vener Dis. 1981;57(2):89–94.

84. Ndowa F, Lusti-Narasimhan M. The threat of untreatable gonorrhoea: implications and consequences for reproductive and sexual morbidity. Reprod Health Matters. 2012;20(40):76–82.

85. Cunningham KA, Beagley KW. Male genital tract chlamydial infection: implications for pathology and infertility. Biol Reprod. 2008;79(2):180–9.

86. Motrich RD, Cuffini C, Oberti JPM, Maccioni M, Rivero VE. Chlamydia trachomatis occurrence and its impact on sperm quality in chronic prostatitis patients. J Infect. 2006;53(3):175–83.

87. Eley A, Pacey AA, Galdiero M, Galdiero M, Galdiero F. Can Chlamydia trachomatis directly damage your sperm? Lancet Infect Dis. 2005;5(1):53–7.

88. Hosseinzadeh S, Eley A, Pacey AA. Semen quality of men with asymptomatic chlamydial infection. J Androl. 2004;25(1):104–9.

89. Vigil P, Morales P, Tapia A, Riquelme R, Salgado AM. Chlamydia trachomatis infection in male partners of infertile couples: incidence and sperm function. Andrologia. 2002;34(3):155–61.

90. Eggert-Kruse W, Neuer A, Clussmann C, Boit R, Geissler W, Rohr G, et al. Seminal antibodies to human 60kd heat shock protein (HSP 60) in male partners of subfertile couples. Hum Reprod. 2002;17(3):726–35.

91. Videau SP, Vivas JC, Salazar N. IgA antibodies to Chlamydia trachomatis and seminal parameters in asymptomatic infertile males. Arch Androl. 2001;46(3):189–95.

92. Gdoura R, Kchaou W, Chaari C, Znazen A, Keskes L, Rebai T, et al. Ureaplasma urealyticum, Ureaplasma parvum, Mycoplasma hominis and Mycoplasma genitalium infections and semen quality of infertile men. BMC Infect Dis. 2007;7:129.

93. Tully JG, Taylor-Robinson D, Cole RM, Rose DL. A newly discovered mycoplasma in the human urogenital tract. Lancet. 1981;1(8233):1288–91.

94. Yoshida T, Maeda S-I, Deguchi T, Ishiko H. Phylogeny-based rapid identification of mycoplasmas and ureaplasmas from urethritis patients. J Clin Microbiol. 2002;40(1):105–10.

95. Xu C, Sun GF, Zhu YF, Wang YF. The correlation of Ureaplasma urealyticum infection with infertility. Andrologia. 1997;29(4):219–26.

96. Megory E, Zuckerman H, Shoham Z, Lunenfeld B. Infections and male fertility. Obstet Gynecol Surv. 1987;42(5):283–90.

97. de Jong Z, Pontonnier F, Plante P, Perie N, Talazac N, Mansat A, et al. Comparison of the incidence of Ureaplasma urealyticum in infertile men and in donors of semen. Eur Urol. 1990;18(2):127–31.

98. Ombelet W, Bosmans E, Janssen M, Cox A, Vlasselaer J, Gyselaers W, et al. Semen parameters in a fertile versus subfertile population: a need for change in the interpretation of semen testing. Hum Reprod. 1997;12(5):987–93.

99. Pajovic B, Radojevic N, Vukovic M, Stjepcevic A. Semen analysis before and after antibiotic treatment of asymptomatic chlamydia- and ureaplasma-related pyospermia. Andrologia. 2013;45(4):266–71.

100. Upadhyaya M, Hibbard BM, Walker SM. The effect of Ureaplasma urealyticum on semen characteristics. Fertil Steril. 1984;41(2):304–8.

101. Wang Y, Liang C-L, Wu J-Q, Xu C, Qin S-X, Gao E-S. Do Ureaplasma urealyticum infections in the genital tract affect semen quality? Asian J Androl. 2006;8(5):562–8.

102. Naessens A, Foulon W, Debrucker P, Devroey P, Lauwers S. Recovery of microorganisms in semen and relationship to semen evaluation. Fertil Steril. 1986;45(1):101–5.

103. Reichart M, Levi H, Kahane I, Bartoov B. Dual energy metabolism-dependent effect of Ureaplasma urealyticum infection on sperm activity. J Androl. 2001;22(3):404–12.

104. Reichart M, Kahane I, Bartoov B. In vivo and in vitro impairment of human and ram sperm nuclear chromatin integrity by sexually transmitted Ureaplasma urealyticum infection. Biol Reprod. 2000;63(4):1041–8.

105. Montagut JM, Leprêtre S, Degoy J, Rousseau M. Ureaplasma in semen and IVF. Hum Reprod. 1991;6(5):727–9.

106. Knox CL, Allan JA, Allan JM, Edirisinghe WR, Stenzel D, Lawrence FA, et al. Ureaplasma parvum and Ureaplasma urealyticum are detected in semen after washing before assisted reproductive technology procedures. Fertil Steril. 2003;80(4):921–9.

107. Deguchi T, Maeda S-I. Mycoplasma genitalium: another important pathogen of nongonococcal urethritis. J Urol. 2002;167(3):1210–7.
108. Kjaergaard N, Kristensen B, Hansen ES, Farholt S, Schønheyder HC, Uldbjerg N, et al. Microbiology of semen specimens from males attending a fertility clinic. APMIS. 1997;105(7):566–70.
109. Rosemond A, Lanotte P, Watt S, Sauget AS, Guerif F, Royère D, et al. [Systematic screening tests for Chlamydia trachomatis, Mycoplasma hominis and Ureaplasma urealyticum in urogenital specimens of infertile couples]. Pathol Biol. 2006;54(3):125–9.
110. Bornman MS, Mahomed MF, Boomker D, Schulenburg GW, Reif S, Crewe-brown HH. [Microbial flora in semen of infertile African men at Garankuwa hospital]. Andrologia. 1990;22(2):118–21.
111. Díaz-García FJ, Herrera-Mendoza AP, Giono-Cerezo S, Guerra-Infante FM. Mycoplasma hominis attaches to and locates intracellularly in human spermatozoa. Hum Reprod. 2006;21(6):1591–8.
112. Andrade-Rocha FT. Ureaplasma urealyticum and Mycoplasma hominis in men attending for routine semen analysis. Prevalence, incidence by age and clinical settings, influence on sperm characteristics, relationship with the leukocyte count and clinical value. Urol Int. 2003;71(4):377–81.
113. Dejucq N, Jegou B. Viruses in the mammalian male genital tract and their effects on the reproductive system. Microbiol Mol Biol Rev. 2001;65(2):208–31.
114. Ochsendorf FR. Sexually transmitted infections: impact on male fertility. Andrologia. 2008;40(2):72–5.
115. Bezold G, Politch JA, Kiviat NB, Kuypers JM, Wolff H, Anderson DJ. Prevalence of sexually transmissible pathogens in semen from asymptomatic male infertility patients with and without leukocytospermia. Fertil Steril. 2007;87(5):1087–97.
116. Kapranos N, Petrakou E, Anastasiadou C, Kotronias D. Detection of herpes simplex virus, cytomegalovirus, and Epstein-Barr virus in the semen of men attending an infertility clinic. Fertil Steril. 2003;79 Suppl 3:1566–70.
117. Yang YS, Ho HN, Chen HF, Chen SU, Shen CY, Chang SF, et al. Cytomegalovirus infection and viral shedding in the genital tract of infertile couples. J Med Virol. 1995;45(2):179–82.
118. Bujan L, Sergerie M, Moinard N, Martinet S, Porte L, Massip P, et al. Decreased semen volume and spermatozoa motility in HIV-1-infected patients under antiretroviral treatment. J Androl. 2007;28(3):444–52.
119. CDC. Monitoring selected national HIV prevention and care objectives by using HIV surveillance data—United States and 6 U.S. Dependent Areas—2010. Center for Disease Control (CDC). 2012. p. 1–27.
120. CDC. Estimated HIV incidence in the United States, 2007 through 2010. Center for Disease Control (CDC). 2012. p. 1–26.
121. Dulioust E, Tachet A, De Almeida M, Finkielsztejn L, Rivalland S, Salmon D, et al. Detection of HIV-1 in seminal plasma and seminal cells of HIV-1 seropositive men. J Reprod Immunol. 1998;41(1–2):27–40.
122. Bandivdekar AH, Velhal SM, Raghavan VP. Identification of CD4-independent HIV receptors on spermatozoa. Am J Reprod Immunol. 2003;50(4):322–7.
123. Shevchuk MM, Pigato JB, Khalife G, Armenakas NA, Fracchia JA. Changing testicular histology in AIDS: its implication for sexual transmission of HIV. Urology. 1999;53(1):203–8.
124. van Leeuwen E, Wit FW, Prins JM, Reiss P, van der Veen F, Repping S. Semen quality remains stable during 96 weeks of untreated human immunodeficiency virus-1 infection. Fertil Steril. 2008;90(3):636–41.
125. Krieger JN, Coombs RW, Collier AC, Koehler JK, Ross SO, Chaloupka K, et al. Fertility parameters in men infected with human immunodeficiency virus. J Infect Dis. 1991;164(3):464–9.
126. Nicopoullos JDM, Almeida PA, Ramsay JWA, Gilling-Smith C. The effect of human immunodeficiency virus on sperm parameters and the outcome of intrauterine insemination following sperm washing. Hum Reprod. 2004;19(10):2289–97.
127. Dulioust E, Du AL, Costagliola D, Guibert J, Kunstmann J-M, Heard I, et al. Semen alterations in HIV-1 infected men. Hum Reprod. 2002;17(8):2112–8.
128. Politch JA, Mayer KH, Abbott AF, Anderson DJ. The effects of disease progression and zidovudine therapy on semen quality in human immunodeficiency virus type 1 seropositive men. Fertil Steril. 1994;61(5):922–8.
129. Dondero F, Rossi T, D'Offizi G, Mazzilli F, Rosso R, Sarandrea N, et al. Semen analysis in HIV seropositive men and in subjects at high risk for HIV infection. Hum Reprod. 1996;11(4):765–8.
130. Crittenden JA, Handelsman DJ, Stewart GJ. Semen analysis in human immunodeficiency virus infection. Fertil Steril. 1992;57(6):1294–9.
131. Muller CH, Coombs RW, Krieger JN. Effects of clinical stage and immunological status on semen analysis results in human immunodeficiency virus type 1-seropositive men. Andrologia. 1998;30 Suppl 1:15–22.
132. Kehl S, Weigel M, Müller D, Gentili M, Hornemann A, Sütterlin M. HIV-infection and modern antiretroviral therapy impair sperm quality. Arch Gynecol Obstet. 2011;284(1):229–33.
133. Taylor S, Ferguson NM, Cane PA, Anderson RM, Pillay D. Dynamics of seminal plasma HIV-1 decline after antiretroviral treatment. AIDS. 2001;15(3):424–6.
134. van Leeuwen E, Wit FW, Repping S, Eeftinck Schattenkerk JKM, Reiss P, van der Veen F, et al. Effects of antiretroviral therapy on semen quality. AIDS. 2008;22(5):637–42.

135. Coombs RW, Lockhart D, Ross SO, Deutsch L, Dragavon J, Diem K, et al. Lower genitourinary tract sources of seminal HIV. J Acquir Immune Defic Syndr. 2006;41(4):430–8.

136. Barboza JM, Medina H, Doria M, Rivero L, Hernandez L, Joshi NV. Use of atomic force microscopy to reveal sperm ultrastructure in HIV-patients on highly active antiretroviral therapy. Arch Androl. 2004;50(2):121–9.

137. Bezold G, Schuster-Grusser A, Lange M, Gall H, Wolff H, Peter RU. Prevalence of human herpesvirus types 1-8 in the semen of infertility patients and correlation with semen parameters. Fertil Steril. 2001;76(2):416–8.

138. el Borai N, Inoue M, Lefèvre C, Naumova EN, Sato B, Yamamura M. Detection of herpes simplex DNA in semen and menstrual blood of individuals attending an infertility clinic. J Obstet Gynaecol Res. 1997;23(1):17–24.

139. Kotronias D, Kapranos N. Detection of herpes simplex virus DNA in human spermatozoa by in situ hybridization technique. In Vivo. 1998;12(4):391–4.

140. el Borai N, Lefèvre C, Inoue M, Naumova EN, Sato K, Suzuki S, et al. Presence of HSV-1 DNA in semen and menstrual blood. J Reprod Immunol. 1998;41(1–2):137–47.

141. Lai YM, Lee JF, Huang HY, Soong YK, Yang FP, Pao CC. The effect of human papillomavirus infection on sperm cell motility. Fertil Steril. 1997;67(6):1152–5.

Psychological Stress and Male Infertility

10

S.C. Basu

Introduction

The Oxford Dictionary defines the word stress as "a state of affair involving demand on physical or mental energy." Stress could be physical and psychological. The psychological stress results from a mental perception in not being able to cope with an untoward situation. It is characterized by a state of disturbed homeostasis that evokes complex physiological and behavioral response. It is generally a natural phenomenon and necessary environmental demand for mobilizing the body resources in an adverse state. Human psychological stress response reflects differences in personality, physical strength, or general health and often varies according to the individual cultural, ethnic, and religious norms [1, 2].

When stress was first studied in the 1950s, the term was used to denote both its causes and the effects. More recently, however, the word stressor has been used for the stimulus that provokes or initiates a stress response. Acute stress developing in course of many day-to-day events evokes adrenergic activation and it is not morbific. Chronic stress, on the other hand, involves heightened intensity

S.C. Basu, MBBS, FRCS (Edinburgh), FRCS (England), FICS, FACS (✉)
Surgery and Urology, Consultant Urologist and Male Infertility Specialist, Fortis C-DOC Healthcare Ltd, B-16, Chirag Enclave, New Delhi 110048, India
e-mail: scbasu@vsnl.com; scibasu@gmail.com

of the stressors, and persistent exposure to them may lead to systemic response disproportionate to the actual adversity. Psychological stress is often a natural outcome of male infertility that acts as a chronic stressor in affected persons [3, 4]. Approximately, 15 % couples are affected by infertility and up to half of these cases arise from male infertility [5].

Infertility is multifaceted and unique to every person challenged with the problem. It is a complicated issue for men, which normally induces them to be the reluctant partner to seek medical advice. Historically, more attention has been focused on treating female infertility than male factor problems. Studies concerning effects on infertile males are few in number and have come to the forefront in the past decade starting in 2001. Not a single article on male infertility appeared in the Psychoanalytic Electronic Publishing archives of the seven primary psychoanalytic journals from 1927 to 2000.

Malik [6] from the Institute of Work, Health, and Organizations (Nottingham University, UK) said, "Men are in fact equally affected by the unfulfilled desire for a child but are less open about their feelings." This could explain the reticence of infertile men to subject themselves to medical examination despite infertility being a conjugal issue. In this regard, perhaps relatively less number of specialists dealing with male reproductive medicine could be an additional factor. Takefman [7] reported in Infertility Awareness Association of Canada website that the American Society of Reproductive Medicine statistics in 2007

S.S. du Plessis et al. (eds.), *Male Infertility: A Complete Guide to Lifestyle and Environmental Factors*, 141
DOI 10.1007/978-1-4939-1040-3_10, © Springer Science+Business Media New York 2014

Table 10.1 Effects of psychological stress

1. Emotional effects—depression, lack of self-esteem, stigma, grief, isolation, etc.
2. Reproductive effects—loss of libido, erectile or ejaculatory dysfunction, deterioration of sperm parameters

had 65 % of its members from the obstetricians and gynecologists, whereas only 10 % constituted urologists or andrologists.

Notwithstanding the paucity of psychological studies on male infertility, it is common knowledge that a significant proportion of infertile men experience a variety of psychological trauma. The manifestations and effects of psychological stress in males with infertility are diverse and variable. Typical manifestations of psychological stress include myriad change in emotional behavior, sexual dysfunction, and decreased fertility. However, the general and reproductive effects of psychological stress are entwined and adversely complementary in any infertile male [8–10].

Often overlooked, psychological stress has a large role in male infertility. Morrow [11] suggested that every sixth couple is infertile and 40 % of infertile individuals experience significant emotional and psychological distress with possible long-term implications. Smith [12] reported findings of a study at the annual meeting of the American Urological Association (AUA) in 2008 that infertile males experience emotional and social distress validating that the male partner of the infertile couple experiences significant psychosocial stress. Psychological stress leads not only to emotional effects but also cast its shadow on the reproduction as shown in Table 10.1.

Effects on Emotional Behavior

Infertility is frequently perceived by the couple as an enormous psychological stress. It seems only logical that a couple failing to achieve the expected goal of reproduction will experience feelings of disappointment, frustration, grief, depression, low self-esteem, and eventual marital problems, which adversely contribute to the psychological stress. If stress leads to infertility,

then infertility leads to more stress. A vicious cycle is formed with what might lead to a dead end.

Infertility is a very private form of grief and often the infertile couple grieves alone mostly without social support. This grief has nothing to focus on as the loss is hidden. The loss of a child wanted albeit in imagination but never conceived, logically is tantamount to a loss much like suffering a miscarriage or a stillborn baby. Isolation or loneliness is another common experience among infertile couples. Most people having children are incapable of comprehending the complex mind-set of an infertile couple and fail to recognize that infertility could be a source of grief [13–15].

A child born from donor insemination or in vitro fertilization (*IVF*) does not change a male mind-set radically although becoming a father might give him some solace. However, it is undeniable that a man's perception about his shortcoming to impregnate his spouse in the natural way can lead to stressful situation. Schover et al. [16] reported one study that concluded 80 % of 100 infertile men developed guilt feelings from their failure to prove manhood with its attendant consequence of not fulfilling partner's desire to have an offspring.

Infertile men could suffer from episodes of depression, anxiety, and sleep disturbance. Furthermore, their feelings of inadequacy might lead to detachment in the marriage from shame, anger, isolation, sense of personal failure, lowering of self-esteem, and loss of libido. Additional psychological disorders like substance abuse, alcohol addiction, and mood disorders are not uncommon occurrence in these men. In one study covering 127 infertile couples, psychological components were found to play a significant role in infertility of unknown etiology, especially in the male partners, which affected their personality and social behavior, and caused anxiety [7, 17, 18].

Self-esteem often is the commonest casualty in male infertility. The feeling of inadequacy as a man dents his self-image, and psychological stress is a natural outcome of this state of mind. The inadequacy in infertile men stems from social ridicule and often results in low self-esteem [19]. Fatherhood is traditionally a sociocultural determinant of masculinity in the Middle East and subcontinent of India, Pakistan, and Bangladesh. Consequently, these societies look down upon men deprived of fatherhood. This stigma leads them to lose their self-esteem and inculcate a belief as a second-grade citizen not being able to prove their masculinity.

In the subcontinent, especially in India, a man's self-esteem takes a beating, when in a joint family a brother younger and marrying later beats him in the race of becoming a father. People are conditioned to assume that they are born fertile and could control the event of pregnancy at will, just as they could postpone having babies by taking contraceptive measures. Depression and hopelessness naturally emerge from the situation that dispossesses them of their so-called control and choice [13].

Miall [20] also found that male infertility was frequently seen as arising from sexual dysfunction and was associated with a higher level of stigma than in females. Moreover, many people assume that infertile men cannot perform sexually. This stigma adds to the heightened insecurity in infertile men. Peronace [17] from the School of Psychology at Cardiff University discoursed that male infertility brings on such a degree of social stigma that it naturally leads to stress and at times a culture of secrecy. The stigma adds to the heightened insecurity in infertile men. Muller, from the University of Mainz, Germany, said, "Sexual dissatisfaction of infertile men could also be related to a withdrawal from sexual activities and hence to even lower chance of conception" [21].

Feelings about fertility and sexual adequacy are interconnected for many men. Couples with long-term infertility report a higher level of depression, low satisfaction with their sex lives, and low level of well-being. The adverse feeling of not being able to satisfy his partner with a child can not only lead to depression but also strain on the sexual relationship. It then becomes a recipe for adversely affecting the man's sense of well-being. The report by Smith [12] at the AUA in 2008 claimed 25 % of patients having high levels of stressful partner relationship, 15 % reported serious issues with their marriage,

and 17 % incidence of treatment of infertility itself becoming the source of significant stress. An infertile man could sometime be beleaguered by the thought of his spouse deserting him for his inability to prove his manhood, and this becomes an additional source of his psychological stress.

With psychological stress, infertile men tend to suppress their emotions and show alexithymic characteristics, which might assume important clinical implications. Alexithymia is characterized by difficulties in describing emotion in words, identifying and communicating emotions. Frequently, alexithymic individuals are unaware of what their feelings are. Psychotherapist Peter Sifneos devised the term alexithymia to describe a state of deficiency in understanding, processing, or describing emotions [22, 23]. There is some evidence that the non-expression of emotion and a tendency to develop somatic complaints have close association [24–28]. Hesse et al. [29] suggested in a study that alexithymia was found to be correlated with impaired understanding and demonstration of affection to the partner. This could let down partner relationship. Furthermore, there is a positive correlation between the alexithymia levels in patients and psychogenic erectile problem [30]. Taylor et al. [31] opined that male infertility may be a symptom or consequence of alexithymia.

Effects on Reproductive Function

Psychological stress is one among many forms of stress that often affect male fertility and reproduction [32]. Chronic psychological stress disrupts male reproductive function that could often negatively influence count, motility and morphology of spermatozoa, and couple fecundability [10]. Besides it causes higher frequency of male sexual disturbances.

Sex is not more than just a physical response and arousal is unquestionably tied to emotions. Stress is a common consequence of modern-day fast life where achievement is the yardstick to material success. A normal male sexual response cycle comprises four interactive, nonlinear stages: desire, arousal, orgasm, and resolution [33] as shown in Table 10.2 and Fig. 10.1a. Orgasm usually coincides with ejaculation, but represents a distinct cognitive and emotional cortical event. Any disruption of this normal cycle may lead to various sexual dysfunctions as shown in Fig. 10.1b.

The most common problems in infertile men are psychosexual disorders like decreased libido, ejaculatory and erectile dysfunctions, orgasmic failure, and deterioration of sperm parameters (Table 10.3). Moreover, there may be disturbed pattern of sexual interaction between partners that leads to mutual discontentment [34].

Table 10.2 Phases of the male sexual cycle

1. Desire (libido)—fantasies, thoughts, feelings
2. Excitement—pleasure and erection
3. Orgasm—emission and ejaculation
4. Resolution—relaxation and refractory period

Table 10.3 Reproductive dysfunctions

1. Loss of libido
2. Erectile dysfunctions
3. Ejaculatory dysfunctions
4. Deterioration of sperm parameters

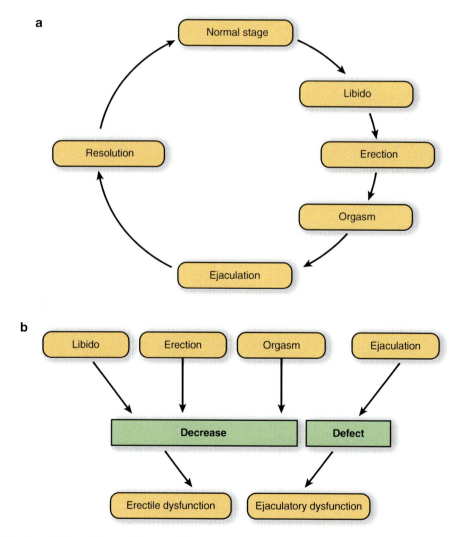

Fig. 10.1 Normal (**a**) and abnormal (**b**) sexual function

Loss of Libido

Stress is known to have a negative influence on the libido. It operates in a cyclical manner. Stress leads to decreased libido with resultant failure to consummate marriage. Depression also suppresses positive feelings and emotions, which inhibit libido and the desire for sexual activity. Most men have experienced either a loss of libido or an inability to maintain an erection during periods of stress. However, these episodes are usually transient, and once the stress factor is eliminated, normal sexual function resumes.

Erectile Dysfunctions

Feelings of stress, depression, guilt, or anxiety in infertile men can cause psychogenic erectile dysfunction that naturally leads to feeling of sexual inadequacy, often a common accompaniment of infertility. Incidentally, erectile dysfunction is much more likely to occur among men with a submissive personality [35].

Causes of Psychological Erectile Failure

The human brain including the CNS has an inbuilt mechanism not only to integrally deal with the initiation of erection but also in suppressing the process. Normally there is a balance between the excitatory and inhibitory impulses, depending on the circumstances [36].

Penile erection has two different underlying mechanisms. The first one is a reflex erection initiated by direct tactile sensation on the penile shaft and the second one or psychogenic erection is the result of erotic or emotional stimulus. The former is mediated by peripheral nerves and the lower spinal cord, whereas the latter uses the limbic system and the brain. A message or impulse is sent following stimulation of the penile shaft to initiate the secretion of nitric oxide (NO) to relax the penile erectile tissue resulting in erection. But if necessary, it could send chemical transmitters to cause constriction of the penile vasculature, thus inhibiting the normal mechanism of erection [37].

Subconscious memory of previous failure to perform completely adequate sexual act often subsequently causes recurrent failure to achieve adequate erection—a phenomenon described as performance anxiety. In this instance, erectile failure results from negative response to psychological reasons like erotic feelings and thoughts in contradistinction to any organic disease.

Stress, depression, guilt, or anxiety in infertile men can cause psychogenic erectile failure that makes the feeling of inadequacy more intense. These emotional reactions may undermine previous belief of being sexually adequate. Consequently it weighs on male minds with resultant mental instability and eventual erectile failure. Most men experience occasional psychological erectile failure due to isolated episodes ascribed to fatigue or stress. Fatigue affects all at certain times and is a common cause of temporary psychological erectile failure. However, once fatigue is reduced, normal sexuality is restored.

If the man reacts to this occasional episode of erectile failure to become more anxious, it could aggravate anxiety. This may culminate in a domino effect ending in more anxiety and more failure, and eventually could lead to persistent performance anxiety and further worsening of self-esteem. The psychological stress of infertility has been shown to affect sperm parameters in significant and demonstrable ways that may further contribute to erectile problems as evidenced by studies showing association between depression and erectile dysfunction [6, 21].

Ejaculatory Dysfunctions

Ejaculation is perhaps the most important sub-event in the erectile response of males. The normal ejaculatory process requires coordination and integration of neurologic, physiologic, anatomic, and psychological events. Any breakdown in the coordination of these events can lead to ejaculatory problems. Abnormal ejaculation could manifest in various forms like premature ejaculation, retrograde ejaculation, delayed ejaculation, or anejaculation. Some of the ejaculatory problems could be ascribed to psychological stress (Fig. 10.2).

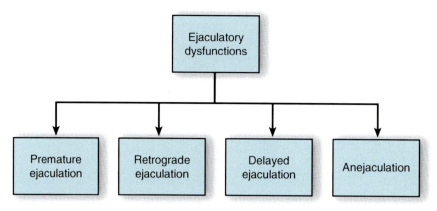

Fig. 10.2 Ejaculatory dysfunctions

Premature Ejaculation

Premature ejaculation (PE) is a common and distressing male sexual dysfunction. Several attempts made over the years to define PE by organizations like WHO (1994), American Psychiatric Association (2000), European Association of Urology (2001), and American Association of Urology (2004) have failed to achieve its holistic and unambiguous definition until that by the International Society of Sexual Medicine (ISSM) in 2009. WHO defined (1994) PE as an inability to delay ejaculation sufficiently to enjoy lovemaking, which manifests as either occurrence of ejaculation before or very soon after the beginning of intercourse (within 15 sec of the beginning of intercourse) or occurrence of ejaculation in the absence of sufficient erection to make intercourse possible. The publication of multidimensional new classification Diagnostic and Statistical Manual of Mental Disorders or DSM-V is now awaited. Some researchers have characterized PE as being psychogenic in origin, while others postulated "biogenic" causes. The proponents of psychogenic theory ascribe PE to anxiety. Some PE types are neurobiologically or medically determined [38–42].

Retrograde Ejaculation

Retrograde ejaculation causing expulsion of semen into the urinary bladder during orgasm is certainly a rare phenomenon that often follows psychological or emotional stress. Probably the underlying pathology could be ascribed to abnormal functioning of the sympathetic system culminating in closure of the posterior sphincter of the urethra during orgasm, thus pushing the semen into the urinary bladder. Frequently, it originates from the result of lesions, like post-prostatectomy, following pelvic operations; diabetes mellitus; bilateral sympathectomy; local vascular disturbances; neurological diseases; and use of different sympatholytic drugs. But in some cases where no organic disease is detected, psychiatric investigations in some of these males have shown extreme animosity and aggressiveness toward the spouse or mental unpreparedness for fatherhood. It is thus logical that in these cases emotional stress possibly precipitates malfunction in the sympathetic system leading to the closure of the posterior sphincter of the urethra during orgasm.

Delayed Ejaculation

Delayed ejaculation is characterized by an extended period of sexual stimulation for a man to reach sexual climax and ejaculate semen. Normally a man can achieve orgasm within 5 min of active thrusting during sexual intercourse. A man with delayed ejaculation either fails to have orgasm at all or achieves it only after prolonged period of intercourse. Most cases of delayed ejaculation present with climaxing and ejaculating only during masturbation, but failing to ejaculate during normal sexual intercourse [43–45].

Both retrograde and delayed ejaculations interfere with the propulsion of the spermatozoa along with the secretion from the seminal vesicles into the posterior urethra. Only examination of the split ejaculate for acid phosphatase and fructose can help in the diagnosis of this condition. It should be emphasized that these ejaculatory dysfunctions are not common.

In some cases, significant differences are noted between semen analysis of specimens obtained by masturbation and after postcoital test. The extreme clinical manifestation of abnormal ejaculation was described as sham ejaculation by Palti [43] which perhaps can be described presently close to delayed ejaculation or retarded ejaculation.

Palti described the clinical manifestation of sham ejaculation, where the affected males showed azoospermia in specimen obtained under extreme emotional stress. But the normal postcoital specimen had near normal or normal semen analysis. This can be attributed to extreme stress causing reduced volume of seminal fluid constituting only the prostatic secretion with absence of spermatozoa. Michael [46] reported that in these cases, there was a significant difference between semen analysis after masturbation and normal postcoital test with no spermatozoa found in postcoital specimen. It was postulated that this is perhaps the result of an abnormal response to the sympathetic stimulus taking place in the seminal vesicles and ampulla of the vas deferens with resultant spastic contraction of the ejaculatory ducts.

Anejaculation

Ejaculatory dysfunction in men, who is unable to ejaculate at all, is described as anejaculation. Anejaculation is different from retrograde ejaculation where the semen with spermatozoa does not travel up to the bladder. It results from inability to ejaculate or persistent difficulty in achieving orgasm despite the presence of normal sexual desire and sexual stimulation.

Effects on Sperm Parameters

Certainly stress can affect sperm production, but it is not consistent and does not follow a definite pattern. Individual men handle stressors differently and their system handles sperm production differently. The effects induced by stress seem to include meiotic and structural alterations in spermatozoa.

Stress can negatively impact on the movement of spermatozoa and reduce their ability to reach the oocyte. Stress makes it difficult for the sperm to actually reach the ovum. A study of a group of 225 infertile men demonstrated that stress was one of the factors that negatively correlated with semen parameters [47]. The study subjects, 80 % of which admitted to being in a stressful professional or personal situation, were associated with abnormal morphology and reduced viability of their spermatozoa. This observation of adverse sperm parameters have been substantiated by Eskiocak et al. [48, 49] indicating that mental stress negatively affected semen quality probably due to injurious component of increased superoxide dismutase (SOD) activities working on the reactive oxygen species (ROS).

In 1,076 men of infertile couples, psychological factors, i.e., exposure to acute stress, coping with stress, the WHO Well-Being Index, and the Zung's Anxiety Scale Inventory scores were assessed by a questionnaire at the time of semen analysis. Regression analyses indicated a significant positive relationship between sperm concentration and the WHO Well-Being Index score, each successive score number accounting for a 7.3 % increase in sperm concentration [50].

Psychological stress interferes with the endocrine and spermatogenetic function of male gonads [9]. Stress-induced hormonal changes depend on the severity and nature of the stressor, duration of exposure to the stressor, and the baseline condition of the body. Negro-Vilar [51] had suggested that the response to stress is not unique to the human race but also manifests in other animals. Blanchard et al. [52] mentioned that chronic or severe stress in animals or humans was associated with decrease in sperm count, motility, and morphology. Depression in infertile males is common and is a contributory factor to cause decreased sperm concentration. In infertile couples, a higher frequency of male sexual disturbances expressed as erectile dysfunction, ejaculatory disorders, loss of libido, and a decrease in the frequency of intercourse is observed. In men excess levels of cortisol, produced under stress, can affect the normal functioning of the reproductive system. Chronic stress can impair testosterone and sperm production, and cause erectile problem.

The forced timing of intercourse synchronizing with the female's ovulation period, as often advised for treating infertility, is associated with psychological pressure, and men may experience inadequate sexual satisfaction. The arduous nature of infertility treatment often compounds the stressful state of an infertile couple, and psychological stress in these patients tends to increase as treatment intensifies and the duration of treatment extends.

It has also been observed that there is an inverse relationship between semen quality and psychological stress in infertile subjects undergoing IVF [53–55]. Some authors observed that stressful situations related to the diagnosis of subfertility or infertility can reduce the pleasure of sex [56]. This aspect has been reiterated by James Smith et al. [12] at the annual meeting of the AUA in 2008 indicating that this type of psychological stress in a couple diagnosed with infertility often causes serious problems with partner relationship.

Oligospermia and Teratospermia

Oligospermia is generally considered to be the result of organic or biological defects during spermatogenesis. Information in the medical literature related to the relationship of psychogenic stress and abnormal spermatogenesis is at best unclear, in contrast to the number of publications on female ovulation disorders and amenorrhea under a similar psychological backdrop. Wolfram [57] and Perloff [58] indicated that emotional stress might lead to oligospermia. Steve [59] had shown that testicular biopsies on men awaiting sentence for rape showed complete spermatogenetic arrest, yet some of the raped women became pregnant, testifying the normal fertility potential in these accused men at the time of the crime. He hypothesized that anxiety and psychological tension was the causative factor for this organic change.

Zondek et al. [60] demonstrated the existence of two types of oligospermia—permanent and periodic. The semen analysis of the latter group showed normal and abnormal sperm parameters alternately. The fact that improvement of sperm parameters sometimes occurred spontaneously or after the use of a placebo supports the theory of the role of psychological factors in this condition. The effects of sperm parameters in psychological stress in 157 volunteers showed that the fecundity of men experiencing stress caused by family bereavement might be temporarily diminished. There is also a significant decline in semen quality of male IVF patients during egg retrieval stages, thereby demonstrating an inverse relationship between semen quality and specific aspects of psychological stress [54, 55].

Appropriate set of controls are often difficult to find in establishing the relationship between psychological stress and male infertility. Most of the investigations performed in the last two decades have not conclusively showed the precise cause and effect in terms of stress and infertility. There are instances where the psychological stress is the result and not the cause of infertility [61]. However, there is now growing evidence that stress always stands as an additional risk factor for infertility even if it is not the primary cause. It is obvious that once infertility and psychological stress coexist, they set up a cascading effect [15].

A review of literature on the psychological background of male infertility caused by gonadal problem reveals two possible hypotheses [62]. One group of articles explored the possibility that infertility may have psychological causes (*psychogenic hypothesis*) and others examined the psychological consequences of infertility (*psychological consequences hypothesis*). The psychogenic hypothesis theory is now abandoned by most researchers. The majority of the studies rejected the theory of stress as a lone factor in the etiology of infertility.

Homeostatic Changes

Any alteration in the human behavioral pattern involves an underlying change in the biochemical, hormonal, cellular, and molecular components in the homeostasis (Table 10.4).

Table 10.4 Homeostatic changes at biochemical, hormonal neurotransmitter, cellular, or molecular levels

1. Biochemical changes—involving L-arginine–NO pathway and oxidative stress on sperms and erectile function
2. Hormonal changes—in hormones involved in HPA axis and HPT axis
3. Neurotransmitter changes
4. Cellular or molecular changes

Biochemical Changes

While investigating the association between psychological stress and semen quality, many studies ignored the biochemical changes accompanying the effect of stress on the L-arginine–NO pathway. The highly reactive free radical NO is synthesized from L-arginine by the isoenzyme nitric oxide synthase (NOS) present in the male reproductive system. Immunohistopathological studies have demonstrated the presence and localization of NOS throughout the male genitourinary tract, especially in the forms of eNOS in the vascular endothelium and nNOS in the neurons.

NO is of critical importance in the physiology of erection by causing relaxation of the vascular and corporal smooth muscle cells of the penile arteries and trabeculae. NO is thought to act centrally in the medial preoptic area and the paraventricular nucleus to modulate sexual behavior, thus exerting effects on the penis. Adequate levels of testosterone from the testes and proper functioning of the pituitary gland are essential for the development of a healthy erectile system.

NO has dual and contrary roles depending on its concentration. Under normal physiological conditions in a no-stress situation the NO concentration is low. It then plays an important and beneficial role in normal sperm production and motility by neutralizing free radicals and thereby prevents the reduction of sperm motility mediated by ROS [63–65]. On the contrary, higher NO concentration under stressful condition has detrimental and cytotoxic effects on the spermatozoa as evidenced by negative correlation with concentration, motility index, and percentage of rapid progressive motility of spermatozoa [66].

Table 10.5 L-Arginine–NO pathway and its implication in stress on sperm parameters

1. L-Arginine is acted upon by NO synthase to produce NO
2. Arginase regulates the activity of NOS. Lower arginase activity is associated with poor sperm parameter
3. NO level under nonstress condition is relatively low—so it can exert beneficial effect on sperm parameters. This effect is helped by NOS inhibitors. Low NO level and NOS inhibitors also play down the ROS activity, thus helping in maintaining normal sperm parameters
4. NO level shows higher value under stress. This has a negative effect on sperm parameters by aggravating ROS activities
5. A negative correlation between seminal plasma NO level and arginase activity during stress indicates its role in the L-arginine–NO pathway
6. The L-arginine–NO pathway, together with arginase and NOS, has thus a role in changing the semen quality under stress

The arginine-depleting enzyme, arginase, plays an important part in the cellular regulatory system affecting NOS activity. NOS inhibitors inhibit the formation of excess NO and prevent the reduction of sperm motility as well as their survival. It was also postulated that arginase may be inhibited by the end products of NO. Elgun et al. [67] have shown that spermatozoa from infertile men with oligospermia have a significantly higher arginase activity than controls. They reported a positive correlation between sperm motility and arginase activity in the infertile group in both seminal plasma and spermatozoa. L-Arginase–NO pathways and its implications in stress and on sperm parameters are summarized in Table 10.5 and Fig. 10.3.

In a similar study, Eskiocak et al. [48] assessed the semen parameters (motility, motility index, and abnormal morphology of spermatozoa), state anxiety scores, NO levels, and arginase activities of seminal plasma during the stress and nonstress periods in 29 healthy volunteer medical students with a gap of 3 months between the two sets of observation. This particular period of interval was specifically chosen to correspond approximately to the 74-day duration of human spermatogenesis and the sperm transit time (WHO-1993).

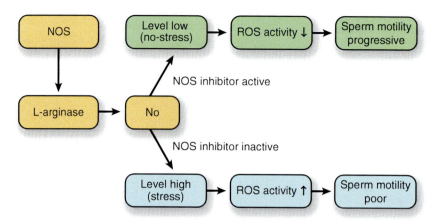

Fig. 10.3 Effects of NO level on ROS and sperm motility. *NO* nitric oxide, *NOS* nitric oxide synthase, *ROS* reactive oxygen species

Table 10.6 Relationship of seminal arginase and NO levels with sperm motility in stress and nonstress periods

	Stress period	Nonstress period
Seminal plasma arginase level	Low	High
NO level	High	Low
Sperm motility	Poor	Progressive

Psychological stress was measured by the widely used State Anxiety Inventory for assessing state or acute anxiety [68].

Eskiocak et al. [48] found that seminal plasma arginase levels were lower, while seminal plasma NO levels were higher during the stress period when compared to the nonstress situation. In addition, Eskiocak et al. [48, 49] investigated the values of antioxidant enzymes like SOD and catalase under stress and nonstress conditions.

During the nonstress period, there was a positive correlation between seminal plasma NO and progressive motility and motility index of spermatozoa. Relationship of seminal plasma arginase and NO levels in relation to the sperm motility in stress and nonstress periods is shown in Table 10.6. The L-arginine–NO pathway, together with arginase and NOS, is thus considered to be involved in semen quality under stress conditions.

The motility of spermatozoa is maintained by high levels of adenosine triphosphate (ATP). NO can reduce ATP levels in cells by inhibiting glycolysis and the electron transport chain. Excessive NO also contributes to the formation of a highly toxic anion peroxynitrite. Peroxynitrite reacts rapidly with proteins, lipids, and DNA and thus acts as destroyer of spermatozoa [48, 69]. Subsequent to ATP depletion and lipid peroxidation of the sperm membrane, motility of spermatozoa is compromised.

Hormonal Changes

Recent research, focusing on hormonal indicators of psychosocial stress, has helped in unraveling knowledge of the pathophysiology of neuroendocrinology for an in-depth assessment of the role of stress in infertility. Any stress, like psychological stress, leads to disturbance of internal homeostasis with resultant changes in the hormonal milieu. Essentially, these changes in the hormone profile are protective mechanisms to help deal with the stress. Depression, a prominent reaction to chronic psychological stress, also leads to an impaired regulation of stress hormones like cortisol (mainly) and norepinephrine (to some extent). The hormonal response to stress is directly proportional to the intensity of the stressor stimulus but varies to a great extent according to the individual man's perception of the stressful event [70].

The central nervous system (brain and spinal cord) plays a crucial role in the body's stress-related

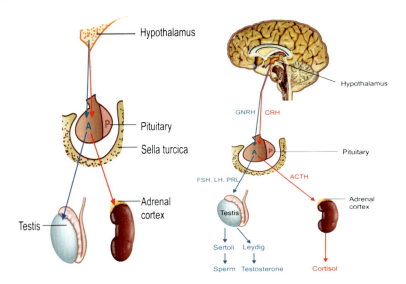

Fig. 10.4 HPA and HPT axes. *HPA* (hypothalamus–pituitary–adrenal) *axis*. Corticotrophin-releasing hormone (CRH) from hypothalamus acts on the anterior pituitary to release adrenocorticotrophic hormone (ACTH), which acts on the adrenal cortex to release cortisol. *HPT* (hypothalamus–pituitary–testis) *axis*. Hypothalamus releases GnRH, which acts on the anterior pituitary to release FSH and LH. FSH gets bound to the receptors on Sertoli cells to regulate spermatogenesis and LH to the receptors on Leydig cells to produce testosterone

mechanisms [71]. The paraventricular nucleus of the hypothalamus is responsible for the integrated response to stress. Besides the pituitary and the adrenal, other parts of the CNS like caudal nuclei, rostral raphe nuclei, and locus coeruleus in the pons, hippocampus, and amygdala take active roles in the biochemical event. The spinal cord performs the critical role in transferring neural impulses from the brain to the other parts of the body. The main components of the stress system are the corticotrophin-releasing hormone (CRH) and locus ceruleus–norepinephrine (LC/NE) autonomic systems and their peripheral effectors, the pituitary–adrenal axis and the limbs of the autonomic system [72].

The biological interaction between stress and infertility is the result of the activation of the hypothalamus–pituitary–adrenal (HPA) axis to set in motion a complex neuroendocrine response. Chronic stress of psychological origin is capable of summoning into action various hormones and cytokines to inhibit the hypothalamic–pituitary–testicular (HPT) axis at various levels with resultant disruption of the reproductive function [73]. The HPA axis constitutes CRH, ACTH (adrenocorticotrophic hormone), and cortisol.

The HPT axis is comprised of GnRH (gonadotrophin-releasing hormone), FSH (follicle-stimulating hormone), LH (luteinizing hormone), PRL (prolactin), and testosterone. HPA and HPT axes are shown in Fig. 10.4.

The effects of stress on reproduction appear to result from multilevel interactions between the hormonal stress response and the hormonal reproductive system represented respectively by the HPA axis and the HPT axis. The hypothalamus stimulated by the stressor inputs secretes CRH that are transported to the pituitary through the hypophyseal portal system to initiate the secretion of ACTH. The pituitary in turn stimulates the adrenal glands to release cortisol. ACTH activates the HPA axis and increases the secretion of cortisol from the adrenal, which is responsible for a number of changes in the body's metabolism. Cortisol is the most important human glucocorticoid.

The stress reaction initially induces activation of the adrenergic system, changes in mental setup, and eventually changes in the functioning of various endocrine glands as well as immune systems. Observations in humans with a background knowledge on animal studies unveil intricate mechanism of secretion of gonadotrophin hormones mainly though CRH and opioids (beta-endorphins). CRH increases the secretion of neuropeptides like ACTH, antidiuretic hormone (ADH), vasoactive intestinal peptide (VIP), and beta-endorphins.

CRH also plays an important role in inhibiting GnRH secretion during stress, while through somatostatin, it also inhibits GH (growth hormone), TRH (thyrotropin-releasing hormone produced by the hypothalamus in medial neurons of the paraventricular nucleus), and thyroid-stimulating hormone (TSH) secretions. As a result, there is suppression of reproductive, growth, and thyroid functions [71]. CRH inhibits the function of neurons that release GnRH directly and indirectly through stimulation of the secretion of beta-endorphins. Stress also inhibits TSH through the action of glucocorticoids on the central nervous system [74], causing its decreased production of TSH and also suppressing peripheral conversion of thyroxin to triiodothyronine. The testicular function may also be modified by prolactin, interferon-g, TNFα (*tumor necrosis factor-alpha*), and NK (*natural killer*) cells [75, 76].

Reduction in semen quality with the underlying mechanism is considered to be related to central impairment of the gonadotrophin drive in psychological stress [9]. In men excess levels of cortisol produced under stress can affect the normal functioning of the reproductive system with hormones like gonadotrophin and prolactin coming into play. Chronically elevated cortisol level is a factor of particular importance for the function of male gonads. Elevated cortisol level centrally acts to inhibit the GnRH by interrupting the intensity of the pulsatile release of pituitary gonadotropins. This may cause hypoandrogenemia [77] as the secretions of FSH, LH, and testosterone are negatively interfered with. This action at times could lead to disruption of spermatogenesis of varying severity, including spermatogenetic arrest. Stress-induced gonadal dysfunction is not restricted to humans, but is observed in all higher animals. However, recent prospective studies have linked a period of psychological stress with reduction in sperm quality to an increase in seminal plasma ROS generation and a reduction in antioxidant protection [48, 49, 77].

Chronic stress might impair testosterone. However, while Swedish authors found a decrease in total testosterone levels during periods of greater mental stress in men, a Danish study contradicted these observations. These results indicate to some possible ambiguity in the relationship between psychological stress and endocrine gonadal function. Incidentally, another Danish study by Hjollund et al. ruled out any demonstrable effect on the reproductive function of men from normal stress encountered in jobs [10, 78–81].

Neurotransmitter Changes

Besides these hormonal interactions, there are simultaneous complementary biochemical events that are enacted by a number of neurotransmitters in chronic psychological stress. All neurotransmitters perform very significant roles in the stress situation. Various stressors induce changes in the secretion of neurotransmitters like somatostatin, neuropeptide Y, catecholamines, adrenal steroids (adrenalin, noradrenalin, and dopamine), beta-endorphins, and serotonin. Endogenous opioids released in the brain in response to these same stressors could be participating in the impairment.

Stimulation of the HPA axis is associated with release of catecholamines. Norepinephrine serves as the primary chemical messenger of the central nervous system's sympathetic component. Transmission of the neurotransmitter serotonin from the caudal nuclei and rostral raphe nuclei is reduced in patients with depression compared to nondepressed controls [70, 82].

Neuropeptide Y is an important regulator of stress reactions through stimulation of neurons that produce CRH, and at the same time, it suppresses the sympathetic system at the central level. During depression, CRH inhibits the function of neurons responsible for the secretion of GnRH directly and indirectly by stimulation of the secretion of beta-endorphins. The increased secretion of beta-endorphins leads to increased secretion of prolactin (PRL) and somatostatin and to decreased secretion of growth hormone (GH). Catecholamines may also inhibit testosterone synthesis at the intratesticular site through auto- and paracrine mechanisms [77].

Kirby et al. have postulated a novel negative regulator of the HPT axis discovered in quail and termed it gonadotrophin inhibitory hormone (GnIH). Furthermore, in primates and rodents, RFamide-related peptides (RFRPs) have been discovered. Only future research would determine whether stress-related GnIH/RFRP's influence on HPT axis will usher in a new concept in stress-related reproductive dysfunction and infertility [83].

Enzymes like SOD and catalase, found in high concentrations in the seminal fluid, play significant roles as oxidant scavengers or enzymatic antioxidants. These enzymatic antioxidants inactivate the superoxide anion and peroxide (H_2O_2) radicals by converting them into water and oxygen. During the period of stress, SOD activities increase significantly compared to the nonstress period, but there is no change in catalase activities [48, 84].

Cellular or Molecular Changes

Currently, psychological distress has attracted attention with regard to its significant negative effects in various pathological conditions. Many studies on animal models have demonstrated that psychological stress produces oxidative stress and increased levels of peroxynitrite. However, the pathological process in a stress-induced oxidative damage is very complicated, so are its resultant effects on the hormonal balance, neurotransmitters, and antioxidants.

Under certain stressed states including that caused by psychological stress, there is a modulation of physiological antioxidant defense mechanisms. Michael J. Forlenza, in his thesis, related to the relationship between psychological stress and oxidative stress from the University of Pittsburgh in 2002, has cited six studies—three on rats and the other three with humans that have directly examined the contribution of stress on oxidative damage of DNA. It could be justifiably argued by extrapolating these results in drawing conclusions that psychological stress induces oxidative stress with its consequent effects on spermatozoa. Irie and colleagues have conducted two studies specifically designed to examine the relationship of psychological factors to oxidative DNA damage [85–90].

The oxidative stress results from imbalances between ROS and the body's antioxidants. It significantly impairs sperm functions and plays a major role in the etiology of male infertility. There are potential harmful effects of high levels of ROS on count, motility, quality, and function of spermatozoa as well as on the sperm nuclear DNA. High levels of ROS is now thought to be involved in these abnormal changes through lipid peroxidation, altered membrane function, and impaired metabolism. Many studies have demonstrated an association of lipid peroxidation with mid-piece abnormality, decreased sperm count and motility, and loss of capacity of the spermatozoa to undergo the acrosome reaction, thereby reducing the chance of fertilization [91, 92].

Modulating Factors for Psychological Stress

The modulating factors of psychological stress involving male infertility are controversial. Often the factors that modify psychological stress could also serve as causative agents. The list of these factors modifying the course of stress reactions in men is virtually unlimited. Race, age, marital status, siblings, educational background, income groups, social environment, and religious background all seem to play their roles.

It is believed that men are perhaps less susceptible to psychological stress than women. A less pronounced tendency to depression and a limited susceptibility to disruption of interpersonal relations are thought to contribute to this phenomenon. Married men report psychological stress less frequently than their unmarried counterparts. Men with higher educational background and belonging to higher-income groups are able to deal with psychological stress better [93, 94]. European males are reported to have a more serious perception of psychological stress that leads to a greater degree of sufferance in comparison to Asians. It has also been shown that the quantitative psychological impact is related to the mutual or reciprocal interaction between the stressor and the coping mechanisms of the individual couple [95–98].

Additional psychological disorders like substance abuse, alcohol addiction, and mood disorders are not uncommon in infertile men with all their attendant deleterious effects. Perhaps these psychologically stressed men find solace in escaping from their depressed state by indulging in these addictions. Chronic alcohol consumption has a detrimental effect on the male reproductive system and affects reproductive organs directly or indirectly. Smoking likewise has been incriminated for ushering in injurious effects on sperms and erectile tissue.

Avicenna, a physician from Bukhara (now in Uzbekistan) in his famous book *The Canon of Medicine*, first described the relationship between obesity and infertility. It took nearly 900 years before the subject found some rational explanations with current studies revealing the detrimental effect of obesity on infertility. The prevalence of depression among infertile men is estimated at 5–15 %. The negative emotions of depression are frequently compensated by compulsive overeating in men with infertility. Particularly during times of high stress, one tends to eat in an attempt to fulfill emotional needs—sometimes referred to as stress or emotional eating [50, 99, 100].

The brain is supposed to play the central role in the activation of stress-induced food intake. The situation is also compounded by the release of serotonin that increases the carbohydrate consumption and discourages physical activities to burn calories. Moreover, depression-related stress increases HPA axis activity, leading to excessive cortisol level that stimulates adiposity [101–103]. Obesity in itself can cause low testosterone level due to peripheral aromatization with its attendant adverse effect on sexual function. Depression, obesity, and infertility could coexist in males with psychological stress, and in combination they naturally aggravate the infertile state.

Many health problems are related to lifestyle factors. The increasing trend in reproductive disorders observed in recent years may be associated at least in part with these factors often compounded by some of the new emergent sedentary lifestyles [104].

Treatment

The treatment of psychological stress-related diseases unlike their organic counterparts assumes different perspectives as the target is metaphysical without any specific organ to aim at. Only a very few medical personnel or psychologists are trained and experienced enough to deal with the complex phenomenon of psychological stress in infertility. Its effective management involves identifying and managing both acute and chronic stress.

Counseling is perhaps singularly the most important step in formulating the treatment of psychological stress to help infertile people [105]. Regardless of which partner is the offender, infertility remains a conjugal problem casting its shadow on both partners. Consequently, treatment of psychological stress-related infertility must have the participation of both partners. Since difficult partner communication is a significant predictor of psychological stress in men, infertility counseling is often an effective remedy [106, 107].

Psychological and behavioral therapy historically has a significant role in the management of PE. A number of drugs like tricyclic antidepressants (clomipramine), and serotonergic (selective serotonin reuptake inhibitors or SSRI) agents like paroxetine, sertraline, etc., have shown varying degrees of success. New drugs like dapoxetine, prilocaine–lidocaine cream, and aerosol spray show promising results in PE. Various antioxidants and anxiolytic agent as subsidiary measures to allay anxiety have beneficial effects in all forms of psychological stress [84].

However, SSRI medicines are known to induce sexual dysfunctions like decreased libido, erectile dysfunction, delayed ejaculation, or anorgasmia. They also have a negative impact on spermatogenesis by inducing DNA fragmentation with resultant changes in motility and concentration [108–111]. The side effects of SSRIs have a reported incidence of 55 % in men according to a questionnaire on sexual dysfunction. Incidentally, a small study has claimed reversal of SSRI-induced sexual dysfunctions using a biennial plant extract of *Lepidium meyenii or maca* [112].

SSRI medicines enhance extracellular levels of the neurotransmitter serotonin (5-hydroxytryptamine or 5-HT) through inhibition of its reuptake into presynaptic the cells. This increases its level in the synaptic cleft available to bind to the postsynaptic 5-HT_2 and 5-HT_3 receptors in the spinal cord. Consequently, serotonin remains in the synaptic gap for a longer period and continually stimulates the receptors of the recipient cell. Increase in the extracellular concentrations of serotonin in the brain decreases dopamine and norepinephrine release from the substantia nigra which leads to sexual dysfunction in various forms [112–115]. At the same time slowing down of sexual stimulation by SSRI is rationally exploited to treat PE [116].

Conclusion

Any stress induces a state of disturbed internal homeostasis, evoking multiple changes in the body. Human psychological stress response is variable depending on the personality, physical, or mental state that is perhaps genetically determined in any individual [117]. Accordingly, the response to infertility differs with individual situations, emotional strength, coping methods, race, and religious belief. It is also important to know that individuals going through treatment for infertility can often suffer from psychological stress. The level of his stress tends to increase as treatment intensifies if its duration extends.

The relationship of psychological stress and infertility is a very difficult field to study. In real life, compared with other stresses such as illness, family problems, or unemployment, infertility possibly plays a less significant role. Infertility acts as a chronic stressor for both male and female partners. No doubt some males perform better under these stressful conditions. But one needs to consider factors like innate personality, coping style of stress, degree of stress, and the support systems in the social environment from the family and friends.

Any stress including psychological stress can lead to infertility, while infertility leads to stress culminating in a perpetuating cycle. However, whether stress causes infertility or infertility causes stress is still debated. The majority of the studies rejected the theory of psychological stress as a lone factor in the overall etiology of infertility, but it certainly acts as an additional risk factor for infertility.

Psychological stress leads to changes in the homeostasis involving various hormones, biochemical status including that of neurotransmitters at cellular and molecular levels. The biochemical changes revolved around L-arginine, NO, NOS, arginine-depleting enzyme, and arginase to influence the sperm parameters in stress and nonstress period. It also leads to the activation of the HPA and HPT axes to initiate complex neuroendocrine response culminating in disorder of the reproductive function with possible oxidative damage at the cellular level of the spermatozoa. Oxidative stress significantly impairs sperm function.

Counseling and behavioral therapy unquestionably are very important in the management. Judicious use of tricyclic antidepressants and SSRI agents could add to efficient management of some of the dysfunctions like PE, notwithstanding some of the specific side effects of SSRI medicines. Various antioxidants and anxiolytic agents also could be added as subsidiary measures in all forms of psychological stress. However, there is a lack of trained and experienced medical personnel or psychologists trained and experienced to deal with the complexities of psychological stress in infertility.

Infertility not only has psychological consequences affecting the couple but also has a societal impact. According to human psychosomatic tenets, every somatic problem has its emotional side. In general, the psychological stress in an infertile male has come into the limelight in only the last two decades. The societal construction of infertility and roles of both partners needs to be given adequate importance in formulating treatment. Counseling, an important method in treatment, needs participation of both partners for its effectiveness.

Quite a few workers endeavored to establish the relationships between psychological stress and male infertility in the last two decades. Yet any unanimous conclusion in this field still remains elusive with many gray areas until carefully designed and conducted longitudinal studies are undertaken.

References

1. Beers MH, Berkow R, editors. The Merck manual of diagnosis and therapy. Whitehouse Station, NJ: Merck Research Laboratories; 2004.
2. Jordan C, Revenson TA. Gender differences in coping with infertility: a meta-analysis. J Behav Med. 1999;22(4):341–58.
3. Lenzi A, Lombardo F, Salacone P, Gandini L, Jannini EA. Stress, sexual dysfunctions, and male infertility. J Endocrinol Invest. 2003;26(3 Suppl):72–6.
4. Pelletier KR. The best alternative medicine, part I, "spirituality and healing". New York: Simon & Schuster; 2002.
5. Johnson AR, Lao S, Wang T, Galanko JA, Zeisel SH. Choline dehydrogenase polymorphism rs12676 is a functional variation and is associated with changes in human sperm cell function. PLoS One. 2012;7(4):e36047. Epub 2012 Apr 27.
6. Malik SH, Coulson N. The male experience of infertility: a thematic analysis of an online infertility support group bulletin board. J Reprod Infant Psychol. 2008;26:18–30.
7. Takefman J. Director of Psychological Services at the McGill Reproductive Centre (MRC). Psychological issues in male factor infertility—IAAC. http://www.iaac.ca. Accessed 30th Oct 2013.
8. Salvador A. Coping with competitive situations in humans. Neurosci Biobehav Rev. 2005;29:195–205.
9. Fenster L, Katz DF, Wyrobek AJ, Pieper C, Rempel DM, Oman D, Swan SH. Effects of psychological stress on human semen quality. Andrology. 1997;18:194–202.
10. Hjollund NH, Bonde JP, Henriksen TB, Giwercman A, Olsen J, Danish First Pregnancy Planner Study Team. Reproductive effects of male psychologic stress. Epidemiology. 2004;15(1):21–7.
11. Morrow KA, Thoreson RW, Penney LL. Predictors of psychological distress among infertility clinic patients. Clin Psychol. 1995;63(1):163–7.
12. Smith JF. Emotional, psychological, and marital stress in male factor infertility. The Annual Meeting of the American Urological Association (AUA)—May 17–22. Orlando, FL: Orange County Convention Center; 2008.
13. Basu SC. Psychological impact of infertility. In: Basu SC, editor. Male reproductive dysfunction. 2nd ed. New Delhi: Jaypee Brothers Medical Publishers; 2011. p. 376–83. Chapter 14.

14. Seibel MM, Taymor ML. Emotional aspects of infertility. Fertil Steril. 1982;37(2):137–45.
15. Schneid-Kofman N, Sheiner E. Does stress effect male infertility?—A debate. Med Sci Monit. 2005;11(8):SR11–3.
16. Schover LR, Richards S, Collins RL. Psychological aspects of donor insemination: evaluation and follow-up of recipient couples. Fertil Steril. 1992;57:583–90.
17. Peronace LA, Boivin J, Schmidt L. Patterns of suffering and social interactions in infertile men: 12 months after unsuccessful treatment. J Psychosom Obstet Gynaecol. 2007;28(2):105–14.
18. Dhaliwal LK, Gupta KR, Gopalan S, Kulhara P. Psychological aspects of infertility due to various causes—prospective study. Int J Fertil Womens Med. 2004;49:44.
19. Wischmann TH. Sexual disorders in infertile couples. J Sex Med. 2010;7(5):1868–76.
20. Miall CE. Community constructs of involuntary childlessness: sympathy, stigma, and social support. Can Rev Sociol. 2008;31:392–421.
21. Muller MJ. Sexual satisfaction in male infertility. Arch Androl. 1999;42:138.
22. Sifneos PE. Clinical observations on some patients suffering from a variety of psychosomatic diseases. Acta Med Psychosom. 1967;7:1–10.
23. Sifneos PE. The prevalence of alexithymic characteristics in psychosomatic patients. Psychother Psychosom. 1973;22:255–62.
24. Bach M, Bach D, Böhmer F, et al. Alexithymia and somatization: relationship to DSM-III-R diagnoses. J Psychosom Res. 1994;38:529–38.
25. Bach M, Bach D, de Zwaan M, et al. Validierung der deutschen Version der 20-Item Toronto-Alexithymie-Skala bei Normalpersonen und psychiatrischen Patienten. Psychother Psychosom Med Psychol. 1996;46:23–8.
26. Bach M, Bach D. Predictive value of alexithymia: a prospective study in somatizing patients. Psychother Psychosom. 1995;64:43–8.
27. Wise TN, Mann LS. The attribution of somatic symptoms in psychiatric outpatients. Compr Psychiatry. 1995;36:407–10.
28. Wise TN, Mann LS, Mitchell JD, et al. Secondary alexithymia: an empirical validation. Compr Psychiatry. 1990;31:284–8.
29. Hesse C, Floyd K. Affectionate experience mediates the effects of alexithymia on mental health and interpersonal relationships. J Soc Pers Relationships. 2008;25(5):793–810.
30. Michetti PM, Rossi R, Bonanno D, Tiesi A, Simonelli C. Male sexuality and regulation of emotions: a study on the association between alexithymia and erectile dysfunction (ED). Int J Impot Res. 2006;18:170–4.
31. Taylor GJ, Bagby RM, Parker JDA. Alexithymia. Cambridge: Cambridge University Press; 1997. 335 p.
32. American Psychiatric Association. Diagnostic and statistical manual of mental disorders. 4th ed.

Washington, DC: American Psychiatric Association; 1994.

33. McGrady AV. Effects of psychological stress on male reproduction: a review. Arch Androl. 1984;13(1):1–7.

34. Sand MS, Fisher W, Rosen R, Heiman J, Eardley I. Erectile dysfunction and constructs of masculinity and quality of life in the multinational Men's Attitudes to Life Events and Sexuality (MALES) study. J Sex Med. 2008;5(3):583–94.

35. Araujo AB, Johannes CB, Feldman HA, Derby CA, McKinlay JB. Relation between psychosocial risk factors and incident erectile dysfunction: prospective results from the Massachusetts Male Aging Study. Am J Epidemiol. 2000;152(6):533–41.

36. Bancroft J. Psychogenic erectile dysfunction. A theoretical approach. Int J Impot Res. 2000; 12:546–8.

37. Lue TF. Causes of erectile dysfunction. Erectile dysfunction. Armenian Health Network. 2006. www.Health.am. Accessed 7 Oct 2007.

38. Sadeghi-Nejad H, Watson R. Continuing medical education: premature ejaculation: current medical treatment and new directions (CME). J Sex Med. 2008;5:1037–50.

39. Mohee A, Eardley I. Medical therapy for premature ejaculation. Ther Adv Urol. 2011;3(5):211–22.

40. Waldinger MD. Premature ejaculation: different pathophysiologies and etiologies determine its treatment. J Sex Marital Ther. 2008;34(1):1–13.

41. Waldinger MD. Recent advances in the classification, neurobiology and treatment of premature ejaculation. Adv Psychosom Med. 2008;29:50–69.

42. Waldinger MD, Schweitzer DH. The use of old and recent DSM definitions of premature ejaculation in observational studies: a contribution to the present debate for a new classification of PE in the DSM-V. Sex Med. 2008;5(5):1079–87.

43. Palti Z. Psychogenic male infertility. Psychosom Med. 1969;31(4):326–30.

44. Knowles DR. Delayed ejaculation. A.D.A.M. Medical Encyclopedia. A.D.A.M. Inc. (2005-06-01). http://www.nlm.nih.gov/medlineplus/ency/article/001954.htm. Accessed 30 Oct 2013.

45. Delvin D. Delayed ejaculation (retarded ejaculation). Net Doctor.co.uk. (2007-06-25). Retrieved 25 Oct 2007. http://www.netdoctor.co.uk. Accessed 30 Oct 2013.

46. Michael M. Male psychogenic subfertility and infertility. Gynecologia. 1956;141:265.

47. Gerhard I, Lenhard K, Eggert-Kruse W, et al. Clinical data which influence semen parameters in infertile men. Hum Reprod. 1992;7:830–7.

48. Eskiocak S, Gozen AS, Kilic AS, Molla S. Association between mental stress & some antioxidant enzymes of seminal plasma. Indian J Med Res. 2005;122(6):491–6.

49. Eskiocak S, Gozen AS, Taskiran A, Kilic AS, Eskiocak M, Gulen S. Effect of psychological stress on the L-arginine-nitric oxide pathway and semen quality. Braz J Med Biol Res. 2006;39(5):581–8.

50. Zorn B, Auger J, Velikonja V, Kolbezen M, Meden-Vrtovec H. Psychological factors in male partners of infertile couples: relationship with semen quality and early miscarriage. Int J Androl. 2008; 31(6):557–64.

51. Negro-Vilar A. Stress and other environmental factors affecting fertility in men and women: overview. Environ Health Perspect. 1993;101 Suppl 2:59–64.

52. Blanchard RJ, McKittrick CR, Blanchard DC. Animal models of social stress: effects on behavior and brain neurochemical systems. Physiol Behav. 2001;73:261–71.

53. Pook M, Krause W, Rohrle B. Coping with infertility: distress and changes in sperm quality. Hum Reprod. 1999;14:1487–92.

54. Boivin J, Shoog-Svanberg A, Andersson L, et al. Distress level in men undergoing intracytoplasmic sperm injection versus in vitro fertilization. Hum Reprod. 1998;13:1403–6.

55. Clarke RN, Klock SC, Geoghegan A, Travassos DE. Relationship between psychological stress and semen quality among in-vitro fertilization patients. Hum Reprod. 1999;14(3):753–8.

56. Reporaki L, Punamaki RL, Unkila-Kallio L, et al. Infertility treatment and marital relationships: a 1-year prospective study among successfully treated ART couples and their controls. Hum Reprod. 2007;22(5):1481–91.

57. Wolfram M. Rev Fr Gynecol Obstet. 1953;48:145.

58. Perloff FW. Obstet Gynecol Latin Am. 1955;13:1.

59. Steve H. Der Einfluss des Nerven System auf Ban und Tdtigkeit der Geschlechtorgane des Menschen. Stuttgart: Thieme; 1952.

60. Zondek B, Bromberg YM, Polishuk KZ. Variations in spermatogenesis of oligospermic men. Nature (London). 1948;161:176.

61. Greil AL. Infertility and psychological distress: a critical review of the literature. Soc Sci Med. 1997;45(11):1679–704.

62. Schenker JG, Meirow D, Schenker E. Stress and human reproduction. Eur J Obstet Gynecol Reprod Biol. 1992;45(1):1–8.

63. Zini A, O'Bryan MK, Schlegel PN. Nitric oxide synthase activity in human seminal plasma. Urology. 2001;58:85–9.

64. Rosselli M, Dubey RK, Imthurn B, et al. Effects of nitric oxide on human spermatozoa: evidence that nitric oxide decreases sperm motility and induces sperm toxicity. Hum Reprod. 1995;10:1786–90.

65. Hallemeesch MM, Lamers WH, Deutz NE. Reduced arginine availability and nitric oxide production. Clin Nutr. 2002;21:273–9.

66. Agarwal A, Makker K, Sharma R. Clinical relevance of oxidative stress in male factor infertility: an update. Am J Reprod Immunol. 2008;59(1):2–11.

67. Elgun S, Kacmaz M, Sen I, et al. Seminal arginase activity in infertility. Urol Res. 2000;28:20–3.

68. Spielberger CD, Gorsuch RL, Lushene RE. STAI manual for the state-trait anxiety inventory (self-evaluation questionnaire). Palo Alto, CA: Consulting Psychologists Press; 1970.

69. Herrero MB, de Lamirande E, Gagnon C. Tyrosine nitration in human spermatozoa: a physiological function of peroxynitrite, the reaction product of nitric oxide and superoxide. Mol Hum Reprod. 2001;7:913–21.
70. Turner-Cobb JM. Psychological and stress hormone correlates in early life: a key to HPA-axis dysregulation and normalization. Stress. 2005;8(1):47–57.
71. Retana-Márquez S, et al. Naltrexone effects on male sexual behavior, corticosterone, and testosterone in stressed male rats. Physiol Behav. 2009;96(2): 333–42.
72. Tsigos C, Chrousos GP. Hypothalamic-pituitary-adrenal axis, neuroendocrine factors and stress. J Psychosom Res. 2002;53(4):865–71.
73. Kyrou I, Tsigos C. Chronic stress, visceral obesity and gonadal dysfunction. Hormones (Athens). 2008;7(4):287–93.
74. Delitala G, Tomasi P, Virdis R. Prolactin, growth hormone and thyrotropin-thyroid hormone secretion during stress states in man. Baillieres Clin Endocrinol Metab. 1987;1(2):391–414.
75. Tsigos C, Kyrou I, Chrousos G. Stress, endocrine physiology and pathophysiology. www.endotext. com. Dartmouth, MA: MDTEXT.COM, INC. 2004. Accessed 30 Oct 2013.
76. Karagiannis A, Harsoulis F. Gonadal dysfunction in systemic diseases. Eur J Endocrinol. 2005;152: 501–13.
77. Jóźków P, Mędraś M. Psychological stress and the function of male gonads. Pol J Endocrinol. 2012; 63(1):44–9.
78. Theorell T, Karasek RA, Eneroth P. Job strain variations in relation to plasma testosterone fluctuations in working men—a longitudinal study. J Intern Med. 1990;227:31–6.
79. Klimek M, Pabian W, Tomaszewska B, et al. Levels of plasma ACTH in men from infertile couples. Neuro Endocrinol Lett. 2005;26:347–50.
80. O'Connor DB, Corona G, Forti G, et al. Assessment of sexual health in aging men in Europe: development and validation of the European Male Ageing Study sexual function questionnaire. J Sex Med. 2008;5:1374–85.
81. Hjollund NH, Bonde JP, Henriksen TB, et al. Job strain and male fertility. Epidemiology. 2004;15: 114–7.
82. Holsboer F, Ising M. Hormone regulation: biological role and translation into therapy. Annu Rev Psychol. 2010;61:81–109.
83. Kirby ED, et al. Stress increases putative gonadotrophin inhibitory hormone and decreases luteinizing hormone in male rats. Proc Natl Acad Sci U S A. 2009;106(27):11324–9.
84. Kefer JC, Agarwal A, Sabanegh E. Role of antioxidants in the treatment of male infertility. Int J Urol. 2009;16(5):449–57.
85. Adachi S, Kawamura K, Takemoto K. Oxidative damage of nuclear DNA in liver of rats exposed to psychological stress. Cancer Res. 1993;53:4153–5.
86. Irie M, Asami S, Nagata S, Ikeda M, Miyata M, Kasai H. Psychosocial factors as a potential trigger of oxidative DNA damage in human leukocytes. Jpn J Cancer Res. 2001;92:367–75.
87. Irie M, Asami S, Nagata S, Miyata M, Kasai H. Classical conditioning of oxidative DNA damage in rats. Neurosci Lett. 2000;288:13–6.
88. Irie M, Asami S, Nagata S, Miyata M, Kasai H. Relationships between perceived workload, stress and oxidative damage. Int Arch Occup Environ Health. 2001;74:153–7.
89. Liu J, Wang X, Shigenaga MK, Yeo HC, Mori A, Ames BN. Immobilization stress causes oxidative damage to lipid, protein, and DNA in the brains of rats. FASEB J. 1996;10:1532–8.
90. Nakajima M, Takeuchi T, Takeshita T, Morimoto K. 8-Hydroxydeoxyguanosine in human leukocyte DNA and daily health practice factors: effects of individual alcohol sensitivity. Environ Health Perspect. 1996;104(12):1336–8.
91. Makker K, Agarwal A. Oxidative stress & male infertility. Indian J Med Res. 2009;129(4):357–67.
92. Cocuzza S, Agarwal A. Clinical relevance of oxidative stress and sperm chromatin damage in male infertility: an evidence based analysis. Int Braz J Urol. 2007;33(5):603–21.
93. Caron J, Liu A. Factors associated with psychological distress in the Canadian population: a comparison of low-income and non low-income sub-groups. Community Ment Health J. 2011;47:318–30.
94. Thapa SB, Hauff E. Gender differences in factors associated with psychological distress among immigrants from low- and middle-income countries-findings from the Oslo Health Study. Soc Psychiatry Psychiatr Epidemiol. 2005;40:78–84.
95. McDonough P, Strohschein L. Age and the gender gap in distress. Women Health. 2003;38:1–20.
96. Jorm AF, Windsor TD, Dear KB, et al. Age group differences in psychological distress: the role of psychosocial risk factors that vary with age. Psychol Med. 2005;35:1253–63.
97. Andrews FM, Abbey A, Halman LJ. Stress from infertility, marriage factors, and subjective well-being of wives and husbands. J Health Soc Behav. 1991;32:238–53.
98. Nelson CJ, Shindel AW, Naughton CK, Ohebshalom M, Mulhall JP. Prevalence and predictors of sexual problems, relationship stress and depression in female partners of infertile couples. J Sex Med. 2008;5:1907–14.
99. Olivius C, Friden B, Borg G, Berg C. Why do couples discontinue in vitro fertilization treatment? A cohort study. Fertil Steril. 2004;81(2):258–61.
100. Fisher RW, Hammarberg K. Psychological and social aspects of infertility in men: an overview of the evidence and implications for psychologically informed clinical care and future research. Asian J Androl. 2012;14(1):121–9.
101. Wurtman J. Depression and weight gain: the serotonin connection. J Affect Disord. 1993;29(2–3):183–92.

102. Adam TC, Epel ES. Stress, eating and the reward system. Physiol Behav. 2007;91(4):449–58.
103. Kim YK, Na KS, Shin KH, Jung HY, Choi SH, Kim JB. Cytokine imbalance in the pathophysiology of major depressive disorder. Prog Neuropsychopharmacol Biol Psychiatry. 2007;31(5):1044–53.
104. Kumar S, Kumari A, Murarka S. Lifestyle factors in deteriorating male reproductive health. Indian J Exp Biol. 2009;47:615–24.
105. Boivin J. A review of psychosocial interventions in infertility. Soc Sci Med. 2003;57(12):2325–41.
106. Van den Broeck U, Emery M, Wischmann T, Thorn P. Counselling in infertility: individual, couple and group interventions. Patient Educ Couns. 2010;81(3):422–8. Epub 2010 Nov 13.
107. Wischmann T. Implications of psychosocial support in infertility—a critical appraisal. J Psychosom Obstet Gynaecol. 2008;29(2):83–90.
108. Coleman, E. Impulsive/compulsive sexual behavior: assessment and treatment. In: Grant JE, Potenza MN, editors. The Oxford handbook of impulse control disorders. New York: Oxford University Press; 2011. p. 385. Chapter 28.
109. Koyuncu H, Serefoglu EC, Ozdemir AT, Hellstrom WJ. Deleterious effects of selective serotonin reuptake inhibitor treatment on semen parameters in patients with lifelong premature ejaculation. Int J Impot Res. 2012;24:171–3.
110. Tanrikut C, Schlegel PN. Antidepressant-associated changes in semen parameters. Urology. 2007;69(1):185.
111. Tanrikut C, Feldman AS, Altemus M, Paduch DA, Schlegel PN. Adverse effect of paroxetine on sperm. Fertil Steril. 2010;94(3):1021–6.
112. Dording CM, Fisher L, Papakostas G, et al. A double-blind, randomized, pilot dose-finding study of maca root (L. meyenii) for the management of SSRI-induced sexual dysfunction. CNS Neurosci Ther. 2008;14(3):182–91.
113. Rosen RC, Lane RG, Menza M. Effects of SSRIs on sexual function: a critical review. J Clin Psychopharmacol. 1999;19:67–85.
114. Montejo AL, Llorca G, Izquierdo JA. Sexual dysfunction with SSRIs: a comparative analysis. In: New research program and abstracts of the 149th Annual Meeting of the American Psychiatric Association; New York, NY. 1996.
115. Monteiro WO, Noshirvani HF, Marks IM, et al. Anorgasmia from clomipramine in obsessive-compulsive disorder: a controlled trial. Br J Psychiatry. 1987;151:107–12.
116. Waldinger MD, Olivier B. Utility of selective serotonin reuptake inhibitors in premature ejaculation". Curr Opin Investig Drugs. 2004;5(7):743–7.
117. Kyrou I, Tsigos C. Stress mechanisms and metabolic complications. Horm Metab Res. 2007;39(6):430–8.

The Impact of Cell Phone, Laptop Computer, and Microwave Oven Usage on Male Fertility

11

John J. McGill and Ashok Agarwal

Introduction

Cell phones, laptops, and microwave ovens have become integral components of modern life. These devices use microwaves, a type of electromagnetic wave (EMW) which can be used to transfer information and also to create heat. The potential effect of EMW radiation on male fertility is controversial and unclear. A possible association with EMW radiation and male infertility may prove most important in subfertile men using laptop computers placed in their laps, in men with cell phone use and storage on either the hip or in a pants pocket, and in men standing in close proximity to active microwave ovens. Current literature on EMW radiation exposure and male reproduction remains controversial, with mixed data from human and animal studies. The potential mechanism of action in biological tissues is poorly understood and the safety of EMWs remains unclear. This chapter will review the current literature on cell phone, laptop computer, and microwave oven EMW radiation effects on the male reproductive system. The potential effects of these technologies may prove to be an important public health issue and potential cause of unexplained male infertility.

Objective/Aims of Chapter

This chapter will focus on microwaves, a type of nonionizing radiation, which includes frequencies used for cell phones, laptop computers, and microwave ovens. The authors will briefly review the biological effects and potential mechanisms of human EMW exposure. The authors will then review the specific literature related to the effects of EMW radiation from cell phones, laptops, and microwave ovens on the male reproductive system. This chapter will emphasize the negative health effects secondary to cell phone radiation, since a majority of current EMW literature related to male reproductive health has been performed using cell phone technology. Topics will also include a review of laptop computer and microwave oven literature. Conventional microwave ovens use a frequency of 2.45 GHz and studies at that frequency will be reviewed as microwave oven literature.

J.J. McGill, MD (✉)
Urology Institute, University Hospitals Case Medical Center, 11100 Euclid Avenue, Lakeside Building, 4th floor, Cleveland, OH 44106, USA
e-mail: johnjmcgill@gmail.com

A. Agarwal, PhD
Center for Reproductive Medicine, Cleveland Clinic Foundation/Glickman Urological and Kidney Institute, 10681 Carnegie Avenue, Cleveland, OH 44195, USA
e-mail: agarwaa@ccf.org

S.S. du Plessis et al. (eds.), *Male Infertility: A Complete Guide to Lifestyle and Environmental Factors*, DOI 10.1007/978-1-4939-1040-3_11, © Springer Science+Business Media New York 2014

General Biological Effects of Electromagnetic Waves: Thermal and Nonthermal

EMW radiation can be absorbed when it interacts with matter, transferring wave energy into a given medium. This absorption process is divided into multiple categories corresponding to different modes of molecular energy storage including thermal and vibrational modes. The thermal mode of energy storage can give off heat by encouraging translational and vibrational movement of atoms in their respective media [1]. The amount of energy from radiation that a tissue will absorb depends primarily on the frequency of exposure but also on the intensity of the beam and duration of exposure. The rate of change of the energy transferred to the material is called the absorbed power or the specific absorption rate (SAR), which is expressed in watts per kilogram (W/kg). An increased SAR correlates with increased tissue radiation absorption, which can be expressed as heated tissue.

The biological effects of nonionizing EMW radiation remain controversial. It is unclear if harmful biological changes can occur in human tissues in the absence of demonstrable thermal effects. Nonthermal effects occur through mechanisms excluding macroscopic heating [1]. This chapter will use the terms thermal and nonthermal to delineate biological effects with and without heat.

Possible Mechanisms of EMW Effects on Male Reproduction

The overall mechanism of EMW effects in the male reproductive system remains unknown, with many potential mechanisms of action. These range from alterations at a tissue level (including the blood-testis barrier (BTB)) down to a subcellular level. Current literature lacks the detailed and exhaustive mechanistic studies of EMW effects within the male reproductive axis necessary to accurately elucidate potential mechanisms of action in male reproductive biology.

Thermal Effects

There are few studies on the thermal effects of EMWs on male reproductive biology. Yan and colleagues measured the surface and core body temperature of rats exposed to cell phone EMWs by placing cell phones 1 cm from each animal and probes near their faces and recta. There was no difference in temperature between face and rectal probes [2]. Conversely, Dasdag and colleagues found an increase in rectal temperature of rats exposed to phones in talk mode [3]. It is unclear if these animals were stressed secondary to audible sound through the phones relative to controls. This study lacked comparison of rectal temperature relative to the remainder of the body (e.g., face). The authors repeated the study later and did not find an association of increased rectal temperature with EMW exposure [4]. Thus, the potential role of thermal effects secondary to cell phone radiation remains undefined.

The United States Federal Communications Commission requires wireless phones to have an SAR < 1.6 W/kg [5]. Mobile phones are typically well below these thresholds. Adverse heating effects occur with an SAR > 4 W/kg; thus, it is unlikely that modern cell phones will have a thermal effect secondary to EMW radiation [6].

Nonthermal Effects

Cell Membrane Injury and the Role of Calcium Ions and Protein Kinase C

Injury to the cell membrane may play a role in the mechanism of EMW-induced cell injury. Excitation of the cell membrane and subsequent formation of large aqueous pores within the membrane is known as electroporation. This coupled with destabilization of the negatively charged plasma membrane and secondary intracellular effects has been implicated in in vitro nerve cell studies [7, 8]. The potentially leaky and unstable plasma membrane may develop subsequent loss of intracellular molecules and ions, including calcium, a known regulator of sperm capacitation and of the acrosome reaction [9, 10]. Calcium plays a critical role in intracellular signal transduction pathways.

Increased calcium efflux may lead to altered intracellular spermatic metabolism.

Calcium ions also regulate protein kinase C (PKC), a regulatory enzyme implicated in a wide range of cellular processes, including cell proliferation, malignancy, and apoptosis [10–12]. PKC, found in sperm flagella, is thought to regulate sperm motility [13], with multiple studies associating EMW exposure with decreased motility [2, 14–19].

Kesari and colleagues [20] found alterations in semen PKC levels, decreased sperm motility, and increased apoptosis in rats exposed to cell phone-emitted EMWs. Given PKC regulates apoptosis and other important cellular functions, alterations may lead to many negative effects in spermatic homeostasis. Since sperm also rely on calcium entry for multiple physiologic functions, including sperm motility, intracellular calcium changes along with alterations in PKC function may explain some of the effects of EMWs on the male reproductive system.

Blood-Testis-Barrier Compromise

Recent studies of EMW radiation have revealed the disrupting effects of EMWs on the integrity of the BTB. The BTB forms tight junctions between Sertoli cells, separating blood and lymph vessels from seminiferous tubules. The BTB is immune privileged, protecting the male germ cell line from recognition by the body's immune system, while protecting the testis from gonadotoxins within the circulatory system.

There are few studies investigating EMW radiation-induced alteration of the BTB and potential testicular damage, but all of these studies use electrical field intensity levels which are higher than those generated by cell phone, laptop, and microwave use. Wang and colleagues exposed mice to electric field intensities at 200 and 400 kV/m and found morphological changes to Sertoli cells at both intensities, respectively [21]. Another study used Evans Blue and lanthanum nitrate tracers to investigate BTB alterations in EMW exposure at 200 kV/m and found increased tracer penetration across the BTB with EMW exposure [22].

A recent study by Hou and colleagues investigated the effect of electromagnetic pulse irradiation at 400 kV/m and noted structural damage to the BTB with increased permeability and many luminal apoptotic spermatogenic cells [23]. Messenger RNA and protein expression levels of occludin, an integral membrane tight junction protein, were significantly decreased. The BTB structure and occludin expression levels showed gradual recovery by 28 days post exposure.

Due to the paucity of EMW radiation and BTB studies, research of the blood-brain barrier (BBB) may help clarify the interaction between the BTB and EMW radiation exposure. The BBB is formed mainly by tight junctions between small capillaries, supported by pericytes. Conversely, the BTB is mainly constituted of specialized junctions between adjacent Sertoli cells near the basement membrane of the seminiferous tubule epithelium [24, 25]. BTB microvasculature may also play a role in barrier function similar to the BBB, as a common antigen to both blood-tissue barriers has been found along BTB microvessels [25]. Thus, these blood-tissue barriers may have similar responses to stress and the development of barrier compromise. Animal and in vitro studies on the effect of EMWs on the BBB have had mixed results, with some studies showing alteration of the BBB and secondary neuropathologic changes [26–28] while others did not show an effect [29–34].

Although the aforementioned BTB studies were performed at high electrical fields, the effects of EMW radiation at lower electrical fields generated by common devices remain unknown and may detrimentally affect male reproductive biology. Ultimately, further studies are needed to elucidate the role of potential BTB compromise after EMW exposure.

Cellular Stress

EMW radiation may induce cellular signal transduction changes and subsequent differential gene and protein expression [35]. Mobile phone radiation has been shown to activate cellular stress responses, with changes to p38MAPK. Functional alteration of this mitogen-activated protein kinase [35] may lead to subsequent downstream activation of stress proteins. This includes heat shock protein 27 (hsp27), a ubiquitously expressed signaling protein in human cells. Hsp27 phosphorylation leads to increased apoptosis and potential increase in BBB permeability [35]. This same increased permeability may occur in the BTB, potentially endangering the male germ cell line. Nevertheless, there are a number of studies which have also shown no clear effect on gene and protein expression secondary to EMW exposure [36, 37]. Thus, it remains unclear if EMW radiation alters intracellular signal transduction pathways.

Oxidative Stress

Oxidative stress occurs when the concentration of sperm reactive oxygen species exceeds total antioxidant capacity. Spermatozoa have a high concentration of plasma membrane polyunsaturated fatty acids which are necessary for many male spermatic functions but also play a role in the production of ROS [37]. Potential polyunsaturated fatty acid production of ROS in the limited volume of spermatic cytoplasm and concentration of cytosolic antioxidant enzymes may leave spermatozoa vulnerable to significant sperm damage secondary to excessive ROS [38, 39]. Men with unexplained infertility often present with significantly higher seminal ROS levels than healthy men [40, 41]. Studies have shown that increased oxidative stress may result from male reproductive exposure to cell phone radiation [15, 16, 18, 42]. This mechanism may include perturbation of the mitochondrial membrane potential (MMP). EMW-induced alteration of the MMP initiates negative effects within the electron transport system and in oxidative phosphorylation, leading to oxidative stress and subsequent induction of apoptosis [43, 44]. This increase in oxidative stress after cell phone exposure may be mitigated by antioxidant treatment [45]. Further studies are required investigating sperm MMP, oxidative stress, and the effects of antioxidants.

DNA Damage

Sperm DNA damage is thought to occur by three mechanisms: DNA strand breaks, oxidative stress, and apoptosis [46]. Direct DNA fragmentation is thought to occur with EMW exposure [47], but it is important to note that DNA fragmentation with EMW exposure may involve more than one mechanism [46]. EMW-induced clastogenic effects (or the ability to fracture chromatin) have been shown in concert with DNA fragmentation in cell phone-exposed rats [48]. Microwaves may also affect cell cycle regulatory enzymes, which may potentially lead to defective cell cycle progression and defective spermatogenesis [48].

Many studies have associated oxidative stress and DNA fragmentation in male infertility, with some studies revealing a reduction of DNA damage with antioxidant therapy [15, 40, 49–52]. Thus, there may be multiple mechanisms of DNA damage secondary to microwave radiation. Given the poor reproductive outcomes associated with increased DNA fragmentation, EMW radiation-induced DNA damage will require detailed and extensive studies to elucidate a potential mechanism of action [53, 54].

Cell Phones and Male Fertility

With the advent of smart phones, mobile phone popularity and use have become widespread constants of modern day life. However, there are limited studies investigating the effects of EMWs on male infertility. Cell phone frequencies in the USA range from 900 to 1,900 MHz (GSM) with some smart phones ranging up to 2.4 GHz. Current US FCC standards limit mobile phone radiation exposure to 1.6 W/kg [5].

How Cell Phones Work

When a cell phone user speaks into a cell phone, sound waves from cell phone speakers go to a transmitter, which convert sound into a sine wave. The transmitter then sends a signal to the cell phone antenna (which sends the signal into space in all directions). The electric sine wave current running through the transmitter circuit also creates an electromagnetic field around it. As electric current moves back and forth, the electromagnetic field continues to build and collapse, forming electromagnetic radiation. This radiation interacts with human tissue and may increase random molecular motion [55, 56].

Increased SAR may lead to increased thermal and nonthermal tissue effects with subsequent perturbation of cell function [57].

Although SAR is determined at a cell phone's maximum power level, the actual SAR value of an active cell phone may be lower [5, 58]. The SAR of a given human tissue depends on multiple factors such as exposed tissue characteristics (thickness, amount of fluid, etc.), proximity of the wireless device to the body while in use, the mode of usage of the device (talk versus standby mode), and the use of hands-free devices (e.g., Bluetooth) [57, 59].

Cell Phone Radiation and Biological Effects

The mechanism of EMW effects in human tissues remains unclear. Currently, EMWs are thought to cause alteration of cell function [57, 59] by initial cell membrane disruption due to passage of electrically shaking current formed from body absorption of EMWs. This cell membrane disruption may affect plasma membrane structures such as NADH oxidase and calcium channels [59], leading to a cascade of cell signaling changes in male reproductive tissues (Fig. 11.1). Other potential effects outside the reproductive system include endothelial dysfunction, skin temperature changes, alterations in the BBB, immune system effects, and nervous system excitability defects [35, 57, 60–62]. Cell phones have been investigated in the central nervous system showing associations with changes in sleep and electroencephalograph patterns, headaches, fatigue, difficulty concentrating, and increased brain glucose metabolism [63–66]. Currently, epidemiological studies show an association between cellular phones and increased risk for glioma, acoustic neuroma, and increased brain tumor mortality [67, 68].

Human Male Reproductive Studies on Cell Phone Effects

Deleterious Effects on Human Semen Quality

There is some evidence associating negative effects on semen analyses with EMW exposure. In an observational study by Agarwal and colleagues, semen analyses of 361 men undergoing infertility evaluation were performed, revealing a decrease in mean sperm motility, viability, and normal morphology, with increasing duration of reported cell phone usage [15]. A similar study performed by Wdowiak et al. examined the semen of men with no phone use, use for 1–2 years, and use for over 2 years, without delineation of daily duration of use. The authors found an exposure-dependent decrease in sperm motility and normal morphology [69]. In these two studies, patients were neither asked about cell phone storage location (pants or shirt pocket versus belt clip) nor type of usage (hands-free versus handheld). Although an observational study by Kilgallon and Simmons revealed a decrease in sperm concentration in men who carried their cell phone in their hip pocket or belt [70], it remains unclear if cell phone exposure is a risk factor for male infertility.

Fejes and colleagues asked men visiting an academic center about cell phone use and habits and found a decrease in motility with increasing reported cell phone use [14]. Gutschi et al. later performed a retrospective study and found no difference in sperm count and a decrease in mean morphology in male cell phone users compared to nonusers [71]. These studies are both limited by their design, since unreported or unknown confounders may obscure delineation of the effects of EMW radiation.

Studies have been performed on neat semen samples with interesting results. Agarwal and colleagues divided semen samples into control and cell phone exposed aliquots. The exposed samples showed a decrease in sperm motility and viability when compared to unexposed aliquots [16]. A similar study by Erogul and colleagues also revealed a decrease in sperm motility [17]. De Iuliis et al. exposed purified human spermatozoa to cell phone radiation overnight with increasing SAR leading to decreased motility [18].

Falzone and colleagues later investigated the effects of cell phone exposure on purified semen samples as well, finding sperm head abnormalities and reduced sperm-zona binding, but no change in the acrosome reaction [72]. This may indicate a relationship between decreased fertilization potential and abnormal morphology with EMW

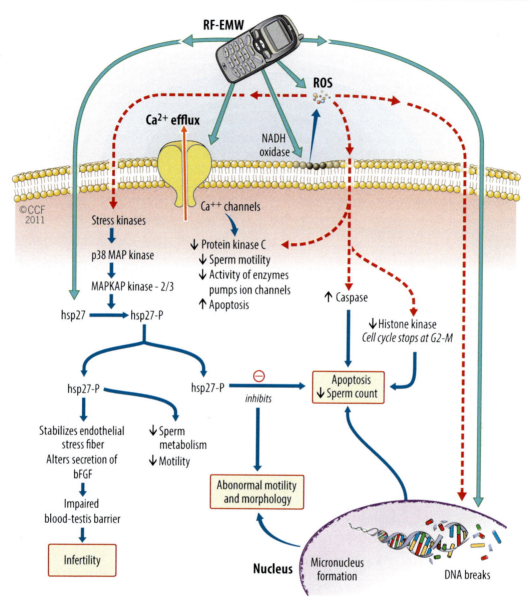

Fig. 11.1 Intracellular effects of cell phone radiation. Cell phone-emitted RF-EMWs can induce many potential subcellular changes. Calcium ion efflux coupled with plasma membrane injury and subsequent induction of ROS production may initiate an intracellular cascade of changes. ROS can negatively impact histone kinase, apoptosis, as well as protein kinase c (PKC). Calcium ion concentration is closely associated with PKC activity, which may be decreased after EMW exposure, leading to a potential decrease in sperm motility and increase in apoptosis. Heat shock proteins (particularly hsp27) may also play a role in EMW-induced intracellular signaling changes including potentially negative effects on the blood-testis barrier and sperm motility. Ultimately, DNA damage can occur with EMW exposure, either via ROS or direct injury [10]. [Reprinted with permission, Cleveland Clinic Center for Medical Art & Photography © 2011-2013. All Rights Reserved]

exposure. By using purified sperm samples, both studies by Falzone and De Iuliis et al. fail to account for the effects of clothing, soft tissues and of other semen components on the absorption of EMWs, which may decrease the effective SAR on human sperm [18, 72].

Human Studies: Male Reproductive Oxidative Stress After Cell Phone Exposure

Oxidative stress (OS) has been implicated as a main contributor to male infertility [15, 73, 74]. OS generated in the testis due to mobile phone exposure leads to accumulation of free radicals and increased ROS levels in sperm, all secondary to high content of polyunsaturated fatty acids [75]. Agarwal and colleagues found elevated ROS with EMW exposure of in vitro neat semen samples [16]. Another in vitro study found increased ROS and 8-hydroxy-2′-deoxyguanasine (8-OH-2G), a marker for oxidative stress [51]. Given the association of OS with DNA fragmentation, EMW radiation effects secondary to OS in human studies require further investigation.

Human Studies: Male Reproductive DNA Damage After Cell Phone Exposure

There are few human studies investigating sperm DNA damage secondary to cell phone radiation. Agarwal and colleagues exposed in vitro semen samples to cell phone EMWs and noted an increase in ROS levels but DNA fragmentation indices showed no significant difference from the unexposed group [16]. De Iuliis and colleagues also noted DNA damage with exposure of human sperm to cell phone EMWs [18]. Furthermore, the authors later found a strong correlation between cell phone radiation-induced oxidative DNA damage and DNA fragmentation, confirmed by a strong association between 8OHdG formation and DNA fragmentation index [51]. Ultimately, though sparse, current literature implicates cell phone radiation as a potential cause of human sperm DNA fragmentation.

Animal Studies on Cell Phone Radiation and Male Reproduction

Deleterious Effects on Animal Semen Quality

A decrease in sperm motility and morphology after cell phone radiation exposure has been shown in multiple rodent studies [20, 42, 76].

Mailankot and colleagues exposed rats to an active 0.9/1.8 GHz mobile phone for 1 h/day for 28 days. Controls were exposed to a mobile phone without a battery for the same duration. The authors found a significant decrease in motile sperm [76]. Yan et al. investigated the effect of cell phones at 1.9 GHz on rats at 1 cm distance from the face of each animal for 6 h/day over a period of 18 weeks at an SAR of 1.18 W/kg. They found an increased number of dead sperm cells and decreased sperm motility [2].

Sperm structural changes after cell phone radiation exposure have also been visualized using electron microscopy. Kesari and colleagues exposed rats for 45 days with 2 h/day of cell phone radiation. The authors found morphological changes in the rat sperm head and midpiece of the sperm mitochondrial sheath [42].

However, current literature does not solely support decreased motility with cell phone EMW exposure. In a recent study, Ozlem Nisbet et al. exposed rats at 900 and 1,800 MHz for 2 h/day over a 90-day period and found an increase in sperm motility in exposed rats relative to controls [77]. Total percentage of abnormal morphology was also lower in exposed animals. These seemingly paradoxical findings reveal a protective effect of cell phone radiation on rat spermatogenesis. Nevertheless, the mechanism of these findings remains unclear.

Animal Studies: Male Reproductive Oxidative Stress After Cell Phone Exposure

OS generated in the testis due to mobile phone exposure has been found in a number of animal studies, although the mechanism of ROS generation secondary to cell phone radiation remains unknown. Mailankot et al. exposed rats to 1 h of cell phone radiation for 28 days and found an increase in lipid peroxidation [76]. Kesari and colleagues studied the effect of mobile phone exposure compared with sham treatment in rats and noted a statistically significant increase in ROS and decrease in antioxidant enzymes in the exposure group [20]. A recent study by Al-Damegh evaluated the effect of treatment of rats with vitamins C and E prior to cell phone

EMW exposure [45]. The authors found increased glutathione peroxidase and glutathione in irradiated rat testicular tissues pretreated with oral antioxidants. In addition, markers of lipid peroxidation (conjugated dienes and hydroperoxides) along with catalase levels were decreased in radiated testicular tissues of vitamin-supplemented animals. These studies reveal a protective effect of pretreatment with vitamins C and E, as displayed by the approximate return to normal values of testicular antioxidants and markers of lipid peroxidation.

Animal Studies: Sperm DNA Damage Secondary to Cell Phone Exposure

Cell phone exposure may also lead to sperm DNA damage. Aitken et al. exposed mice to EMWs at a frequency of 900 MHz for 12 h/day for 1 week and showed evidence of DNA damage to epididymal spermatozoa [6]. Kesari and colleagues investigated cell phone EMW-induced clastogenic activity (ability to fracture chromatin) and DNA fragmentation in exposed rats [48]. The authors found an increase in DNA fragmentation as well as an increase in micronucleated polychromatic erythrocytes, a measure of chromatin fragmentation. Histone kinase, an enzyme which regulates chromatin condensation throughout the cell cycle, was also evaluated, with EMW exposure leading to decreased histone kinase activity. Decreased histone kinase activity would potentially lead to defective cell cycle progression and ultimately defective spermatogenesis [48]. However, it remains unclear how EMWs affect histone kinase and induce clastogenic activity.

Many human and animal studies have associated oxidative stress and sperm DNA fragmentation in male infertility, further supported by a reduction of DNA damage with oral antioxidants [40, 49–52]. Semen samples with elevated levels of DNA damage are often associated with poor reproductive outcomes, including decreased pregnancy rates, embryo cleavage, and embryo quality [53, 54]. Given the association of ROS and potential secondary DNA fragmentation, the effect of EMWs on sperm DNA fragmentation levels is an important and understudied topic.

Animal Studies: Male Reproductive Cell Phone Exposure and Apoptosis

Recent studies have investigated a possible link between cell phone exposure and apoptosis. Dasdag and colleagues investigated the effect of cell phone radiation on activated caspase 3 levels, a direct measure of apoptosis. The authors exposed 14 rats to 900 MHz radiation over 10 months for 2 h/day and measured active testicular caspase 3 levels and did not find an association between EMW exposure and increased caspase 3 levels [78]. However, Kesari et al. found an increase in semen apoptotic cells on flow cytometry with cell phone exposure [20]. A later study by Kesari and colleagues supported this finding, with increased caspase-3 activity found in EMW-exposed animals compared to controls [42].

Animal Studies: Male Reproductive Histopathological Changes After Cell Phone Exposure

There are multiple studies using rodent models to investigate the testicular histopathological changes secondary to cell phone exposure. Meo and colleagues exposed rats to cell phone exposure for 60 min and found 18.75 % hypospermatogenesis and 18.75 % maturation arrest in the testes of exposed rats [79]. Dasdag and colleagues exposed rats to cell phone radiation for 2 h/day and revealed a decrease in seminiferous tubular diameter [3]. However, follow-up studies by the same authors did not reproduce seminiferous tubule changes [4, 78], despite using generally higher SARs (0.52 and 0.07–0.57 W/kg versus 0.141 W/kg) compared to the earliest study.

In another study, investigators exposed rats to cellular phones for 15, 30, and 60 min with frequencies ranging from 900/1,800/1,900 MHz at 2-W peak power and an SAR of 0.9 W/kg [45]. The rats were exposed at a distance of 50 cm between the phone and the rats. Controls included unexposed and exposed rats. Two additional cohorts were given a 2-week pretreatment of vitamin C or E. Rat seminiferous tubules were widened with cell phone exposure, accompanied by the absence of spermatozoa within the lumen, but a significant regenerative effect was noted on histopathological analysis of antioxidant pre-treated animals.

To add, Celik and colleagues investigated the light and electron microscopic changes on rat testes after 3 months of cell phone exposure at an SAR of 1.58 W/kg. Exposed rat testes revealed vacuolization in the cytoplasm and development of large lipid droplets in Sertoli cells, along with other extracellular matrix changes [80]. Ultimately, EMW radiation may cause testicular histopathological changes. Consistent reproducibility of histopathological changes will depend on development of a standardized exposure protocol.

Male Reproductive Hormonal Studies in Animals and Humans

Leydig cells account for the majority of total body testosterone, which is necessary for spermatogenesis. Leydig cell function may be affected by EMW exposure, although there are few studies investigating testosterone levels in animals. Meo and colleagues found a stepwise decrease in testosterone levels with increasing duration of cell phone exposure [81]. This supports the findings of Wang et al., who demonstrated a decrease in serum testosterone coupled with Leydig cell mitochondrial swelling and other cellular changes in EMW-exposed mice [82]. Zhou and colleagues also found a decrease in serum testosterone in EMW-exposed rats along with alterations in Leydig cell steroidogenesis [83]. Ozguner et al. studied testicular histology, testosterone, LH, and FSH levels in EMW-exposed rats, showing a decrease in seminiferous tubule diameter and testosterone levels but no other hormonal or histopathological changes [84].

Nevertheless, current animal literature does not unanimously support lower testosterone levels after EMW radiation exposure. Interestingly, some studies have found an increase in testosterone levels, specifically at 24 h and 2 weeks post EMW exposure [77, 85]. Thus, testosterone may have a rebound effect in certain instances of EMW exposure. Further studies are necessary to elucidate the mechanism of cell phone radiation-induced hormonal alterations within animal testes, given the effects of cell phone radiation are evident, but remain poorly understood.

Cell Phone Effects on the Pituitary Gland

The risk of negative pituitary gland effects secondary to cell phone exposure is of interest, given their intracranial location and increasing global use of cell phones. However, there is little literature on the effects of pituitary gland exposure to cell phone radiation. A population based case control study of 291 cases and 630 controls investigated the risk of pituitary tumor development and did not reveal any association of cellular phone use and pituitary tumor risk [86]. Other studies of pituitary gland function after cell phone exposure have not revealed any significant disturbance in human pituitary endocrine function [87, 88]. Ultimately, although there are few studies on the effect of cell phone radiation on pituitary gland function, there does not appear to be an association between increased cell phone exposure and perturbation of pituitary function.

Laptop Computers and Male Fertility

Laptop computer use has increased dramatically in recent years and is an essential component of everyday life for many people. Many portable computers are placed in the operators lap during use of Wi-Fi, which is generally set at a frequency of 2.4 GHz. As with other nonionizing radiation devices, exposure is dependent upon the distance of the device antenna from the exposed tissues. However, there is a limited amount of data regarding the potential adverse reproductive health effects of Wi-Fi use of laptop computers. The few and limited studies to date focus on two aspects of laptop and Wi-Fi use: thermal and non-thermal effects.

Laptops and Thermal Effects on Male Reproduction

Thermal toxicity has been implicated in male infertility [89, 90] and may also play a role in male laptop use. Sheynkin and colleagues [91] studied scrotal hyperthermia in laptop computer use by young men of reproductive age in a seated position with a laptop balanced on their legs. The authors found an approximately 3 °C increase with 60 min of seated laptop computer use. The authors repeated the study with variation in leg position and found an increase in temperature of all participants by approximately 30 min [92]. However, these studies did not investigate semen analyses or pregnancy outcomes of study participants. Thus, it remains unclear if an increase in scrotal temperature with laptop use is clinically relevant.

Given human spermatogenesis is temperature dependent, with the male scrotum typically 1–2 °C below core body temperature, scrotal hyperthermia may disturb intratesticular oxidative balance, leading to potential oxidative stress, cell apoptosis, and compromised sperm DNA integrity [93, 94]. Current literature lacks any studies investigating thermal toxicity secondary to EMWs from Wi-Fi use of laptops. Further studies are needed to delineate the male reproductive consequences of laptop computer thermal output, as well as possible thermal effects secondary to EMWs.

Laptops and Nonthermal Effects on Male Reproduction

Due to the paucity of available literature, the potential nonthermal effects of EMWs in laptop computers remain unclear. Oni et al. performed an in vitro pilot study investigating the effects of EMWs from Wi-Fi on ejaculated semen samples [95]. Samples from ten donors were split and unexposed samples were compared to samples placed 60 cm from each laptop for 1 h. The authors found a decrease in sperm motility and morphology with laptop Wi-Fi exposure. However, the unexposed aliquots were not placed near laptop computers with Wi-Fi turned off. The scientific relevance of a 60 cm distance and 1 h duration of exposure is unclear. Overall, it is difficult to differentiate the potential thermal effects of laptop exposure from the nonthermal effects of EMW in this study.

In a similar study, Avendano and colleagues [96] evaluated semen samples of 29 donors and exposed them to Wi-Fi connected laptop computers with a 3 cm distance. The authors aliquoted each sample into two fractions: the exposed fraction was placed in dishes under the laptop for 4 h. The second fraction was treated as a control and was not placed near a computer or other electronic devices. An air conditioning system was placed under the laptop to homogenize the temperature at 25 °C above each sample. The authors reported a significant decrease in progressive motility and nonmotile sperm and increased DNA fragmentation index in laptop exposed samples.

This study did not have an adequate control, given the nonexposed fraction was not placed under a laptop with Wi-Fi off. The study also lacked adequate control for temperature, since this was not measured and it is unclear if the temperature of the experimental area was homogenized [97, 98]. In addition, although the laptops were all placed 3 cm from each exposed sample, location of the antennae is not reported, which would significantly affect the strength of the electromagnetic field under the laptop. The authors also included three teratozoospermic semen samples within their cohort, which may have biased study outcomes [98]. Given the pervasive use of laptop computers in men of reproductive age, further studies are warranted to clarify the potential effects of laptop exposure in male reproductive health.

Microwaves and Male Fertility

Microwave ovens use the formation of an electromagnetic field to create a thermal effect through random molecular motion. Cell phones and laptops are a subset of microwaves, using a similar range of frequency along the EMW spectrum. However, conventional microwave ovens typically operate at a slightly higher frequency than most cell phones, at approximately 2.45 GHz and power ranging from 0.5 to 2 kW [99].

As microwaves are absorbed in tissue, heat is produced which warms and cooks the tissue. However, the nonthermal effects of microwaves remain unknown. The effect of leakage of electromagnetic radiation from microwave ovens may have negative health effects. Currently, US Food and Drug Administration regulations limit operational microwave oven leakage to 5 mW/cm^2 at any point within a 2 in. distance from the oven [100].

To date, there are no studies related to microwave oven leakage and male reproductive health. However, there are animal studies using the 2.45 GHz frequency commonly used in commercial microwave ovens. Kesari and colleagues found a decrease in antioxidant enzymes and histone kinase with a concomitant increase in apoptosis after exposing rodents to EMWs at 2.45 GHz [101]. A later study by Kumar and colleagues reported increased apoptosis in rodents exposed to microwaves at 2.45 GHz EMW radiation, with a significant decrease in testosterone, increase in both caspase levels and sperm creatine kinase, a measure of sperm quality and immaturity [102, 103].

Saygin and colleagues exposed rats at 2.45 GHz and an SAR of 3.21 W/kg for 1 h/day over a 28-day period and found a decrease in the number of Leydig cells in exposed animals and increased levels of the Bax apoptosis genes and caspase-8 apoptosis enzyme [104]. However, Leydig cell number was increased with increasing exposure in a preceding study by Kim et al. [105]. The authors exposed animals at 2.45 GHz at an SAR of 1.4 W/kg for either 1 or 2 h/day for 45 days and found a dose-dependent increase in the number of Leydig cells after exposure. Epididymal sperm counts trended downward and there were no histopathological changes found with exposure.

This variation in affect on Leydig cell number may relate to the different SAR levels (3.21 W/kg versus 1.4 W/kg) in each study, with the higher SAR leading to a decrease in Leydig cell number. A lower SAR may lead to a compensatory hyperplastic effect in an attempt to restore normal spermatogenesis. This may potentially precede a decrease in Leydig cell number, as seen at a higher SAR by Saygin and colleagues [104]. Variation in SAR may ultimately affect fertilization rates [106]. Overall, although 2.45 GHz EMW exposure appears to effect male reproductive biology, the mechanism of action remains unclear.

Discussion

Cell phone, laptop, and microwave EMW radiation exposure may be a possible cause of unexplained male infertility. Although studies have shown adverse effects of EMW exposure in the male reproductive system (Fig. 11.2), current research on the effects of EMW radiation on male reproductive health has been limited by inadequate study design and methods. Observational and in vitro studies preclude pathologic studies of male reproductive tissues. Observational studies also disallow elucidation of the true chronicity and amount of EMW exposure since these studies are subject to recall bias [107]. Reported cell phone usage may be affected by current cell phone use and may not reflect remote or recent changes in cell phone usage.

EMW animal studies are limited by the models chosen (mouse and rat) given the small size of the animal's testes, their nonpendulous scrota, and the ability of their testes to freely ascend through the inguinal canal into the abdomen. The rodent model does not accurately mimic human EMW absorption from cellular phones, given the tissues and distance between the antenna of the phone are not comparable. Current animal studies are also limited by inconsistent placement of cell phone antennae, with cell phones placed either on the cage, in the cage, or near the face of exposed rodents without any mention of antennae location or standardization of cell phone location relative to exposed animal testes.

Previous studies are also limited by the cell phone frequencies chosen, with most being below 1,800/1,900 MHz, which is more commonly used today. Irrespective of frequency difference, some studies did not reveal any correlation between EMW and cell phone exposure [108, 109]. These studies were very similar in design to aforementioned studies which reported an association between EMW and male fertility.

Computational analysis may play a significant role in EMW research in the future. Using two-dimensional modeling, Mouradi and colleagues calculated a distance of 0.8–1.8 cm as the distance from the testes needed to have an impact on male spermatozoa [110]. However, three-dimensional modeling will ultimately be necessary to account for the contours and shape of male genital soft tissues. Because previous rodent models are inadequate and results are inconsistent [2–4, 20, 78, 108, 109], these studies can never be directly applied to humans. Until an adequate animal model is found, computational studies may play a key role in proving a stronger

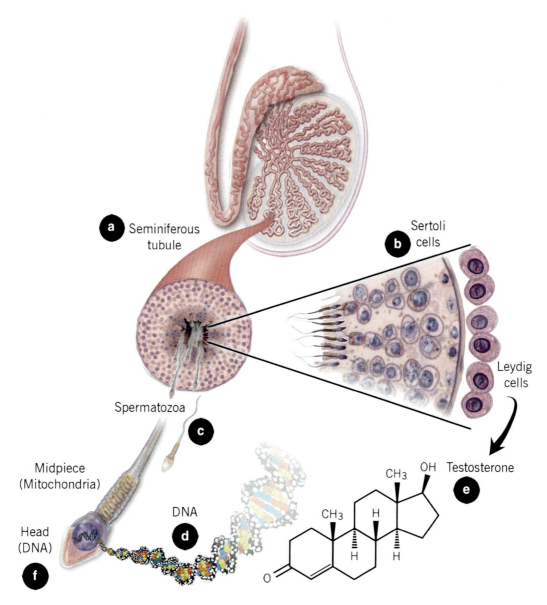

Fig. 11.2 Potential effects of cellular phone EMW toxicity in the male reproductive system. (**a**) Seminiferous tubule—↓diameter, structural abnormalities, hypospermatogenesis, and maturation arrest. (**b**) Sertoli cells—structural changes. (**c**) Spermatozoa—↓concentration, ↓viability, ↓motility, ↓morphology, ↑oxidative stress. (**d**) DNA—↑DNA damage. (**e**) Testosterone—↓testosterone. (**f**) Sperm—head—↑sperm head abnormalities, ↓sperm-zona binding. [Reprinted with permission, Cleveland Clinic Center for Medical Art & Photography © 2011-2013. All Rights Reserved]

association between adverse reproductive effects and EMW exposure.

In addition, the current studies at microwave oven frequency do not mimic microwave oven use in humans, given real exposure is likely from EMW leakage rather than direct EMW exposure. To add, the thermal and nonthermal effects of laptop exposure remain unknown. Nevertheless, EMW exposure and abnormalities in the human male reproductive axis appear to be strongly associated (Fig. 11.1) and early studies have begun elucidation of a possible mechanism of action (Fig. 11.2). The inherent weaknesses of available study designs and paucity of data mitigate any substantive gains in our knowledge on EMW effects on human testes. Conclusive data regarding cell phone, laptop, and microwave oven usage are needed to clarify the risks associated with EMW exposure in subfertile men.

Conclusion

Overall, current studies are unable to suggest a true mechanism of EMW radiation effects on the male reproductive axis. Although some molecular markers and oxidative stress have been inconsistently implicated, the mechanism of possible cell EMW effects remains unknown. Inadequate and variable study designs are major mitigators of study reproducibility, leaving the potential deleterious effects of EMW radiation unproven. An improved animal model with histopathologic, molecular, and hormonal studies is needed to elucidate a true mechanism of EMW radiation injury in the male reproductive system. Future studies may be aided by three-dimensional computational modeling, which may help to safely and reproducibly assess the effects of varying EMW exposure and frequencies on male reproductive potential.

Until further studies are obtained using a standardized study protocol with a known radiation dosage which accounts for cell phone distance, frequency, SAR, and duration of exposure, no significant conclusions can be made regarding EMW exposure in unexplained male infertility. Although current literature lacks definitive evidence associating male infertility with cell phone exposure, limitation of exposure to the possible harmful effects of cell phone, laptop, and microwave ovens is recommended. Subfertile men should avoid placement of laptop computers in the lap during use and limit Bluetooth cell phone use, with cell phones turned off while near genitalia. Subfertile men should also avoid close proximity to microwave ovens during use. Given the EMW association with ROS, there may later be a role for antioxidant therapy in men with subfertility and increased EMW exposure. It remains unknown if subfertile men with extensive EMW damage to testes will require assisted reproductive technology (ART) and what the outcomes

will be. Carefully designed study protocols are needed to establish conclusive evidence of the potential negative effects of EMW radiation in the male reproductive system.

References

1. Habash RW, Bansal R, Krewski D, Alhafid HT. Thermal therapy, part 1: an introduction to thermal therapy. Crit Rev Biomed Eng. 2006;34(6): 459–89.
2. Yan JG, Agresti M, Bruce T, Yan YH, Granlund A, Matloub HS. Effects of cellular phone emissions on sperm motility in rats. Fertil Steril. 2007;88(4): 957–64.
3. Dasdag S, Ketani MA, Akdag Z, Ersay AR, Sari I, Demirtas OC, et al. Whole-body microwave exposure emitted by cellular phones and testicular function of rats. Urol Res. 1999;27(3):219–23.
4. Dasdag S, Zulkuf Akdag M, Aksen F, Yilmaz F, Bashan M, Mutlu Dasdag M, et al. Whole body exposure of rats to microwaves emitted from a cell phone does not affect the testes. Bioelectromagnetics. 2003;24(3):182–8.
5. Cell phones and specific absorption rate [Internet]. 2013 June 4. FCC.gov. Accessed 4 June 2013 [updated 2013 June 4; cited 2013 June 4]. http://www.fcc.gov/encyclopedia/cell-phones-and-specific-absorption-rate
6. Aitken RJ, Bennetts LE, Sawyer D, Wiklendt AM, King BV. Impact of radio frequency electromagnetic radiation on DNA integrity in the male germline. Int J Androl. 2005;28(3):171–9.
7. Ha BY. Stabilization and destabilization of cell membranes by multivalent ions. Phys Rev E Stat Nonlin Soft Matter Phys. 2001;64(5 Pt 1):051902.
8. Blackman CF, Benane SG, Kinney LS, Joines WT, House DE. Effects of ELF fields on calcium-ion efflux from brain tissue in vitro. Radiat Res. 1982; 92(3):510–20.
9. Abou-haila A, Tulsiani DR. Signal transduction pathways that regulate sperm capacitation and the acrosome reaction. Arch Biochem Biophys. 2009; 485(1):72–81.
10. Hamada A, Singh A, Agarwal A. Cell phones and their impact on male fertility: fact or fiction. Open Reprod Sci J. 2011;5(3):125–37.
11. Zhao M, Xia L, Chen GQ. Protein kinase cdelta in apoptosis: a brief overview. Arch Immunol Ther Exp (Warsz). 2012;60(5):361–72.
12. Griner EM, Kazanietz MG. Protein kinase C and other diacylglycerol effectors in cancer. Nat Rev Cancer. 2007;7(4):281–94.
13. Kalive M, Faust JJ, Koeneman BA, Capco DG. Involvement of the PKC family in regulation of early development. Mol Reprod Dev. 2010;77(2): 95–104.

14. Fejes I, Zavaczki Z, Szollosi J, Koloszar S, Daru J, Kovacs L, et al. Is there a relationship between cell phone use and semen quality? Arch Androl. 2005; 51(5):385–93.
15. Agarwal A, Deepinder F, Sharma RK, Ranga G, Li J. Effect of cell phone usage on semen analysis in men attending infertility clinic: an observational study. Fertil Steril. 2008;89(1):124–8.
16. Agarwal A, Desai NR, Makker K, Varghese A, Mouradi R, Sabanegh E, et al. Effects of radiofrequency electromagnetic waves (RF-EMW) from cellular phones on human ejaculated semen: an in vitro pilot study. Fertil Steril. 2009;92(4):1318–25.
17. Erogul O, Oztas E, Yildirim I, Kir T, Aydur E, Komesli G, et al. Effects of electromagnetic radiation from a cellular phone on human sperm motility: an in vitro study. Arch Med Res. 2006;37(7):840–3.
18. De Iuliis GN, Newey RJ, King BV, Aitken RJ. Mobile phone radiation induces reactive oxygen species production and DNA damage in human spermatozoa in vitro. PLoS One. 2009;4(7):e6446.
19. Mahfouz R, Sharma R, Thiyagarajan A, Kale V, Gupta S, Sabanegh E, et al. Semen characteristics and sperm DNA fragmentation in infertile men with low and high levels of seminal reactive oxygen species. Fertil Steril. 2010;94(6):2141–6.
20. Kesari KK, Kumar S, Behari J. Mobile phone usage and male infertility in Wistar rats. Indian J Exp Biol. 2010;48(10):987–92.
21. Wang XW, Ding GR, Shi CH, Zeng LH, Liu JY, Li J, et al. Mechanisms involved in the blood-testis barrier increased permeability induced by EMP. Toxicology. 2010;276(1):58–63.
22. Wang XW, Ding GR, Shi CH, Zhao T, Zhang J, Zeng LH, et al. Effect of electromagnetic pulse exposure on permeability of blood-testicle barrier in mice. Biomed Environ Sci. 2008;21(3):218–21.
23. Hou WG, Zhao J, Li Z, Li W, Li T, Xiong LZ, et al. Effects of electromagnetic pulse irradiation on the mouse blood-testicle barrier. Urology. 2012;80(1):225 e1–6.
24. Cheng CY, Mruk DD. The blood-testis barrier and its implications for male contraception. Pharmacol Rev. 2012;64(1):16–64.
25. Ghabriel MN, Lu JJ, Hermanis G, Zhu C, Setchell BP. Expression of a blood-brain barrier-specific antigen in the reproductive tract of the male rat. Reproduction. 2002;123(3):389–97.
26. Eberhardt JL, Persson BR, Brun AE, Salford LG, Malmgren LO. Blood-brain barrier permeability and nerve cell damage in rat brain 14 and 28 days after exposure to microwaves from GSM mobile phones. Electromagn Biol Med. 2008;27(3):215–29.
27. Salford LG, Brun AE, Eberhardt JL, Malmgren L, Persson BR. Nerve cell damage in mammalian brain after exposure to microwaves from GSM mobile phones. Environ Health Perspect. 2003;111(7): 881–3; discussion A408.
28. Fritze K, Sommer C, Schmitz B, Mies G, Hossmann KA, Kiessling M, et al. Effect of global system for mobile communication (GSM) microwave exposure on blood-brain barrier permeability in rat. Acta Neuropathol. 1997;94(5):465–70.
29. Grafstrom G, Nittby H, Brun A, Malmgren L, Persson BR, Salford LG, et al. Histopathological examinations of rat brains after long-term exposure to GSM-900 mobile phone radiation. Brain Res Bull. 2008;77(5):257–63.
30. Finnie JW, Blumbergs PC, Manavis J, Utteridge TD, Gebski V, Davies RA, et al. Effect of long-term mobile communication microwave exposure on vascular permeability in mouse brain. Pathology. 2002; 34(4):344–7.
31. Franke H, Ringelstein EB, Stogbauer F. Electromagnetic fields (GSM 1800) do not alter blood-brain barrier permeability to sucrose in models in vitro with high barrier tightness. Bioelectromagnetics. 2005;26(7):529–35.
32. Franke H, Streckert J, Bitz A, Goeke J, Hansen V, Ringelstein EB, et al. Effects of Universal Mobile Telecommunications System (UMTS) electromagnetic fields on the blood-brain barrier in vitro. Radiat Res. 2005;164(3):258–69.
33. Kuribayashi M, Wang J, Fujiwara O, Doi Y, Nabae K, Tamano S, et al. Lack of effects of 1439 MHz electromagnetic near field exposure on the blood-brain barrier in immature and young rats. Bioelectromagnetics. 2005;26(7):578–88.
34. de Gannes FP, Billaudel B, Taxile M, Haro E, Ruffie G, Leveque P, et al. Effects of head-only exposure of rats to GSM-900 on blood-brain barrier permeability and neuronal degeneration. Radiat Res. 2009;172(3): 359–67.
35. Leszczynski D, Joenvaara S, Reivinen J, Kuokka R. Non-thermal activation of the hsp27/p38MAPK stress pathway by mobile phone radiation in human endothelial cells: molecular mechanism for cancer- and blood-brain barrier-related effects. Differentiation. 2002;70(2–3):120–9.
36. McNamee JP, Chauhan V. Radiofrequency radiation and gene/protein expression: a review. Radiat Res. 2009;172(3):265–87.
37. Cotgreave IA. Biological stress responses to radio frequency electromagnetic radiation: are mobile phones really so (heat) shocking? Arch Biochem Biophys. 2005;435(1):227–40.
38. Henkel R. The impact of oxidants on sperm function. Andrologia. 2005;37(6):205–6.
39. Aitken RJ, Baker MA, De Iuliis GN, Nixon B. New insights into sperm physiology and pathology. Handb Exp Pharmacol. 2010;198:99–115.
40. Moustafa MH, Sharma RK, Thornton J, Mascha E, Abdel-Hafez MA, Thomas Jr AJ, et al. Relationship between ROS production, apoptosis and DNA denaturation in spermatozoa from patients examined for infertility. Hum Reprod. 2004;19(1):129–38.
41. Pasqualotto FF, Sharma RK, Kobayashi H, Nelson DR, Thomas Jr AJ, Agarwal A. Oxidative stress in normospermic men undergoing infertility evaluation. J Androl. 2001;22(2):316–22.

42. Kesari KK, Behari J. Evidence for mobile phone radiation exposure effects on reproductive pattern of male rats: role of ROS. Electromagn Biol Med. 2012;31(3):213–22.

43. Turrens JF. Mitochondrial formation of reactive oxygen species. J Physiol. 2003;552(Pt 2):335–44.

44. Jin Z, Zong C, Jiang B, Zhou Z, Tong J, Cao Y. The effect of combined exposure of 900 MHz radiofrequency fields and doxorubicin in HL-60 cells. PLoS One. 2012;7(9):e46102.

45. Al-Damegh MA. Rat testicular impairment induced by electromagnetic radiation from a conventional cellular telephone and the protective effects of the antioxidants vitamins C and E. Clinics (Sao Paulo). 2012;67(7):785–92.

46. Aitken RJ, De Iuliis GN. On the possible origins of DNA damage in human spermatozoa. Mol Hum Reprod. 2010;16(1):3–13.

47. Blank M, Goodman R. Electromagnetic fields may act directly on DNA. J Cell Biochem. 1999;75(3): 369–74.

48. Kesari KK, Kumar S, Behari J. Effects of radiofrequency electromagnetic wave exposure from cellular phones on the reproductive pattern in male Wistar rats. Appl Biochem Biotechnol. 2011;164(4): 546–59.

49. Tamburrino L, Marchiani S, Montoya M, Elia Marino F, Natali I, Cambi M, et al. Mechanisms and clinical correlates of sperm DNA damage. Asian J Androl. 2012;14(1):24–31.

50. Greco E, Iacobelli M, Rienzi L, Ubaldi F, Ferrero S, Tesarik J. Reduction of the incidence of sperm DNA fragmentation by oral antioxidant treatment. J Androl. 2005;26(3):349–53.

51. De Iuliis GN, Thomson LK, Mitchell LA, Finnie JM, Koppers AJ, Hedges A, et al. DNA damage in human spermatozoa is highly correlated with the efficiency of chromatin remodeling and the formation of 8-hydroxy-2′-deoxyguanosine, a marker of oxidative stress. Biol Reprod. 2009;81(3):517–24.

52. Oger I, Da Cruz C, Panteix G, Menezo Y. Evaluating human sperm DNA integrity: relationship between 8-hydroxydeoxyguanosine quantification and the sperm chromatin structure assay. Zygote. 2003;11(4): 367–71.

53. Agarwal A, Said TM. Role of sperm chromatin abnormalities and DNA damage in male infertility. Hum Reprod Update. 2003;9(4):331–45.

54. Sharma RK, Said T, Agarwal A. Sperm DNA damage and its clinical relevance in assessing reproductive outcome. Asian J Androl. 2004;6(2):139–48.

55. Privateline.com: Digital wireless basics: frequencies [Internet]. Accessed 22 July 2012. http://www.privateline.com/PCS/Frequencies.htm

56. How cell-phone radiation works [Internet]. Accessed 22 July 2012. http://www.howstuffworks.com/cell-phone-radiation.html

57. Deepinder F, Makker K, Agarwal A. Cell phones and male infertility: dissecting the relationship. Reprod Biomed Online. 2007;15(3):266–70.

58. Cleveland Jr JR, Sylvar DM, Ulcek JL. Evaluating compliance with FCC guidelines for human exposure to radiofrequency electromagnetic fields. August 1997 [Internet]. Accessed 22 July 2012. http://www.fcc.gov/Bureaus/Engineering_Technology/Documents/bulletins/oet65/oet65.pdf

59. Desai NR, Kesari KK, Agarwal A. Pathophysiology of cell phone radiation: oxidative stress and carcinogenesis with focus on male reproductive system. Reprod Biol Endocrinol. 2009;7:114.

60. Straume A, Oftedal G, Johnsson A. Skin temperature increase caused by a mobile phone: a methodological infrared camera study. Bioelectromagnetics. 2005;26(6):510–9.

61. Friedman J, Kraus S, Hauptman Y, Schiff Y, Seger R. Mechanism of short-term ERK activation by electromagnetic fields at mobile phone frequencies. Biochem J. 2007;405(3):559–68.

62. D'Costa H, Trueman G, Tang L, Abdel-rahman U, Abdel-rahman W, Ong K, et al. Human brain wave activity during exposure to radiofrequency field emissions from mobile phones. Australas Phys Eng Sci Med. 2003;26(4):162–7.

63. Kramarenko AV, Tan U. Effects of high-frequency electromagnetic fields on human EEG: a brain mapping study. Int J Neurosci. 2003;113(7):1007–19.

64. Oftedal G, Wilen J, Sandstrom M, Mild KH. Symptoms experienced in connection with mobile phone use. Occup Med (Lond). 2000;50(4):237–45.

65. Hillert L, Akerstedt T, Lowden A, Wiholm C, Kuster N, Ebert S, et al. The effects of 884 MHz GSM wireless communication signals on headache and other symptoms: an experimental provocation study. Bioelectromagnetics. 2008;29(3):185–96.

66. Volkow ND, Tomasi D, Wang GJ, Vaska P, Fowler JS, Telang F, et al. Effects of cell phone radiofrequency signal exposure on brain glucose metabolism. JAMA. 2011;305(8):808–13.

67. Hardell L, Carlberg M, Hansson MK. Use of mobile phones and cordless phones is associated with increased risk for glioma and acoustic neuroma. Pathophysiology. 2013;20(2):85–110.

68. Roosli M, Michel G, Kuehni CE, Spoerri A. Cellular telephone use and time trends in brain tumour mortality in Switzerland from 1969 to 2002. Eur J Cancer Prev. 2007;16(1):77–82.

69. Wdowiak A, Wdowiak L, Wiktor H. Evaluation of the effect of using mobile phones on male fertility. Ann Agric Environ Med. 2007;14(1):169–72.

70. Kilgallon SJ, Simmons LW. Image content influences men's semen quality. Biol Lett. 2005;1(3): 253–5.

71. Gutschi T, Mohamad Al-Ali B, Shamloul R, Pummer K, Trummer H. Impact of cell phone use on men's semen parameters. Andrologia. 2011;43(5):312–6.

72. Falzone N, Huyser C, Becker P, Leszczynski D, Franken DR. The effect of pulsed 900-MHz GSM mobile phone radiation on the acrosome reaction, head morphometry and zona binding of human spermatozoa. Int J Androl. 2011;34(1):20–6.

73. Agarwal A, Saleh RA, Bedaiwy MA. Role of reactive oxygen species in the pathophysiology of human reproduction. Fertil Steril. 2003;79(4):829–43.

74. Shen HM, Chia SE, Ong CN. Evaluation of oxidative DNA damage in human sperm and its association with male infertility. J Androl. 1999;20(6):718–23.

75. Aitken RJ, Baker MA. Oxidative stress, sperm survival and fertility control. Mol Cell Endocrinol. 2006;250(1–2):66–9.

76. Mailankot M, Kunnath AP, Jayalekshmi H, Koduru B, Valsalan R. Radio frequency electromagnetic radiation (RF-EMR) from GSM (0.9/1.8GHz) mobile phones induces oxidative stress and reduces sperm motility in rats. Clinics (Sao Paulo). 2009; 64(6):561–5.

77. Ozlem Nisbet H, Nisbet C, Akar A, Cevik M, Karayigit MO. Effects of exposure to electromagnetic field (1.8/0.9 GHz) on testicular function and structure in growing rats. Res Vet Sci. 2012;93(2): 1001–5.

78. Dasdag S, Akdag MZ, Ulukaya E, Uzunlar AK, Yegin D. Mobile phone exposure does not induce apoptosis on spermatogenesis in rats. Arch Med Res. 2008;39(1):40–4.

79. Meo SA, Arif M, Rashied S, Khan MM, Vohra MS, Usmani AM, et al. Hypospermatogenesis and spermatozoa maturation arrest in rats induced by mobile phone radiation. J Coll Physicians Surg Pak. 2011; 21(5):262–5.

80. Celik S, Aridogan IA, Izol V, Erdogan S, Polat S, Doran S. An evaluation of the effects of long-term cell phone use on the testes via light and electron microscope analysis. Urology. 2012;79(2):346–50.

81. Meo SA, Al-Drees AM, Husain S, Khan MM, Imran MB. Effects of mobile phone radiation on serum testosterone in Wistar albino rats. Saudi Med J. 2010;31(8):869–73.

82. Wang SM, Wang DW, Peng RY, Gao YB, Yang Y, Hu WH, et al. [Effect of electromagnetic pulse irradiation on structure and function of Leydig cells in mice]. Zhonghua Nan Ke Xue. 2003;9(5):327–30.

83. Zhou W, Wang XB, Yang JQ, Liu Y, Zhang GB. [Influence of electromagnetic irradiation on P450scc mRNA expression in rat testis tissues and protective effect of the shield]. Zhonghua Nan Ke Xue. 2005;11(4):269–71.

84. Ozguner M, Koyu A, Cesur G, Ural M, Ozguner F, Gokcimen A, et al. Biological and morphological effects on the reproductive organ of rats after exposure to electromagnetic field. Saudi Med J. 2005; 26(3):405–10.

85. Forgacs Z, Somosy Z, Kubinyi G, Bakos J, Hudak A, Surjan A, et al. Effect of whole-body 1800 MHz GSM-like microwave exposure on testicular steroidogenesis and histology in mice. Reprod Toxicol. 2006;22(1):111–7.

86. Schoemaker MJ, Swerdlow AJ. Risk of pituitary tumors in cellular phone users: a case-control study. Epidemiology. 2009;20(3):348–54.

87. de Seze R, Fabbro-Peray P, Miro L. GSM radiocellular telephones do not disturb the secretion of antepituitary hormones in humans. Bioelectromagnetics. 1998;19(5):271–8.

88. Djeridane Y, Touitou Y, de Seze R. Influence of electromagnetic fields emitted by GSM-900 cellular telephones on the circadian patterns of gonadal, adrenal and pituitary hormones in men. Radiat Res. 2008;169(3):337–43.

89. Dada R, Gupta NP, Kucheria K. Spermatogenic arrest in men with testicular hyperthermia. Teratog Carcinog Mutagen. 2003;Suppl 1:235–43.

90. Ahmad G, Moinard N, Esquerre-Lamare C, Mieusset R, Bujan L. Mild induced testicular and epididymal hyperthermia alters sperm chromatin integrity in men. Fertil Steril. 2012;97(3):546–53.

91. Sheynkin Y, Jung M, Yoo P, Schulsinger D, Komaroff E. Increase in scrotal temperature in laptop computer users. Hum Reprod. 2005;20(2):452–5.

92. Sheynkin Y, Welliver R, Winer A, Hajimirzaee F, Ahn H, Lee K. Protection from scrotal hyperthermia in laptop computer users. Fertil Steril. 2010;95(2):647–51.

93. Banks S, King SA, Irvine DS, Saunders PT. Impact of a mild scrotal heat stress on DNA integrity in murine spermatozoa. Reproduction. 2005;129(4): 505–14.

94. Shiraishi K, Takihara H, Matsuyama H. Elevated scrotal temperature, but not varicocele grade, reflects testicular oxidative stress-mediated apoptosis. World J Urol. 2009;28(3):359–64.

95. Oni O, Amuda D, Gilbert C. Effects of radiofrequency radiation from WiFi devices on human ejaculated semen. Int J Res Rev Appl Sci. 2011;19: 292–4.

96. Avendano C, Mata A, Sanchez Sarmiento CA, Doncel GF. Use of laptop computers connected to internet through Wi-Fi decreases human sperm motility and increases sperm DNA fragmentation. Fertil Steril. 2012;97(1):39–45.e2.

97. Dore JF, Chignol MC. Laptop computers with Wi-Fi decrease human sperm motility and increase sperm DNA fragmentation. Fertil Steril. 2012;97(4):e12; author reply e3.

98. Choy JT, Brannigan RE. Words of wisdom. Re: Use of laptop computers connected to Internet through Wi-Fi decreases human sperm motility and increases sperm DNA fragmentation. Eur Urol. 2012;62(6): 1196–7.

99. Alhekail ZO. Electromagnetic radiation from microwave ovens. J Radiol Prot. 2001;21(3):251–8.

100. Microwave oven radiation. [Internet]. Accessed 7 Mar 2013. [Updated 2013 Mar 7; cited 2013 Mar 7]. http://www.fda.gov/Radiation-EmittingProducts/ RadiationEmittingProductsandProcedures/ HomeBusinessandEntertainment/ucm142616.htm

101. Kesari KK, Behari J. Microwave exposure affecting reproductive system in male rats. Appl Biochem Biotechnol. 2010;162(2):416–28.

102. Kumar S, Kesari KK, Behari J. The therapeutic effect of a pulsed electromagnetic field on the reproductive patterns of male Wistar rats exposed to a 2.45-GHz microwave field. Clinics (Sao Paulo). 2011;66(7):1237–45.
103. Hallak J, Sharma RK, Pasqualotto FF, Ranganathan P, Thomas Jr AJ, Agarwal A. Creatine kinase as an indicator of sperm quality and maturity in men with oligospermia. Urology. 2001;58(3): 446–51.
104. Saygin M, Caliskan S, Karahan N, Koyu A, Gumral N, Uguz A. Testicular apoptosis and histopathological changes induced by a 2.45 GHz electromagnetic field. Toxicol Ind Health. 2011; 27(5):455–63.
105. Kim JY, Kim HT, Moon KH, Shin HJ. Long-term exposure of rats to 2.45 GHz electromagnetic field: effects on reproductive function. Korean J Urol. 2007;48:1308–14.
106. Cleary SF, Liu LM, Graham R, East J. In vitro fertilization of mouse ova by spermatozoa exposed isothermally to radio-frequency radiation. Bioelectromagnetics. 1989;10(4):361 9.
107. Jepsen P, Johnsen SP, Gillman MW, Sorensen HT. Interpretation of observational studies. Heart. 2004;90(8):956–60.
108. Lee HJ, Pack JK, Kim TH, Kim N, Choi SY, Lee JS, et al. The lack of histological changes of CDMA cellular phone-based radio frequency on rat testis. Bioelectromagnetics. 2010;31(7):528–34.
109. Imai N, Kawabe M, Hikage T, Nojima T, Takahashi S, Shirai T. Effects on rat testis of 1.95-GHz W-CDMA for IMT-2000 cellular phones. Syst Biol Reprod Med. 2011;57(4):204–9.
110. Mouradi R, Desai N, Erdemir A, Agarwal A. The use of FDTD in establishing in vitro experimentation conditions representative of lifelike cell phone radiation on the spermatozoa. Health Phys. 2012;102(1):54–62.

Part II

Occupational Exposure

Pesticides and Heavy Metal Toxicity

12

Lidia Mínguez-Alarcón, Jaime Mendiola, and Alberto M. Torres-Cantero

Introduction

There is evidence in the literature that male reproductive function has deteriorated significantly in the past 50 years [1]. A later review, which included 47 additional studies, confirmed that sperm concentration has declined, being the role of decline more pronounced in Europe (−2.3 %) than in the USA (−0.8 %) or other countries (−0.2 %) [2].

However, even within geographical regions there are important intercountry differences. In a cross-sectional study, the Finnish and Estonian men had higher total sperm counts, sperm concentrations, and number of normal sperm than the Norwegian and Danish men [3]. This variation has been supported by other studies with men who were not selected because of fertility or infertility [4–8]. Besides, there are significant intra-country variations. Swan et al. suggested that sperm concentration and motility might be reduced in semirural and agricultural areas compared to urban and less agriculturally intensive areas [9].

Semen quality differences could be related to lifestyle factors and dietary patterns [10–12],

L. Mínguez-Alarcón, PhD (✉) • J. Mendiola, PhD
A.M. Torres-Cantero, MD, DrPH
Department of Preventive Medicine and Public Health, School of Medicine, University of Murcia, Campus de Espinardo, Espinardo, 30100 Murcia, Spain
e-mail: minguezalarcon@gmail.com; jaime.mendiola@um.es; amtorres@um.es

prenatal exposures [13, 14], and occupational and environmental exposures [15–17].

The objective of this chapter is to summarize the negative impact of pesticides and heavy metal exposures on adult male reproductive function.

Pesticides and Impairment of Adult Male Reproductive Function

Pesticides are an important group of environmental pollutants used in intensive agriculture for protection against diseases and pests caused by weeds (herbicides), insects (insecticides), and fungi (fungicides) [18] (Table 12.1). According to their chemical composition, there are two main types of pesticides: organochlorine and organophosphate pesticides. Organochlorines contain at least one covalently bonded chlorine atom in their chemical structure, while organophosphates have a carbon–phosphorus bond in their configuration. They both may impair reproductive male function through disruption of the endocrine axis [19].

In general, pesticides could adversely affect human semen parameters due to their hormonal activity on spermatogenesis. At the mitotic or meiotic level, those compounds may decrease sperm counts. With regard to postmeiotic processes and epididymal sperm maturation, those chemicals may impair sperm motility [20, 21]. Some pesticides are able to bind estrogen receptors because of their estrogen-like characteristics [22]. It has also been shown that the effect of pesticides, with either antiandrogenic or estrogenic properties, on male

S.S. du Plessis et al. (eds.), *Male Infertility: A Complete Guide to Lifestyle and Environmental Factors*,
DOI 10.1007/978-1-4939-1040-3_12, © Springer Science+Business Media New York 2014

Table 12.1 Main products where pesticides can be found

	Type	Uses
Organochlorine pesticides	Dichlorodiphenyltrichloroethane (DDT)	In pharmaceutical drugs against malaria and as insecticide
	Polychlorinated biphenyls (PCB)	In paints and cements as plasticizers, stabilizing additives in flexible PVC coatings, of electrical wiring and electronic components, pesticide extenders, cutting oils, reactive flame retardants, lubricating oils, hydraulic fluids, adhesives, wood floor, paints, de-dusting agents, water-proofing compounds, casting agents, vacuum pump fluids, fixatives in microscopy, surgical implants, and in carbonless copy paper
	Carbaryl	In agriculture as insecticide and in veterinary as drug
	Chlordane	In agriculture as powerful pesticide
	1,2-Dibromo-3-chloropropane (DBCP)	In the synthesis of organic chemicals as an intermediate and in agriculture as nematocide and insecticide
Organophosphate pesticides	Chlorpyrifos	In cotton, corn, almonds, and fruit trees agriculture mainly as insecticide
	Paraquat	In plant protection products as herbicide
	Malathion	In agriculture as pesticide and in medical care for treatment of pediculosis and scabies
	Diethylthiophosphate (DETP)	In many food crops as insecticide
	Dimethylphosphate (DMP)	In insecticides
	Ethylphosphate (EP)	In plastics, solvents, and pesticides
	Methamidophos	In Chinese ricefields as insecticide and in poisoning
Other compounds included in pesticides	Phthalates	In nutritional supplements, adhesives and glues, agricultural adjuvants, building materials, personal-care products, medical devices, detergents and surfactants, packaging, children's toys, modeling clay, waxes, paints, printing inks and coatings, pharmaceuticals, food products, textiles, soft plastics. In household applications, personal-care items, modern electronics and medical applications, and PVC
	Abamectin	In products as insecticide, acaricide, and nematicide

reproductive health, may be related to an alteration of the gonadotropin-releasing hormone (GnRH) or a disruption of the production of the gonadotropin hormones by the pituitary gland [23, 24].

Although the current chapter refers to adult function, it is worth mentioning that prenatal (fetal/maternal) exposure may have significant effects later in life. The testicular dysgenesis syndrome (TDS) hypothesis suggests that disturbed testicular development in fetal life may result in one or more postnatal reproductive disorders, with fetal exposure to pesticides being one of the main risk factors [13, 25–28]. Several other human observational studies have reported that genital malformations (including cryptorchidism or hypospadias) may be related to parental pesticide exposure [29–33].

Organochlorine Pesticides

Dichlorodiphenyltrichloroethane (DDT) is one of the most commonly used persistent organochlorine pesticides and its insecticidal qualities were discovered in 1939 (Table 12.1). In the early 1970s, DDT was banned due to its high toxicity and long-term persistence. However, DDT continues to be used today as an antimalarial in several regions of Africa and Asia [34]. Isomer forms like *p,p'*-DDT and *o,p'*-DDT or its metabolites dichlorodiphenyldichloroethylene (DDE) and dichlorodiphenyldichloroethane (DDD) [34] can also be found.

Several reports have examined the associations between DDT exposure and human semen parameters among fertile men around the world [35–37]. In 2006, Toft and colleagues suggested that higher levels of DDE exposure may be associated with impaired sperm motility in 798 fertile men of four European countries (Poland, Ukraine, Greenland, and Sweden) [35]. In America, a cross-sectional study conducted with 116 young men from Mexico reported a positive association between plasma p,p'-DDE levels and sperm tail defects and a negative association with sperm motility [36]. Similarly, in South Africa, lipid-adjusted serum p,p'-DDE concentration was inversely associated with sperm volume and total sperm count in 303 healthy males between 18 and 40 years old [37].

The association between DDT exposure and human semen parameters has been investigated in infertile or subfertile men as well [38–40]. Hauser and colleagues found no association between serum p,p'-DDE concentration and semen volume, sperm concentration, motility, or morphology in 212 male partners of subfertile couples attending the Massachusetts General Hospital Andrology Laboratory [38, 39]. However, a study conducted in India with 45 cases and 45 controls concluded that concentrations of p,p'-DDE, p,p'-DDD, and total DDT were higher in seminal fluid of men with male factor infertility (cases) compared with controls [40].

With regard to testicular germ cell tumors (TGCT), only one case–control study have found a statistically significant association with p,p'-DDE exposures using pre-diagnostic serum samples ($p < 0.01$) [41]. Other studies using similar samples reported a borderline association between increasing p,p'-DDE exposures and TGCT ($p = 0.07$) [42].

Polychlorinated biphenyls (PCBs) are a family of synthetic, persistent, lipophilic organochlorine pesticides found in the environment (Table 12.1). The general population is exposed to this compound on a daily basis due to the ingestion of contaminated foods [39]. Richthoff et al. analyzed the relationship between serum PCBs and semen parameters in 305 presumed-fertile military recruits between 18 and 21 years old from Sweden [43]. Total PCB concentration was inversely correlated with sperm motility, but was not associated with sperm volume, concentration, and total sperm count. Similarly, serum PCB-153 (an individual PCB congener) concentration has been weakly associated with sperm motility, but no relationship was seen with other sperm parameters (sperm volume, concentration, and total count) among Swedish fishermen [44].

In a cross-sectional study including 212 male partners of subfertile couples attending an infertility clinic, Hauser and colleagues reported a statistically significant negative association between serum levels of PCB-138 (another individual PCB congener) and sperm concentration, motility, and morphology [38].

Carbaryl is a nonpersistent-organochlorine pesticide used to protect residential lawns and gardens from insects (Table 12.1). This compound may impair sperm parameters and male reproductive hormone concentrations [45]. A study conducted between 2000 and 2003 with 272 male partners of couples attending a Massachusetts infertility clinic concluded that men with low urine concentrations of 1-naphtol (a urinary metabolite of carbaryl) were more likely to have sperm concentration and sperm motility ($p < 0.05$) above the WHO reference values [46]. Furthermore, the same research group published a latter article finding a suggestive inverse association between urinary concentrations of 1-naphtol and circulating serum estradiol levels ($p = 0.09$) [47], a steroid hormone that inhibits testicular apoptosis much more effectively than testosterone [48].

Carbaryl was also related with sperm quality in a case–control study conducted among Chinese men, but in this case, the organochlorine pesticide was measured in the ambient air of the workplace [49]. Seminal volume and sperm motility were significantly lower ($p < 0.05$) in the case group (air-exposed pesticide) compared with the controls (non-air-exposed pesticide).

Nonachlor is a derived compound of an organochlorine pesticide named chlordane (Table 12.1). Its half-life in the human body is 10–20 years [50]. Some articles have reported a positive relationship with the presence of TCGT [41, 42, 51]. It is less commercialized than the other organochlorine pesticides, though.

In 1979, a study investigating the association between the exposures to another organochlorine pesticide, the 1,2-dibromo-3-chloropropane

(DBCP), and semen quality was published [52]. Out of the 142 non-vasectomized men providing semen samples, 107 and 35 had and had not been exposed to DBCP, respectively. The authors concluded that there were more percentage of azoospermic and severely oligozoospermic cases in the group of exposed men compared with the nonexposed.

Organophosphate Pesticides

Chlorpyrifos is one of the most commonly used insecticides in homes, and more than 90 % of males in the US population had urine samples with detectable levels of 3.5.6.-trichloro-2-pyridinol (TCPY), the major urinary metabolite of this insecticide [53] (Table 12.1). A study conducted by Meeker and colleagues in a Massachusetts infertility clinic assessed the relationship between urinary levels of TCPY and semen parameters [47]. They reported that men in the medium and high TCPY tertiles were more likely to have below-reference sperm concentration and motility [46] (p value for trend=0.01), compared with men in the lowest TCPY tertile. In addition, there was an inverse association between urinary TCPY concentrations and serum estradiol levels [47]. Although estradiol is mainly a female hormone, it has been demonstrated that estradiol plays an important role in male reproductive health. Estradiol is produced in the testes and it has been shown to inhibit testicular apoptosis much more effectively than testosterone, for instance [48].

Another example of a potential negative impact of this group of chemicals on semen quality was found in Sabah, Malaysia [54]. A cross-sectional study was conducted including 152 farmers (which 62 have been exposed to either paraquat or malathion or both organophosphate pesticides) to explore the relation between the exposure to these compounds and semen quality. The exposed workers presented significantly lower sperm concentration, volume, count, and motility ($p<0.005$) and higher percent of teratozoospermia, compared with nonexposed farmers.

Diethylthiophosphate (DETP) is a specific organophosphate insecticide metabolite that has been associated with decreased sperm concentration among exposed men of an agricultural region of China [55]. Somewhat similar results have been reported in other areas. For example, the same research group also found a relationship between another organophosphate metabolite measured in urine, dimethylphosphate (DMP), and semen quality impairment in environmentally exposed men from China [56]. Another study conducted in Peru looked at the relationship between urinary levels of DETP, DMP, and thiophosphate metabolites (Table 12.1) and semen quality as well [57]. The study recruited 31 exposed and 31 nonexposed men (between 20 and 60 years old) to these organophosphate metabolites. A significant reduction of semen volume was found in the exposed group compared with controls (nonexposed men) [57].

Ethylparathion and methamidophos are organophosphate pesticides with restricted use due to their toxicity [53] (Table 12.1). Giving their circumstances, human exposure through diet or drinking water is very low. However, Padungtod and colleagues reported a significant lower sperm concentration and motility among Chinese workers exposed to ethylparathion and methamidophos compared with nonexposed workers, but there were no differences in sperm morphology [58].

In Mexico, a longitudinal follow-up study of 52 male volunteers, between the ages of 18–55, performing agricultural work was carried out [59]. Semen parameters and several urinary organophosphate levels (DETP, DMP, etc.) were assessed. The results showed a significant decrease in total sperm count among subjects with the highest (compared with the lowest) concentrations of urinary organophosphate levels.

Other Compounds Included in Pesticides

Phthalates are a family of industrial chemicals that are part of the ingredients of fragrances, adhesives and glues, building materials, personal-care products, detergents, paints, pharmaceuticals, food products, textiles, and agricultural adjuvants, including pesticides.

Phthalates are endocrine-disrupting compounds and its antiandrogenic effects are well known [60–62].

The most widely used phthalates are the di-(2-ethylhexyl) phthalate (DEHP), the diisodecyl phthalate (DIDP), and the diisononyl phthalate (DINP) [63]. Several cross-sectional studies have reported a negative relationship between phthalates and male semen quality around the world [64–72].

Duty and coworkers conducted a study including 168 men who were part of subfertile couples at the Massachusetts General Hospital Andrology Laboratory between January 2000 and April 2001. They examined the associations between 8 urinary phthalate metabolites and the participants' semen quality [65]. The authors reported two negative and significant dose–response relationships, one between the levels of monobutyl phthalate and sperm concentration as well as motility and another one between levels of monobenzyl phthalate and sperm concentration. The same research group also evaluated another outcome, sperm DNA damage, in relationship with environmental exposures of phthalates measured in urine [66]. The main results showed a significant positive association between urinary concentrations of one phthalate (monoethyl phthalate) and DNA sperm damage in the same study population.

Other articles from the same research group reported similar results in that particular population [67, 68]. For example, a dose–response negative association between urinary levels of monobutyl phthalate and sperm concentration and motility was found [67]. Besides, a positive relationship between urine concentration of monobutyl phthalate and DNA sperm damage was also shown [68].

In 2005, Duty and coworkers conducted another study among 295 male partners of subfertile couples at the same Hospital between 1999 and 2003. In this case, they explored the association between environmental levels of phthalates and altered reproductive hormone levels. They found associations between urinary phthalate metabolite concentrations and altered levels of inhibin B and FSH, but the hormone concentrations did not change in the expected patterns [69].

Pan et al. studied adult men occupationally exposed to phthalates showing that exposure to DEHP and dibutyl phthalate (DBP) was negatively associated with free testosterone serum levels [70]. In a Swedish population of young men, Jönsson et al. reported an inverse association between urinary monoethyl phthalate (MEP) concentration and LH values in 234 young Swedish men, although no association was found between other phthalate metabolites and other reproductive hormones [71].

Hauser and collaborators [39] studied the associations between both PCBs and phthalate metabolites and human semen quality, especially sperm motility. The study included 303 men who were partners in subfertile couples attending an infertility clinic between January 2000 and April 2003. For example, after adjusting for important covariates (age and abstinence time), for below-reference sperm motility, there was a greater than additive interaction between monobutyl phthalate (MBP) and PCB-153 and a suggestive interaction between MBP and sum of PCBs. Due to the potential public health implications of interactions between these two ubiquitous types of compounds, the authors suggested that further studies are warranted to confirm these results and identify possible mechanisms of interactions [39].

Meeker and collaborators also investigated the relationships between phthalate metabolites and serum reproductive hormones and extended their previous study [69] by including a bigger sample size [73]. In a male population attending an infertility clinic, the authors reported an association between increased urinary concentration of mono(2-ethylhexyl) phthalate (MEHP) with decreased testosterone, estradiol, and free androgen index levels, showing that exposure to DEHP might be associated with altered steroid hormones in these men [73]. Recently, Mendiola et al. [74] investigated these associations in a population of fertile men. Both Meeker et al. and Mendiola et al. reported a significant inverse association between FAI levels and urinary concentrations of several DEHP metabolites [73–75].

For example, another non-organochlorine and non-organophosphate pesticide is abamectin, which is used as acaricide and nematicide [76]. In Turkey, a study evaluating the relationship between abamectin exposure and semen quality among occupationally exposed farm workers was conducted [77]. The main results were that exposed men had significantly lower sperm motility than the nonexposed ones ($p < 0.05$).

Heavy Metals and Male Reproductive Disorders

The human population could be exposed to heavy metals at trace concentrations usually through intake of contaminated water and food or contact with contaminated air or soil [78]. However, heavy metal exposures do not have the same effect in each individual [79]. Several heavy metals—mainly lead (Pb) and cadmium (Cd)—are considered reproductive toxicants and may adversely affect the male reproductive system causing hypothalamic–pituitary–gonadal axis disruption or directly affecting spermatogenesis, resulting in impaired semen quality [80].

One of the main mechanisms of heavy metal toxicity is the inhibition of some enzyme activity due to molecular mechanisms [81–84]. For example, the creatine kinase (CK) enzyme is widely distributed in cells which require large amounts of energy, like spermatozoa. Its main function is to provide an ATP "buffer" system [85, 86]. For its activity, the presence of Mg^{2+} and sulfhydryl (SH) groups at the CK active site is necessary [87]. Several heavy metals may reduce CK activity in human sperm through displacement of Mg^{2+} in its active site. Moreover, heavy metals could also act as competitive inhibitors of the human sperm CK enzyme [88].

Cadmium

The predominant commercial use of cadmium is battery manufacturing [53]. Other uses include pigment production, coatings and plating, plastic stabilizers, and nonferrous alloys (Table 12.2). Cadmium has been recognized for its toxic effects on semen quality [78, 89–91].

In 2006, Akinloye and colleagues published an article on the relationship between cadmium exposure and infertility among normozoospermic, oligozoospermic, and azoospermic men from Nigeria [89]. Men with the highest concentrations of Cd in seminal plasma (65 µg/dL) presented lower values of sperm counts and motile sperms. There was also a positive correlation between Cd concentrations and serum FSH levels ($p < 0.05$).

Telisman et al. conducted a study looking at semen quality and serum reproductive hormones in 149 healthy male industrial workers between 20 and 43 years of age of Zagreb, Croatia. They found an impairment of the sperm morphology (head pathologic sperms) even with low concentrations of cadmium (<1 µg/dL) measured in whole blood [90].

Table 12.2 Main products where heavy metals can be found

	Type	Uses
Heavy metals	Cadmium (Cd)	In battery manufacturing, pigment production, coatings and plating, plastic stabilizers, and nonferrous alloys
	Lead (Pb)	In storage batteries, solders, metal alloys, plastics, leaded glass, ceramic glazes, ammunition, gasoline, and residential paints
	Mercury (Hg)	In cosmetics (mascaras,) medicine (thermometers), and laboratories (mercury-vapor lamps) and as dental amalgam
	Manganese (Mn)	In fireworks, dry batteries, gasoline, cosmetics, paint pigments, and medical image agent
	Arsenic (As)	In medicine as treatments for syphilis, psoriasis, cancers, and mental disorders and as a cosmetic to lighten complexion. In alloys like semiconductors, in homicidal poisons, and in paint pigments and for tanning animal hides
	Molybdenum (Mo)	In metal alloys as corrosion inhibitors, hydrogenation catalysts, and lubricants; in hospital laboratories like chemical reagents; in batteries as semiconductor; and in pigments for ceramics, inks, and paints

A study including different populations (infertility patients, artificial insemination donors, and general population volunteers) was conducted by Benoff and colleagues in the USA between 1995 and 2000, obtaining somewhat similar results. They found that sperm concentration, motility, and morphology were affected even with low seminal plasma concentrations of cadmium (0.028 µg/dL) [91]. Similarly, low concentrations of cadmium in seminal plasma (0.085 µg/dl) were moderately associated with low sperm motility in a case–control study including 61 Spanish men attending infertility clinics [78].

Lead

Elemental lead is a soft, malleable, dense, blue-gray metal that occurs naturally in soils and rocks [53]. It can be found in storage batteries, solders, metal alloys, plastics, leaded glass, ceramic glazes, ammunition, etc. (Table 12.2). In the past, lead was added to gasoline and residential paints and used in soldering the seams of food cans. Lead was used in plumbing for centuries and may still be present.

There is considerable agreement that high or even moderate concentrations of lead may cause fertility problems in humans [78, 92, 93]. A cross-sectional study was conducted on male partners of 57 infertile couples attending a tertiary infertility center in Dhaka (Bangladesh) in order to explore the relationship between blood lead concentrations and sperm parameters [92]. They concluded that a concentration of >40 µg/dL of lead in blood was associated with a significant decline of sperm count. In addition, they observed a significant lower motility and morphology with >35 µg/dL of blood lead [92].

Telisman and colleagues also studied the relation between blood lead concentrations and semen quality among 98 subjects with slight to moderate occupational exposure to lead and other reference group with 51 subjects [90]. The exposed subjects showed significantly lower sperm density and motility associated with higher lead concentrations in blood (36.7 µg/dL).

Hernández-Ochoa and coworkers evaluated environmental-lead effects on semen quality and sperm chromatin. Lead concentrations were assessed in seminal fluid, spermatozoa, and blood as biomarkers of exposure for urban men from Mexico [93]. Impairment of certain sperm parameters (motility, normal morphology, and sperm concentration) was found, but only at low lead concentrations in seminal fluid (0.2 µg/dL).

Mendiola et al. also explored the relationship between lead exposure and semen quality in a case–control study carried out in Southern Spain. They found an inverse relationship between motility and levels of lead in seminal fluid (2.93 µg/dL) [78].

Other Metals

Various heavy metals have also been related with semen quality impairment [94–97] (Table 12.2).

Mercury is used, for example, in cosmetics (mascaras), medicine (thermometers), and laboratories (mercury-vapor lamps), but inhalation of elemental mercury volatilized from dental amalgam was a major source of mercury exposure in the general population [39]. Mercury exposure may also result in semen quality alteration [71]. Choy et al. [94] compared blood mercury concentrations of infertile couples with those of fertile couples in a case–control study conducted in Hong Kong. High concentrations of total mercury (inorganic and organic) measured in whole blood (geometric mean: 40.6 mmol/L) were significantly associated with below WHO reference values [46] for all sperm parameters. Another investigation from the same research group reported that seminal fluid mercury concentrations were correlated with abnormal sperm morphology, as well as with abnormal sperm motion, in subfertile males in Hong Kong, China [98].

From a mechanistic point of view, in vitro studies have shown that SH groups in the membrane, head, midpiece, and tail of the sperm are sites of mercury binding [99]. Therefore, mitochondrial functional integrity, DNA synthesis in mitotic spindles, or the microtubule sliding assembly of the sperm motor apparatus are all potential targets of mercury toxicity [100]. Besides, several studies have reported that the Sertoli and Leydig cells in the testis, as well as those outside the testis, such as in the epididymis, are also diverse targets of mercury toxicity [101].

A population-based study investigating the role of manganese exposure (heavy metal found in drinking water and gasoline, etc.) on semen quality was conducted on Chinese men [95]. The authors reported that high serum manganese levels appeared to have harmful effects on sperm morphology and motility among healthy men with nonoccupational exposure to manganese [95].

Also in China, a cross-sectional study of 96 men attending an infertility clinic between 2009 and 2010 was conducted in order to explore the associations between urinary concentrations of arsenic and semen quality [96]. Urinary concentrations of an arsenic specie (dimethylarsinous, DMA) above the median were significantly associated with below-reference sperm concentrations ($p=0.02$) after adjusting for important covariates (age, body mass index, abstinence, smoking, and drinking habits) [96].

Molybdenum is present in drinking water and foods in low concentrations and it is used as corrosion inhibitors, hydrogenation catalysts, lubricants, and chemical reagents in hospital laboratories and semiconductor in batteries and in pigments for ceramics, inks, and paints [53]. Meeker and coworkers conducted a study including 219 males of two infertility clinics of Michigan in order to explore the relationship between environmental metal exposures and male reproductive function. Significant associations and dose-dependent relationships between molybdenum concentrations in blood and low sperm concentration and morphology were found [97].

Conclusions

Many toxic chemicals as pesticides and heavy metals have been associated with an impairment of male reproductive function. The negative effects of these compounds have been related to the main sperm parameters (sperm concentration, morphology, motility, volume, and total sperm count), DNA sperm damage, as well as alterations of the reproductive hormone concentrations. Fortunately, some of these injurious substances have been banned in most countries and even globally. However, further studies are warranted to explore and confirm the potential damage of current commercial chemical substances, and their mixtures, on human reproductive health.

References

1. Carlsen E, Giwercman A, Keiding N, Skakkebaek NE. Evidence for decreasing quality of semen during the past 50 years. BMJ. 1992;305(6854):609–13.
2. Swan SH, Elkin EP, Fenster L. The question of declining sperm density revisited: an analysis of 101 studies published 1934–1996. Environ Health Perspect. 2000;108(10):961–6.
3. Jørgensen N, Carlsen E, Nermoen I, Punab M, Suominen J, Andersen AG, et al. East-West gradient in semen quality in the Nordic–Baltic area: a study of men from the general population in Denmark, Norway, Estonia and Finland. Hum Reprod. 2002;17(8):2199–208.
4. Jørgensen N, Andersen AG, Eustache F, Irvine DS, Suominen J, Petersen JH, et al. Regional differences in semen quality in Europe. Hum Reprod. 2001;16(5):1012–9.
5. Punab M, Zilaitiene B, Jorgensen N, Horte A, Matulevicius V, Peetsalu A, et al. Regional differences in semen qualities in the Baltic region. Int J Androl. 2002;25(4):243–52.
6. Richthoff J, Rylander L, Hagmar L, Malm J, Giwercman A. Higher sperm counts in Southern Sweden compared with Denmark. Hum Reprod. 2002;17(9):2468–73.
7. Paasch U, Salzbrunn A, Glander HJ, Plambeck K, Salzbrunn H, Grunewald S, et al. Semen quality in sub-fertile range for a significant proportion of young men from the general German population: a co-ordinated, controlled study of 791 men from Hamburg and Leipzig. Int J Androl. 2008;31(2):93–102.
8. Mendiola J, Jørgensen N, Mínguez-Alarcón L, Sarabia-Cos L, López-Espín JJ, Vivero-Salmerón G, et al. Sperm counts may have declined in young university students in Southern Spain. Andrology. 2013;1(3):408–13.
9. Swan SH, Brazil C, Drobnis EZ, Liu F, Kruse RL, Hatch M, et al. Geographic differences in semen quality of fertile U.S. males. Environ Health Perspect. 2003;111(4):414–20.

10. Belcheva A, Ivanova-Kicheva M, Tzvetkova P, Marinov M. Effects of cigarette smoking on sperm plasma membrane integrity and DNA fragmentation. Int J Androl. 2004;27(5):296–300.
11. Agarwal A, Deepinder F, Sharma RK, Ranga G, Li J. Effect of cell phone usage on semen analysis in men attending infertility clinic: an observational study. Fertil Steril. 2008;89(1):124–8.
12. Mínguez-Alarcón L, Mendiola J, López-Espín JJ, Sarabia-Cos L, Vivero-Salmerón G, Vioque J, et al. Dietary intake of antioxidant nutrients is associated with semen quality in young university students. Hum Reprod. 2012;27(9):2807–14.
13. Skakkebæk NE, Rajpert-De Meyts E, Main KM. Testicular dysgenesis syndrome: an increasingly common developmental disorder with environmental aspects. Hum Reprod. 2001;16(5):972–8.
14. Ramlau-Hansen CH, Thulstrup AM, Storgaard L, Toft G, Olsen J, Bonde JP. Is prenatal exposure to tobacco smoking a cause of poor semen quality? A follow-up study. Am J Epidemiol. 2007;165(12):1372–9.
15. Wagner U, Schlebusch H, Van der Ven H, Van der Ven K, et al. Accumulation of pollutants in the genital tract of sterility patients. J Clin Chem Clin Biochem. 1999;28(10):683–8.
16. Benoff S, Jacob A, Hurley IR. Male infertility and environmental exposure to lead and cadmium. Hum Reprod Update. 2000;6(2):107–21.
17. Jensen TK, Bonde JP, Joffe M. The influence of occupational exposure on male reproductive function. Occup Med (London). 2006;56(8):544–53.
18. Casida JE. Pest toxicology: the primary mechanisms of pesticide action. Chem Res Toxicol. 2009;22(4):609–19.
19. Toppari J, Larsen JC, Christiansen P, Giwercman A, Grandjean P, Guillette Jr LJ, et al. Male reproductive health and environmental xenoestrogens. Environ Health Perspect. 1996;104 Suppl 4:741–803.
20. Bush B, Bennett AH, Snow JT. Polychlorobiphenyl congeners, p, p'-DDE, and sperm function in humans. Arch Environ Contam Toxicol. 1986;15:333–41.
21. Tuohimaa P, Wichmann L. Sperm production of men working under heavy metal or organic solvent exposure. In: Hemminki K, Sorsa M, Vainio H, editors. Occupational hazards and reproduction. Washington, DC: Hemisphere Publishing Corp; 1985. p. 73–9.
22. Korach KS, Sarver P, Chae K, McLachlan JA, McKinney JD. Estrogen receptor-binding activity of polychlorinated hydroxybiphenyls: conformationally restricted structural probes. Mol Pharmacol. 1988;33:120–6.
23. Jansen HT, Cooke PS, Porcelli J, Liu TC, Hansen LG. Estrogenic and antiestrogenic actions of PCBs in the female rat: in vitro and in vivo studies. Reprod Toxicol. 1993;7:237–48.
24. Kelce WR, Stone CR, Laws SC, Gray LE, Kemppainen JA, Wilson EM. Persistent DDT metabolite p, p'-DDE is a potent androgen receptor antagonist. Nature. 1995;375:581–5.
25. Carbone P, Giordano F, Nori F, Mantovani A, Taruscio D, Lauria L, et al. Cryptorchidism and hypospadias in the Sicilian district of Ragusa and the use of pesticides. Reprod Toxicol. 2006;22:8–12.
26. Carbone P, Giordano F, Nori F, Mantovani A, Taruscio D, Lauria L, et al. The possible role of endocrine disrupting chemicals in the aetiology of cryptorchidism and hypospadias: a population-based case-control study in rural Sicily. Int J Androl. 2007;30:3–13.
27. Kristensen P, Irgens LM, Andersen A, Bye AS, Sundheim L. Birth defects among offspring of Norwegian farmers, 1967-1991. Epidemiology. 1997;8:537–44.
28. Damgaard IN, Skakkebaek NE, Toppari J, Virtanen HE, Shen H, Schramm KW, Petersen JH, Jensen TK, Main KM. Persistent pesticides in human breast milk and cryptorchidism. Environ Health Perspect. 2006;114:1133–8.
29. Fernandez MF, Olmos B, Granada A, López-Espinosa MJ, Molina-Molina JM, Fernandez JM, Cruz M, Olea-Serrano F, Olea N. Human exposure to endocrine-disrupting chemicals and prenatal risk factors for cryptorchidism and hypospadias: a nested case-control study. Environ Health Perspect. 2007;115 Suppl 1:8–14.
30. Garcia-Rodriguez J, Garcia-Martin M, Nogueras-Ocana M, de Dios L-d-C J, Espigares GM, Olea N, Lardelli-Claret P. Exposure to pesticides and cryptorchidism: geographical evidence of a possible association. Environ Health Perspect. 1996;104:1090–5.
31. Gaspari L, Paris F, Jandel C, Kalfa N, Orsini M, Daures JP, Sultan C. Prenatal environmental risk factors for genital malformations in a population of 1442 French male newborns: a nested casecontrol study. Hum Reprod. 2011;26:3155–62.
32. Weidner IS, Moller H, Jensen TK, Skakkebaek NE. Risk factors for cryptorchidism and hypospadias. J Urol. 1999;161:1606–9.
33. Rocheleau CM, Romitti PA, Dennis LK. Pesticides and hypospadias: a meta-analysis. J Pediatr Urol. 2009;5:17–24.
34. Cook MB, Trabert B, McGlynn KA. Organochlorine compounds and testicular dysgenesis syndrome: human data. Int J Androl. 2011;34(4 Pt 2):e68–84.
35. Toft G, Rignell-Hydbom A, Tyrkiel E, Shvets M, Giwercman A, Lindh CH, et al. Semen quality and exposure to persistent organochlorine pollutants. Epidemiology. 2006;17(4):450–8.
36. De Jager C, Farias P, Barraza-Villarreal A, Avila MH, Ayotte P, Dewailly E, et al. Reduced seminal parameters associated with environmental DDT exposure and p, p'-DDE concentrations in men in Chiapas, Mexico: a cross-sectional study. J Androl. 2006;27(1):16–27.
37. Aneck-Hahn NH, Schulenburg GW, Bornman MS, Farias P, de Jager C. Impaired semen quality associated with environmental DDT exposure in young men living in a malaria area in the Limpopo Province, South Africa. J Androl. 2007;28(3):423–34.

38. Hauser R, Chen Z, Pothier L, Ryan L, Altshul L. The relationship between human semen parameters and environmental exposure to polychlorinated biphenyls and p, p'-DDE. Environ Health Perspect. 2003;111(12):1505–11.
39. Hauser R, Williams P, Altshul L, Calafat AM. Evidence of interaction between polychlorinated biphenyls and phthalates in relation to human sperm motility. Environ Health Perspect. 2005; 113(4):425–30.
40. Pant N, Mathur N, Banerjee AK, Srivastava SP, Saxena DK. Correlation of chlorinated pesticides concentration in semen with seminal vesicle and prostatic markers. Reprod Toxicol. 2004;19(2):209–14.
41. McGlynn KA, Quraishi SM, Graubard BI, Weber JP, Rubertone MV, Erickson RL. Persistent organochlorine pesticides and risk of testicular germ cell tumors. J Natl Cancer Inst. 2008;100(9):663–71.
42. Purdue MP, Engel LS, Langseth H, Needham LL, Andersen A, Barr DB, et al. Prediagnostic serum concentrations of organochlorine compounds and risk of testicular germ cell tumors. Environ Health Perspect. 2009;117(10):1514–9.
43. Richthoff J, Rylander L, Jonsson BA, Akesson H, Hagmar L, Nilsson-Ehle P, et al. Serum levels of 2,2′,4,4′,5,5′-hexachlorobiphenyl (CB-153) in relation to markers of reproductive function in young males from the general Swedish population. Environ Health Perspect. 2003;111(4):409–13.
44. Rignell-Hydbom A, Rylander L, Giwercman A, Jonsson BA, Nilsson-Ehle P, Hagmar L. Exposure to CB-153 and p, p'-DDE and male reproductive function. Hum Reprod. 2004;19(9):2066–75.
45. Meeker JD, Ryan L, Barr DB, Herrick RF, Bennett DH, Bravo R, et al. The relationship of urinary metabolites of carbaryl/naphthalene and chlorpyrifos with human semen quality. Environ Health Perspect. 2004;112(17):1665–70.
46. World Health Organization (WHO). Laboratory manual for the examination of human semen and semen-cervical mucus interaction. 4th ed. Cambridge: Cambridge University Press; 1999.
47. Meeker JD, Ravi SR, Barr DB, Hauser R. Circulating estradiol in men is inversely related to urinary metabolites of nonpersistent insecticides. Reprod Toxicol. 2008;25(2):184–91.
48. Pentikäinen V, Erkkilä K, Suomalainen L, Parvinen M, Dunkel L. Estradiol acts as a germ cell survival factor in the human testis in vitro. J Clin Endocrinol Metab. 2000;85(5):2057–67.
49. Tan LF, Sun XZ, Li YN, Ji JM, Wang QL, Chen LS, et al. Effects of carbaryl production exposure on the sperm and semen quality of occupational male workers. Zhonghua Lao Dong Wei Sheng Zhi Ye Bing Za Zhi. 2005;23(2):87–90.
50. Dearth MA, Hites RA. Complete analysis of technical chlordane using negative ionization mass spectrometry. Environ Sci Technol. 1991;25:245–54.
51. Hardell L, Van Bavel B, Lindstrom G, Carlberg M, Dreifaldt AC, Wijkstrom H, et al. Increased concentrations of polychlorinated biphenyls, hexachlorobenzene, and chlordanes in mothers of men with testicular cancer. Environ Health Perspect. 2003; 111(7):930–4.
52. Whorton D, Milby TH, Krauss RM, Stubbs HA. Testicular function in DBCP exposed pesticide workers. J Occup Med. 1979;21(3):161–6.
53. Centers for Disease Control and Prevention (CDC). Fourth national report on human exposure to environmental chemicals. Washington, DC. 2013. http://www.cdc.gov/exposurereport/. Accessed 29 Oct 2013.
54. Hossain F, Ali O, D'Souza UJ, Naing DK. Effects of pesticide use on semen quality among farmers in rural areas of Sabah, Malaysia. J Occup Health. 2010;52(6):353–60.
55. Perry MJ, Venners SA, Barr DB, Xu X. Environmental pyrethroid and organophosphorus insecticide exposures and sperm concentration. Reprod Toxicol. 2007;23(1):113–8.
56. Perry MJ, Venners SA, Chen X, Liu X, Tang G, Xing H, et al. Organophosphorous pesticide exposures and sperm quality. Reprod Toxicol. 2011;31(1):75–9.
57. Yucra S, Gasco M, Rubio J, Gonzales GF. Semen quality in Peruvian pesticide applicators: association between urinary organophosphate metabolites and semen parameters. Environ Health. 2008;7:59.
58. Padungtod C, Savitz DA, Overstreet JW, Christiani DC, Ryan LM, Xu X. Occupational pesticide exposure and semen quality among Chinese workers. J Occup Environ Med. 2000;42(10):982–92.
59. Recio-Vega R, Ocampo-Gómez G, Borja-Aburto VH, Moran-Martínez J, Cebrian-Garcia ME. Organophosphorus pesticide exposure decreases sperm quality: association between sperm parameters and urinary pesticide levels. J Appl Toxicol. 2008;28(5):674–80.
60. Gray Jr LE, Ostby J, Furr J, Price M, Veeramachaneni DN, Parks L. Perinatal exposure to the phthalates DEHP, BBP, and DINP, but not DEP, DMP, or DOTP, alters sexual differentiation of the male rat. Toxicol Sci. 2000;58(2):350–65.
61. Foster PM. Disruption of reproductive development in male rat offspring following in utero exposure to phthalate esters. Int J Androl. 2006;29(1):140–7.
62. Swan SH. Environmental phthalate exposure in relation to reproductive outcomes and other health endpoints in humans. Environ Res. 2008;108(2): 177–84.
63. Api AM. Toxicological profile of diethyl phthalate: a vehicle for fragrance and cosmetic ingredients. Food Chem Toxicol. 2001;39(2):97–108.
64. Wirth JJ, Rossano MG, Potter R, Puscheck E, Daly DC, Paneth N, et al. A pilot study associating urinary concentrations of phthalate metabolites and semen quality. Syst Biol Reprod Med. 2008;54(3): 143–54.
65. Duty SM, Silva MJ, Barr DB, Brock JW, Ryan L, Chen Z, et al. Phthalate exposure and human semen parameters. Epidemiology. 2003;14:269–77.

66. Duty SM, Singh NP, Silva MJ, Barr DB, Brock JW, Ryan L, et al. The relationship between environmental exposures to phthalates and DNA damage in human sperm using the neutral comet assay. Environ Health Perspect. 2003;111(9):1164–9.
67. Hauser R, Meeker JD, Duty S, Silva MJ, Calafat AM. Altered semen quality in relation to urinary concentrations of phthalate monoester and oxidative metabolites. Epidemiology. 2006;17(6):682–91.
68. Hauser R, Meeker JD, Singh NP, Silva MJ, Ryan L, Duty S, et al. DNA damage in human sperm is related to urinary levels of phthalate monoester and oxidative metabolites. Hum Reprod. 2007;22(3): 688–95.
69. Duty SM, Calafat AM, Silva MJ, Ryan L, Hauser R. Phthalate exposure and reproductive hormones in adult men. Hum Reprod. 2005;20(3):604–10.
70. Pant N, Shukla M, Patel KD, Shukla Y, Mathur N, Gupta YK, et al. Correlation of phthalate exposures with semen quality. Toxicol Appl Pharmacol. 2008;231(1):112–6.
71. Jönsson AG, Richthoff J, Rylander L, Giwercman A, Lars H. Urinary phthalate metabolites and biomarkers of reproductive function in young men. Epidemiology. 2005;16(4):487–93.
72. Zhang Y, Zheng L, Chen B. Phthalate exposure and human semen quality in Shanghai: a cross-sectional study. Biomed Environ Sci. 2006;19(3):205–9.
73. Meeker JD, Calafat AM, Hauser R. Urinary metabolites of di(2-ethylhexyl) phthalate are associated with decreased steroid hormone levels in adult men. J Androl. 2009;30(3):287–97.
74. Mendiola J, Jørgensen N, Andersson AM, Calafat AM, Silva MJ, Redmon JB, et al. Associations between urinary metabolites of di(2-ethylhexyl) phthalate and reproductive hormones in fertile men. Int J Androl. 2011;34(4):369–78.
75. Mendiola J, Meeker JD, Jørgensen N, Andersson AM, Liu F, Calafat AM, et al. Urinary concentrations of di(2-ethylhexyl) phthalate metabolites and serum reproductive hormones: pooled analysis of fertile and infertile men. J Androl. 2012;33(3): 488–98.
76. Burg RW, Miller BM, Baker EE, Birnbaum J, Currie SA, Hartman R, et al. Avermectins, new family of potent anthelmintic agents: producing organism and fermentation. Antimicrob Agents Chemother. 1979;15(3):361–7.
77. Celik-Ozenci C, Tasatargil A, Tekcan M, Sati L, Gungor E, Isbir M, et al. Effect of abamectin exposure on semen parameters indicative of reduced sperm maturity: a study on farmworkers in Antalya (Turkey). Andrologia. 2012;44(6):388–95.
78. Mendiola J, Moreno JM, Roca M, Vergara-Juárez N, Martínez-García MJ, García-Sánchez A, et al. Relationships between heavy metal concentrations in three different body fluids and male reproductive parameters: a pilot study. Environ Health. 2011;10(1):6.
79. Mínguez-Alarcón L, Mendiola J, Roca M, López-Espín JJ, Guillén JJ, Moreno JM, et al. Correlations

between different heavy metals in diverse body fluids: studies of human semen quality. Adv Urol. 2012; 2012:420893. doi:10.1155/2012/420893.
80. Wyrobek AJ, Schrader SM, Perreault SD, Fenster L, Huszar G, Katz DF, et al. Assessment of reproductive disorders and birth defects in communities near hazardous chemical sites. III. Guidelines for field studies of male reproductive disorders. Reprod Toxicol. 1997;11(2–3):243–59.
81. Shinozaki T, Pritzker KP. Regulation of alkaline phosphatase: implications for calcium pyrophosphate dehydrate crystal dissolution and other alkaline phosphatase functions. J Rheumatol. 1996; 23:677–83.
82. Waalkes MP. Cadmium carcinogenesis in review. J Inorg Biochem. 2000;79:241–4.
83. Ghaffari MA, Abroumand M, Motlagh B. In vitro inhibition of human sperm creatine kinase by nicotine, cotinine and cadmium, as a mechanism in smoker men infertility. Int J Fertil Steril. 2008; 2:125–30.
84. Farian M, Brandao R, deLara FS, Pagliosa LB, Soares FA, Souza DO, et al. Profile of non-protein thiols, lipid peroxidation and δ-aminolevulinate dehydrogenase activity in mouse kidney and liver in response to acute exposure to mercuric chloride and sodium Selenite. Toxicology. 2003;184:179–87.
85. Ellington WR. Evolution and physiological roles of phosphagen system. Annu Rev Physiol. 2001;63:289–325.
86. Miyaji K, Kaneko S, Ishikawa H, Aoyaqi T, Hayakawa K, Hata M. Creatine kinase isoforms in the seminal plasma and the purified human sperm. Arch Androl. 2001;46:127–34.
87. Lowe G, Sproat BS. Evidence for an associative mechanism in the phosphoryl transfer step catalyzed by rabbit muscle creatine kinase. J Biol Chem. 1980;255:3944–51.
88. Ghaffari MA, Motlagh B. In vitro effect of lead, silver, tin, mercury, indium and bismuth on human sperm creatine kinase activity: a presumable mechanism for men infertility. Iran Biomed J. 2011;15:38–43.
89. Akinloye O, Arowojolu AO, Shittu OB, Anetor JI. Cadmium toxicity: a possible cause of male infertility in Nigeria. Reprod Biol. 2006;6(1):17–30.
90. Telisman S, Cvitkovic P, Jurasovic J, Pizent A, Gavella M, Rocic B. Semen quality and reproductive endocrine function in relation to biomarkers of lead, cadmium, zinc and copper in men. Environ Health Perspect. 2000;108(1):45–53.
91. Benoff S, Hauser R, Marmar JL, Hurley IR, Napolitano B, Centola GM. Cadmium concentrations in blood and seminal plasma: correlations with sperm number and motility in three male populations (infertility patients, artificial insemination donors, and unselected volunteers). Mol Med. 2009;15(7–8):248–62.
92. Fatima P, Debnath BC, Hossain MM, Rahman D, Banu J, Begum SA, et al. Relationship of blood and

semen lead level with semen parameter. Mymensingh Med J. 2010;19(3):405–14.

93. Hernández-Ochoa I, García-Vargas G, López-Carrillo L, Rubio-Andrade M, Morán-Martínez J, Cebrián ME, et al. Low lead environmental exposure alters semen quality and sperm chromatin condensation in northern Mexico. Reprod Toxicol. 2005; 20(2):221–8.

94. Choy CM, Lam CW, Cheung LT, Briton-Jones CM, Cheung LP, Haines CJ. Infertility, blood mercury concentrations and dietary seafood consumption: a case-control study. BJOG. 2002;109(10): 1121–5.

95. Li Y, Wu J, Zhou W, Gao E. Effects of manganese on routine semen quality parameters: results from a population-based study in China. BMC Public Health. 2012;12:919.

96. Xu W, Bao H, Liu F, Liu L, Zhu YG, She J, et al. Environmental exposure to arsenic may reduce human semen quality: associations derived from a Chinese cross-sectional study. Environ Health. 2012;11:46.

97. Meeker JD, Rossano MG, Protas B, Diamond MP, Puscheck E, Daly D, et al. Cadmium, lead, and other metals in relation to semen quality: human evidence for molybdenum as a male reproductive toxicant. Environ Health Perspect. 2008;116(11):1473–9.

98. Choy CM, Yeung QS, Briton-Jones CM, Cheung CK, Lam CW, Haines CJ. Relationship between semen parameters and mercury concentrations in blood and in seminal fluid from subfertile males in Hong Kong. Fertil Steril. 2002;78:426–8.

99. Mohamed MK, Lee WI, Mottet NK, Burbacher TM. Laser lightscattering study of the toxic effects of methylmercury on sperm motility. J Androl. 1986;7:11–5.

100. Vogel DG, Margolis RL, Mottet NK. Effects of methyl mercury binding to microtubules. Toxicol Appl Pharmacol. 1985;80:473–86.

101. Ernst E, Moller-Madsen B, Danscher G. Ultrastructural demonstration of mercury in Sertoli and Leydig cells of the rat following methylmercuric chloride or mercuric chloride treatment. Reprod Toxicol. 1991;5:205–9.

Endocrine Disruptors and Male Infertility

13

Riana Bornman and Natalie Aneck-Hahn

Introduction

A healthy endocrine system is necessary for good reproductive health. Currently there is an increasing trend of endocrine-related disorders in humans. The speed at which this has occurred, rules out genetic factors as the sole cause. Environmental and other non-genetic factors, including chemical exposures may be responsible and associations are emerging, linking these endocrine disrupting chemicals (EDCs) to male reproductive health (MRH).

The objective of this chapter is to define an EDC, discuss some mechanisms of action as well as to give examples of EDCs and their sources. With this in mind, such chemicals will be linked to lifestyle factors and MRH.

What Are Endocrine Disrupting Chemicals (EDCs)?

Definition of an EDC

"An endocrine disruptor is an exogenous substance or mixture that alters function(s) of the endocrine system and consequently causes

R. Bornman, MBChB, PhD
N. Aneck-Hahn, DTech (✉)
Department of Urology, University of Pretoria,
Room 71213, Steve Biko Academic Hospital,
Malherbe Street, Pretoria 0001, South Africa
e-mail: Natalie.aneck-hahn@up.ac.za

adverse health effects in an intact organism, or its progeny, or (sub) populations". The same applies to a potential endocrine disruptor [1, 2].

Mechanisms and Mode of Action

The role of hormone action in development and adult physiology needs consideration to understand the potential health consequences on human or wildlife populations, in experimental systems or human epidemiology. Chemicals can disrupt hormone action in two possible ways: (1) direct action on a hormone receptor protein complex or (2) a direct action on a specific protein that regulates some aspect of hormone delivery to the right place at the right time, e.g. delivery to its normal target cells or tissue. Therefore, a chemical could block the synthesis of a hormone (antagonist), resulting in an increase or decrease of the blood hormone level. This could cause a similar effect as a result of disease or genetic defects, which either leads to stimulation or inhibition of the hormone action. However, if the chemical interacts directly with the hormone receptor (agonist) the effects could be quite complex and would follow the mechanisms for hormone receptor interaction [2].

EDCs interfere with hormone action and can consequently produce adverse health effects in humans and wildlife. This most likely includes all hormonal systems, from the development and function of the reproductive organs, to the adult onset of diabetes or cardiovascular disease [2].

S.S. du Plessis et al. (eds.), *Male Infertility: A Complete Guide to Lifestyle and Environmental Factors*,
DOI 10.1007/978-1-4939-1040-3_13, © Springer Science+Business Media New York 2014

The majority of studies have focused primarily on chemicals that interact with the estrogen, androgen and thyroid hormone systems. With some exceptions, hormone receptors have a high affinity for their natural ligand, but typically a much lower affinity for endocrine disruptors [2]. The ability to bind to the receptor is not the same as the ability to cause effects (i.e. potency) [2, 3]. There are also tissue- or cell-specific differences in effects of endocrine disruptors and some endocrine disruptors have affinities similar or greater than that of the natural ligand [2].

Endocrine System

Hypothalamic–Pituitary–Gonadal HPG Axis

Sex determination is genetically determined in humans mainly by the sex-determining region Y (SRY) gene on the short arm of the Y chromosome. Once gonadal sex is determined, the foetal Leydig cells produce testosterone, which induces development of the internal genitalia and after conversion to dihydrotestosterone (DHT), masculinises the external genitalia. Transinguinal descent is controlled by testosterone, whereas insulin-like-3, also produced by the Leydig cells, promotes trans-abdominal testis descent into the scrotum. The foetal Sertoli cells produce Müllerian-inhibiting substance (MIS), which prevents the Müllerian ducts from further development and it keeps the early germ cells dormant in the testis. Any disruption of these developmental pathways commonly results in either birth defects or intersex disorders.

The hormonal feedback relationships within the HPG axis are established during foetal development. Around the 12th year, puberty begins when the hypothalamus starts to generate Gonadotropin-releasing Hormone (GnRH) pulses, which stimulates the secretion of luteinizing hormone (LH) and follicle-stimulating hormone (FSH) from the anterior pituitary. GnRH secretion shows rhythmic patterns namely seasonal (peaking in the spring); circadian (diurnal, higher testosterone levels during the early morning hours); and pulsatile (GnRH peaking ~ every 90–120 min). Puberty is initiated at a critical growth, weight and nutritional status, and is possibly triggered by kisspeptin (formerly metastin), melatonin and leptin [4].

The primary binding site of FSH is on Sertoli cells where it stimulates the production of androgen-binding protein (ABP), transferrin, lactate, ceruloplasmin, clusterin, plasminogen activator, prostaglandins and growth factors. Through these FSH-mediated factors, seminiferous tubule growth is stimulated and sperm production is initiated. In humans, at puberty, FSH is essential for the initiation of spermatogenesis; while it stimulates quantitatively normal levels of spermatogenesis in the adult [5]. Sertoli cells also produce inhibin and activin. Inhibin inhibits FSH release by its negative feedback on the pituitary and hypothalamus. Activin, a testis protein with close structural homology to transforming growth factor-β (TGF-β), exerts a stimulatory effect on FSH secretion [6].

LH binds to the Leydig cells to induce testosterone production. Testosterone is converted in most peripheral tissues, except in the testis and skeletal muscle, to DHT by the action of 5α-reductase or to estradiol through the action of aromatases. Testosterone feedback occurs mainly at the level of the hypothalamus, whereas estrogen's feedback is at the level of the pituitary [7]. It appears as if testosterone is the primary regulator of LH secretion, while estradiol (along with inhibin from Sertoli cells) is the predominant regulator of FSH secretion [8].

Prolactin, also an anterior pituitary hormone, is responsible for stimulating milk synthesis during pregnancy and lactation in women. The physiological role of prolactin in men is not clear, but it may help to sustain normal, high intra-testicular testosterone levels and enhance the effects of androgens on the growth and secretions of the male accessory sex glands [9, 10]. Patients with hyperprolactinemia often present with lack of libido as the primary symptom.

Vulnerable Periods

Developing organs are particularly sensitive to fluctuations in hormone levels, and subsequently exposure to EDCs during critical window periods of development may cause irreversible effects. These affects may not be obvious at birth, but only become evident in adulthood. Currently critical developmental periods include during foetal development, perinatal life, childhood and puberty. However, there may be other developmental windows of increased susceptibility that will need to be addressed such as delayed effects manifesting with ageing are not included either and needs further research [11–13].

Dose-Response Relationships

EDCs challenge traditional concepts in toxicology, particularly the common saying of "the dose makes the poison". EDCs can have effects at low doses that are not predicted by effects at higher doses. Natural hormones act at extremely low serum concentrations, usually in the pico- to nanomolar range, while EDCs can act in nano- to micromolar range, but some even show activity at picomolar levels [2, 14]. Natural hormones and EDCs produce non-linear dose-responses; the simplest form is a sigmoidal shape. The non-linear dose response occurs because hormones act on receptors, which are limited in number and the response itself can become saturated [2]. However, hormones and EDCs can also produce non-monotonic dose-responses (NMDRs), in which the slope of the curve changes sign from positive to negative or vice versa at some point over the course of the dose-response curve [14]. With regard to EDCs, low dose exposure and NMDR curves are inter-related concepts [14].

Low Dose-Response

The National Toxicology Program (NTP) evaluated the scientific evidence on low dose effects and NMDR relationships for EDCs in mammalian species [15]. The NTP defined low dose effects as "biologic changes that occur in the range of human exposures or at doses lower than those typically used in the standard testing paradigm of the USA Environmental Protection Agency (EPA) for evaluating reproductive and developmental toxicity". The panel of experts verified that low dose effects were observed for a multitude of endpoints for specific EDCs that included diethylstilbestrol (DES), genistein, methoxychlor and nonylphenol (NP) [14, 15]. In the review by Vandenberg et al. [14] the authors give a number of examples of low dose effect studies on Bisphenol-A (BPA).

Non-monotonic Dose-Response Curves

Non-monotonic dose response curves (NMDRCs) are often a U-shape or inverted U-shape, also sometimes referred to as biphasic dose response curves because responses show ascending and descending phases in relation to dose [2, 14]. For example, foetal mice were exposed to low or high doses of the synthetic estrogen, DES, and their adult prostate weights were relatively low, while intermediate doses of DES resulted in significantly heavier prostates [16]. NMDRs have been reported in both animal and cell cultures for more than a dozen natural hormones and more than 60 EDCs, recent research has suggested that this can be extrapolated to population levels. As yet, the mechanisms to explain these non-monotonic effects at the population level have not yet been identified, it is important to know that these dose response characteristics are expected due to hormone action and endocrine disruption [2].

Mixture Effects

Humans and wildlife are exposed to mixtures of multiple EDCs [17] as opposed to single/individual chemicals. There is good evidence that several EDCs can work together to produce combined effects [18]. When evaluating the toxicity of chemicals their effects are usually considered in isolation with "tolerable" doses derived from data on one single chemical. These assumptions are flawed when exposure is to a mixture of chemicals. This is especially the case when the chemicals involved contribute to the same effect, for example the combined action between estradiol and other chemicals capable of mimicking the hormone's action [2]. The "something from nothing" concept implies that EDCs combined in sufficient numbers and concentrations produce substantial estrogenic effects that on their own do not elicit measurable effects; or may even lead to doubling the effects of the hormone [19].

Sources of Exposure

An individual's aggregate EDC exposure or EDC exposure profile is determined by how much contact they have with each pathway of exposure, which in turn is affected by the individual's lifestyle choices [20].

Occupational

It is important that a patient consulting for infertility is screened for his occupational and environmental history. For example, work in agricultural or pest control sectors that routinely use pesticides increase an individual's aggregate exposure to EDC pesticides [20–23]. Other examples of occupations with probable exposure include electricians, workers in the plastics industry, electricians, painters, cleaners, printers, hairdressers, dentists, textile and laboratory workers. A useful summary is found in Van Togeren et al.'s publication indicating examples of occupation with the potential substance [23]. Children are also at risk from occupational exposure, an example of this is where one or both parents worked in agriculture or who lived near farms growing soya or maize. These children had far higher exposure levels of organophosphate pesticides than children from non-agricultural families used as controls [24].

Non-occupational

We are inadvertently exposed to EDCs. One of the most common important routes of exposure is the use of pesticides in the home environment [25, 26]. Pesticides like the organophosphates, carbamates and pyrethroids have replaced the older organochlorines for residential pesticide control [27]. Whyatt et al., found that pesticide use can be correlated with one or more housing problems, e.g. peeling or flaking paint, holes in ceilings and walls, water damage, leaking pipes, visible mould and lack of heating or electricity in the preceding 6 months [20, 27]. Another example of exposure could be phthalate dust particles found in vinyl tiles and furniture coverings [28]. When assessing variations in exposure values and health effects to a particular chemical, emphasis on individual lifestyle factors should be considered [28].

Recreational

Travel and recreation also provide a number of potential routes of exposure. When travelling in aircraft between certain countries to prevent the spread of insects and disease vectors pyrethroids are routinely sprayed inside the aircraft cabin [20, 29]. In this case both passengers and flight crew are exposed to these compounds [30]. Gardeners, pet owners and household do-it-yourself projects often use EDC pesticides or impregnated products such as gardens sprays, flea collars, wood preservatives and wall paper pastes, and glues [20, 31–33]. Other recreational activities that may be responsible for exposures include applications of EDCs to maintain golf courses, sports fields or nearby agricultural activities [34, 35].

Lifestyle Related

People who consume a diet containing a high proportion of organic food have less pesticide exposure from food residues than those who do not [36, 37]. Children on organic had lower pesticide exposures than those fed conventional diets [36]. People who consume oily fish, meat and dairy products are likely to receive a higher dose of the older and more persistent compounds, such as organochlorines, due to the bioaccumulation of some persistent lipophilic pesticides such as dichlorodiphenyldichloroethane (DDE) and other dichlorodiphenyltrichloroethane (DDT) breakdown products in the fat, than people who eat predominantly vegetable-based diets [38, 39]. Infants and children receive disproportionately large exposures to some organochlorines and newer less persistent pesticides from dietary sources because their diets generally contain a lot of fruit and vegetable products. They also eat more per unit bodyweight than adults [40].

Major Chemicals of Concern

Persistent Organic Pollutants

Persistent organic pollutants (POPs) are organic compounds that are often halogenated and characterized by low water solubility and high lipid solubility. To varying degrees, they resist photolytic, biological, and chemical degradation [41]. The majority of the POPs in the Stockholm Convention (http://chm.pops.int) are known as EDCs. Due to their estrogenic or anti-androgenic activity, they may have disrupting effects on male reproductive activity [42]. These include the following chemicals DDT, dieldrin, toxaphene, chlordane and several industrial chemical products and by-products, including polychlorinated biphenyls (PCBs), dioxins and furans [41]. POPs (e.g. PCBs and DDT) have been banned in many countries for several decades, but are still global pollutants because of their persistence. This presents a challenge with regard to limiting exposure to humans and wildlife [2] and future monitoring.

Polychlorinated Biphenyls

PCBs were produced from 1929 until the 1980s to use as sealants in building, insulating agents in transformer oils and capacitators and heat transfer agents [2]. PCBs are part of a group of synthetic organic chemicals containing about 200 individual compounds/congeners [43]. PCB exposure was also linked to semen quality and especially reduced sperm motility [44–48].

DDT, DDE

DDT is a persistent, widespread environmental contaminant found in most regions of the world and at high concentrations in countries where it is still used for malaria vector control [2]. DDT has been banned in the USA, Western Europe, Japan and many other countries since the early 1970s [49]. The Stockholm Convention has given exemption for the production and public health use of DDT for indoor residual spraying for malaria vector control, mainly because of the absence of equally effective and efficient alternatives [2].

Technical-grade DDT is a mixture of p,p'-DDT (~85 %), o,p'-DDT (~15 %) and o,o'-DDT (trace amounts), with both p,p'-DDT and o,p'-DDT having estrogenic activity. The persistent metabolite p,p'-dichlorodiphenyl-dichloroethylene (p,p'-DDE), also a widespread environmental contaminant [50], is anti-androgenic by inhibitive binding to androgen receptors [51] and has been shown to inhibit the action of testosterone [52–54]. The hypothesis is that p,p'-DDE interacts in an additive or multiplicative way with other DDT compounds as an endocrine-disruptive environmental pollutant [50].

Alkylphenols

Alkylphenolethoxylates (APEs) are widely used surfactants in domestic and industrial products. They are found in domestic detergents, pesticide formulations and industrial products. Octylphenolethoxylates (OPEs) and nonylphenolethoxylates (NPEs) are two of the most common surfactants in the marketplace. These compounds and their metabolites such as nonylphenol (NP), octylphenol (OP) and alkylphenolmono- to tri-ethoxylates (NPE1, NPE2 and NPE3) are commonly found in wastewater discharges and in sewage treatment plant (STP) effluents [55]. These metabolites are more toxic than the parent compounds and interact with the estrogen receptor and are able to mimic natural hormones [56–59]. In a South African study, atypical germ cells were encountered in the testes of wild eland, although detailed morphological examination for carcinoma in situ (CIS) was not possible. Testicular microlithiasis and neoplastic lesions were also reported in these animals, while at the same high body burdens of environmental pollutants, in particular, alkylphenols were measured [60].

Nonylphenol

Nonylphenol (NP) is used in the manufacturing of surfactants and plastics [61]. It is found in food, food packaging materials, cleaning products, skin care products, environmental water samples and drinking water [61–63]. The toxic effects of NP on aquatic life were first reported by Giger and co-workers [64], while Soto et al. [56] observed its capability to induce breast tumour cell proliferation. NP was found to mimic the natural hormone 17β-estradiol by competing for the binding site of the estrogen receptor. The environmental impacts of NP include feminization of aquatic organisms and decreased male fertility [56]. The European Union banned NP in 2003 because of its high toxicity to invertebrates and estrogenic activity in vertebrates [65].

Bisphenol-A

As early as 1936 Dodds and Lawson reported on the estrogenic properties of BPA (2,2-bis-(4-hydroxyphenyl)propane). Today BPA is produced in excess of six billion pounds per year [66]. It is found in the resin lining of metal cans, dental sealants [66] and in many plastic consumer products including toys, water pipes, drinking containers, eyeglass lenses, sports safety equipment, medical equipment, tubing and consumer electronics [14, 67].

A limited number of epidemiological studies, investigating the exposure of BPA, are referred to in the World Health Organization (WHO) review on the Toxicological and Health effects of BPA [68]. These studies investigated the association of urinary BPA concentrations with semen quality. They varied in their sample population: men who were partners of pregnant women in the USA (i.e. fertile men) [69], male partners in infertile couples that were patients in an infertility clinic [69, 70] and workers with occupational exposure to BPA in China [71]. All three studies reported associations of increased urinary BPA concentration with one or more measures of reduced semen quality. With the limited human and toxicological evidence, further studies on the association of BPA with semen quality are recommended.

Phthalates

Phthalates are industrial chemicals used as solvents, additives and plasticizers (compounds that increase the flexibility and resilience of plastic products) in vinyl flooring, adhesives, detergents, lubricating oils, solvents, automotive plastics, plastic clothing, personal care products, medical equipment and pharmaceuticals, plastic bags, garden hoses, inflatable products and children's toys [72]. There are a number of compounds in this group which includes dimethyl phthalate (DMP), diethyl phthalate (DEP), dibutyl phthalate (DBP), dicyclohexylphthalate (DCHP), di-*n*-octyl phthalate (DOP), di-2-ethylhexyl phthalate (DEHP), di-isononyl phthalate (DiNP) and benzylbutyl phthalate (BzBP), which is commonly called butyl benzyl phthalate (BBP) [72, 73].

Exposure to phthalates is consistent as they are ubiquitous in the environment. A possible reason for this may be due to the fact that as plasticizers they are required to remain unbound to plastic, thereby facilitating leaching of the chemical into the surrounding environment [74]. Exposure occurs through ingestion, inhalation, dermal and direct contact routes [73].

In the USA, the National Health and Nutrition Examination survey conducted between 1999 and 2000, found that more than 75 % of the population sampled had four phthalate metabolites present in their urine; MEP, MEHP, mono-benzyl phthalate (MBzP) and mono-*n*-butyl phthalate (MBP) [75]. Phillips and Tanphaichitr [43] reviewed several human studies that investigated phthalate exposure and semen quality. These studies investigating phthalate levels and semen quality [46, 76, 77] suggest that the effects are on sperm morphology and motility, rather than on total sperm numbers. Urinary phthalate metabolite measurements indicated a level of exposure, but may not reflect exposure of the testicular and reproductive tissue compartments [43].

Insecticides/Pesticides

The generic term "pesticide" refers to a broad range of structurally unrelated compounds with different mechanisms of action, biological targets and target pests [43, 78]. Pesticides cover a wide variety of compounds with different targets (e.g. herbicides, fungicides and insecticides) and chemical compositions [42]. They are used to protect crops, landscape and in the control of pest populations. Human exposure occurs during occupational use and from environmental contamination of food, water and air. The persistence and bioaccumulation ability of pesticides use years ago have led to the development of compounds with a shorter half life [42].

There are currently chemical mixtures available to control insects, weeds, fungi or other pests that are non-persistent pesticides as opposed to persistent pesticides that have been banned from use in most countries (e.g. OC pesticides such as DDT). Three common classes of non-persistent pesticides are used; organophosphates, carbamates, and pyrethroids, although environmentally non-persistent extensive use results in the general population being exposed at low levels [79]. Studies have suggested associations between non-persistent pesticide exposure, mostly occupational, involving simultaneous exposure to several pesticides and reduced semen quality [79].

Organophosphate Insecticides

A small study on male partners of pregnant women [80], found elevated odds ratios for poorer semen quality in relation to urinary concentrations of alachlormercapturate, 2-isopropoxy-4-methylpyrimidinol (diazinon metabolite), atrazine mercapturate, 1-naphthol (carbaryl and naphthalene metabolite) and 3,5,6-trichloro-2-pyridinol (chlorpyrifos metabolite).

Metals

A number of metals and metalloids are known endocrine disruptors responsible for disrupting a whole host of hormone pathways. Metals are present in rocks, soil, ground and surface water but are also used in commercial products or are released into the environment during mining and metal smelting, the production of electricity using fossil fuels and waste incineration. Cadmium, arsenic, lead and mercury have all been identified as metals with endocrine-disruptive properties. Metal exposure can target the following steroid receptor pathways: estrogen, progesterone, testosterone, corticosteroids and mineralocorticoids. They can also target the

receptors for retinoic acid, thyroid hormone and peroxisome proliferators (PPAR) [2].

Other Potential/Suspected EDCs

Biocides

Approximately 350 tons of triclosan [81], commercially known as Irgasan DP 300 or Irgacare MP, are presently used annually as an antimicrobial substance in many products in Europe. Increased demand and successful marketing of hygiene products for household use has increased the market for the use of triclosan as an antimicrobial agent. It is found in toothpaste, mouthwash, soaps, as well as in household cleaners and even in textiles, such as sportswear, bed linen, shoes and carpets [82].

In aquatic environments, triclosan attaches mainly to the surface of suspended solids and sediments and it also bioaccumulates in organisms. There are not many studies on the effects of triclosan; however, it disrupts steroidogenic enzymes involved in the production of testosterone and estrogen. This may lead to reduced reproductive success in both males and females [2].

Male Reproductive Health Effects (Including Possible Explanations for Different Results)

Interference with male sex determination and sexual differentiation (masculinisation) is a key concern for "endocrine disruption", especially as the masculinisation process is completely hormone dependent. Moreover, testicular development during masculinisation is partly hormone dependent and may possibly also be at risk area for endocrine disrupter exposure [83].

Hypospadias

Insufficient male hormone and/or an imbalance between female and male hormones (more estrogen than androgen) during critical developmental periods trigger male reproductive endocrine disorders. These may affect sexual differentiation (malformations such as cryptorchidism and hypospadias) and/or maturation during puberty [84–86]. Cryptorchidism and hypospadias also share risk factors such as being small-for-gestational age factors [87–89]. The imbalance and subsequent adverse effects may not be present at birth, but only become evident later in life. These disorders often occur simultaneously and Skakkebæk et al. [90] suggested that the increasing occurrence of hypospadias, undescended testes (UDT), male infertility and testicular cancer may reflect a single underlying condition, termed testicular dysgenesis syndrome (TDS) [91].

Hypospadias develop when there is incomplete closure of the urethral folds leaving a split on the penis and the opening on the underside of the penis or in the perineum instead of at the tip [92]. In distal hypospadias the urethra opens on the glans or corona of the penis. These may be missed, because a physiological phimosis at birth may hide the abnormality until such time as the foreskin can be retracted behind the glans [87]. There is concern that the incidence of hypospadias has increased in various regions of Australia, Europe and the USA [88, 93, 94].

The sad outcome after DES was used to treat threatening miscarriage in pregnant women and resulted in genital malformations, including hypospadias and cryptorchidism, was a wakeup call to consider and address the impact of foetal exposure to hormone active substances (endocrine disruption; reviewed by Toppari et al. [84]). The sons born after in utero DES exposure have a higher prevalence of hypospadias than other men, suggestive of possible trans-generational effects via epigenetic mechanisms [95–97].

Maternal, but not paternal occupational exposures, showed an elevated, marginally significant risk to develop hypospadias [98]. Sons born to mothers on vegetarian diets had an increased risk of hypospadias [99], while they had a decreased risk if the mothers had fish or meat during pregnancy [100]. In a large case–control study of boys operated on for hypospadias, Christensen et al. [101], demonstrated that frequent consumption of high fat dairy products (milk, butter) during pregnancy instead of rarely or never choosing the organic alternative was associated with increased odds of hypospadias. Subfertility and the use of assisted reproductive techniques increase the risk of hypospadias [102–106].

The risk associated with exposure to pharmaceutical sex steroids other than DES is not clear. Although the risk of hypospadias was associated with the use of progestins [107, 108], a later meta-analysis could not demonstrate any association between exposures to sex steroids (excluding DES) during the first trimester [109]. Progestins are available on the US market as prevention for threatening miscarriage and should offer an opportunity to clarify a possible role of progestin in hypospadias [110]. Anti-androgenic pesticides and fungicides are of concern in animal models, but as of yet their role and effect is not clear in humans.

Undescended Testes

Congenital cryptorchidism or UDT is the most common birth defect in newborn boys. The incidence is between 1 and 9 % [2] and it has increased in many countries [87]. The cryptorchid testis may be non-palpable (abdominal) or high scrotal and must be distinguished from retractile testis [111]. The higher intra-abdominal temperature is toxic to germ cells and any other position than normal may render it more prone to injury. UDT may be part of complex disorders and various chromosomal abnormalities [87], but maternal exposure to DES and polybrominated diphenyl ethers (PBDEs) and pesticides, except for DDE and DDT, and PCBs have been associated [2]. No associations were found with exposure to individual pesticides, emphasizing the need to include mixture assessment in epidemiological and laboratory investigations as all humans are exposed to various chemicals at the same time [2, 87].

Approximately 90 % of untreated men with bilateral cryptorchidism develop azoospermia and men with unilateral UDT also have unpredictable fertility [112]. Surgical correction of bilateral cryptorchidism in boys between the ages of 10 months and 4 years result in normal sperm count in 76 % of cases compared to 26 % when boys were surgically treated between the ages of 4 and 14 years [113]. The risk to develop testicular cancer is 4–6-fold higher in men with cryptorchidism [89, 114] and three times higher in boys with unilateral cryptorchidism than in their respective counterparts [115]. Corrective surgery for UDT (orchidopexy) makes it more easily palpable, but does not lower the cancer risk [87].

Testicular Cancer

Testicular cancer is a relatively rare cancer, but it is the most prevalent cancer in young men and, therefore, scrotal examination of men in an infertility setting is crucial. The highest rates are documented in industrialized countries, predominantly in western and northern Europe as well as Australia and New Zealand [2]. Furthermore, the prevalence of testicular cancer has doubled in the last 40 years, mainly in Caucasians. Reports documented that both seminomas and non-seminomas increased by 1–6 % per annum. These trends are influenced by birth cohort, with increasing risk for each generation of men born from the 1920s until the 1960s. For some of the high risk countries, it appears that the rate of increase has slowed over time and in several countries the most recent testicular cancer incidence rates have decreased slightly [2].

The specific pathophysiology of testicular germ cell tumours (TGCTs) is not clear, but there is ample evidence that in CIS testis, the precursor cells for all types of TGCTs arise during foetal development and is called the foetal origin of TGCTs [116]. CIS seems to develop when Sertoli and Leydig cells, during development, failed to orchestrate the normal differentiation of the primordial germ cells into spermatogonia [116, 117]. These failures may not only result in TGCTs, but also in impaired spermatogenesis, cryptorchidism, hypospadias and other disorders of sexual development [85].

Male Infertility

Male infertility may be attributed to a number of causes [43], which includes genetic and congenital abnormalities, infection, multi-systemic diseases, varicocele and others; however, most cases have no known etiology [43]. Exposure to environmental chemicals contained in pesticides, food sources, plastics, electronics and other synthetic materials are the suggested causes for the global changes in semen quality [118].

In infertile men the majority of cases of poor semen quality are not linked to cryptorchidism and hypospadias. Recent evidence from studies of anogenital distance (AGD) in men indicate that poorer semen quality is associated with a shorter AGD, indicating that the low sperm count in some cases could have a prenatal origin, even if it is not accompanied by undescended testis and/or hypospadias [119, 120].

Sperm Count

A low sperm count (oligozoospermia) increases the likelihood of a male being infertile, especially if his female partner also shows reduced fertility [121]. In 1992, a meta-analysis published by Carlson et al., indicated that sperm counts had declined by approximately half. This was reinforced by even more studies [80]; however it also resulted in much debate [11, 122]. A coordinated prospective study of young men (18–25 years) in seven European countries found the average sperm count to be low, with 20–25 % below 20 million/mL [123–126]. Geographical variations were also seen between countries and different parts of the same country [2, 127]. The question of declining sperm count continues to elicit controversial debate [122, 128].

Adult EDC studies investigating adverse effects on sperm production are useful in that the exposure and effect are concurrent [11, 129, 130]. Studying adult effects theoretically allows insight into which EDCs can affect the foetal testis and the potential relevance to TDS [11]. Caution should be exercised when extrapolating from one to the other as spermatogenesis does not occur in the foetal testes and the EDC effects may be fundamentally different from those that occur in adulthood [11]. Once exposure ceases, the EDC effects on the adult testis are likely to "self-correct", especially if they involve hormonal changes. For foetal EDC effects, the opposite is generally considered to be the case [11].

A significant amount of toxicology data based on laboratory and wildlife animal studies showing that exposure to certain EDCs is associated with reproductive toxicity, that included abnormalities of the male reproductive tract (cryptorchidism, hypospadias), reduced semen quality and impaired fertility in the adult can be found in Phillips and Tanchaiphitr's review [43]. Lifestyle factors such as cocaine [131], anabolic steroids [132, 133], alcohol [133, 134] and tobacco [135, 136] exposure may also lower sperm counts resulting in impaired fertility [137].

Sperm Motility

Sperm motility is believed to be one of the most important semen parameters correlated with fertility [138–140].

A number of epidemiological studies have been published examining the effects of DDT and metabolite exposure on MRH supporting the hypothesis that DDT exposure is related to reduced semen quality. A study of 195 Swedish fishermen showed a weak inverse association between serum p,p'-DDE and sperm motility [141]. A study in Mexico of non-occupationally DDT exposed men in a malaria endemic area found an association between higher p,p'-DDE plasma levels (mean unadjusted p,p'-DDE: 245 µg/L; mean lipid adjusted: 45 µg/g) and reduced sperm motility [142]. A similar study in the Limpopo Province in South Africa found that levels of p,p'-DDE, which were 5 times higher than those in the Mexico study (mean lipid adjusted: 215.47 µg/g), resulted in lower semen volume, total sperm count, progressive motility and viability [138]. In another study it was found that p,p'-DDT serum levels of a group of occupationally exposed DDT male Malaria Control Centre workers were negatively associated with sperm motility and sperm count [143]. These findings were similar to other PCB studies [44–46].

Sperm Morphology

The WHO [144] states that the fertilization rates in vitro will be reduced if the morphology is less than 15% normal forms. Disruption during spermatogenesis can result in impairment of sperm condensation, motility and morphology [138, 142, 145]. In a randomized controlled study of men with unexplained infertility, there was a negative correlation between seminal plasma phthalate ester concentration and sperm morphology [76]. Similarly, reductions in sperm motility and morphology exhibited a dose dependence on urinary MBP levels and MBzP levels in infertility patients. Urinary levels of monomethyl phthalate (MMP; 7.5 ng/mL) were weakly associated with poor sperm morphology [146]. The study investigating occupational DDT exposure reported a mean normal morphology score of 2.5 ± 1.8 %, with 84 % of the morphology scores being below the WHO (1992) and Tygerberg strict criteria [143]. In non-occupationally exposed men a significantly high proportion of the participants presented with teratozoospermia (99.5 %), and the mean normal morphology was 4.13 ± 2.70 %, also well below the WHO (1999) reference range. Cytotoxic effects, such as the production of superoxide anion and activation of various intracellular signal transduction pathways, might explain the significant decrease in normal morphology [76].

DNA Damage

There are detrimental developmental consequences due to environmentally mediated DNA damage to spermatozoa which can lead to impaired embryonic development, abortion and the induction of abnormalities in the offspring such as childhood or testicular cancer [147]. Aitken et al. [147] emphasized that damage to a father's sperm—either genetic, affecting the DNA sequence itself, or otherwise perturbing DNA function through epigenetic mechanisms—can be responsible for diseases in his offspring, as well as being itself a cause of infertility or early loss of pregnancy. The increased rates of childhood cancers as a result of heavy paternal smoking [148] are thought to be mediated by oxidative damage to the DNA in the father's sperm and thereby affect the health and well-being of the ensuing children [147]. Over exposure to reactive oxygen species results in oxidative injury, excites oxygen-containing molecules, generated as a by-product of cell metabolism and the intracellular processing can attack and damage DNA [147] leading to infertility [149].

Testicular Dysgenesis Syndrome

TGCT often occurs in subjects with hypospadias, cryptorchidism and/or low semen quality, suggesting these are risk factors for one another [111, 150]. These pathologies were linked together as a single underlying disorder, termed TDS, which originates during foetal life [151, 152] and is caused by chemical exposures. Research in rodent models is particularly helpful to identify chemicals that interfere with male reproductive development. It also aided in the discovery of the male programming window and demonstrated the irreversible nature of the subsequent events. The male offspring produced by these studies has demonstrated that all of the constituent elements of TDS can be induced in the rat, as in men, with the exception of TGCTs. These models should be particularly useful for assessment of anti-androgenic pesticides and fungicides.

Prostate Cancer

Many prostate cancers can be detected in an early curable stage by digital rectal examination (DRE), which should be performed in every male for infertility evaluation and especially in men older than 40 years of age. Prostate cancer is the second most common cause of male cancer deaths after age 55 years and the most common cause of cancer deaths in men older than 70 years [153]. The estimated lifetime risk of disease is 16.72 %, with a lifetime risk of death at 2.57 %, with African-Americans at highest risk [154].

The increased availability of prostate-specific antigen (PSA) for routine screening of prostate cancer may partly explain the trend [155]. Changes in prostate cancer incidence among migrant populations and studies of twins show that environmental factors, including diet and chemical exposures, also contribute to prostate cancer risk [156, 157]. Unhealthy western lifestyles such as smoking and physical inactivity and consumption of calorie-dense food may be particularly detrimental [158]. Although estrogens and androgens play a role in normal prostate development [159], estrogen exposure during foetal life sensitizes the prostate to the development of hyperplasia and cancer later in life (reviewed by [160, 161]). Epidemiological studies have identified occupational chemical exposure during pesticide application in agriculture [162, 163], and pesticide manufacture [164] as issues of concern.

Some PCB congeners, including CB-138, -153 and -180 [165, 166] and cadmium exposure have been linked to prostate cancer in several, but not all epidemiological studies [157, 167–169]. However, arsenic exposure is strongly associated with prostate cancer [170, 171]. The exact mechanism by which these chemicals induce carcinogenesis is not clear, but in view of the discussion above on the effects of estrogen, androgen and anti-androgen on the prostate, similar effects from these chemicals seem likely.

Foetal Onset of Adulthood Disease

The concept of TDS is based on the premise that the associated symptoms have a common origin in foetal development, and that the extent and severity to which they are manifested is dependent on the degree to which normal developmental processes have been perturbed. In addition, it assumes that any perturbations occurring during the male programming window are irreversible and have lifelong implications for the affected individual and, potentially, also for their offspring. Although there is good evidence that each of the diseases comprising TDS have strong genetic components, Skakkebæk et al. [90] noted that the majority of baby boys born with these symptoms lacked the expected genetic aberrations, indicating that environmental factors must play an important role in the etiology of these phenomena. Hormonal perturbations, arising from EDC exposures, have been widely implicated in the causation of TDS in humans, and also in the widespread reports of reproductive dysgenesis in wildlife, between which there are obvious parallels, as well as clear distinctions.

General Health Effects That May Affect MRH

Systemic diseases and ejaculatory dysfunction may be partly or entirely the cause of impaired male fertility. Certain medications may have a further negative effect on sperm function. If the physician is content to make a diagnosis on the semen analysis report without listening to the patient and taking a thorough history or looking for specific signs (examination), significant conditions may be overlooked. Unfortunately, this may lead not only to inappropriate management, but also to the loss of an opportunity to make a difference to the short- and long-term prognosis of both reproductive and general health.

Discussion and Conclusions

Key Points

The concept of endocrine disruption is no longer limited to estrogenic, androgenic and thyroid pathways. As it becomes clear that some chemicals can also interfere with metabolism, fat storage, bone development and the immune system, indicating that all endocrine systems can and will be affected by EDCs. We need further research to more comprehensively assess how EDCs affect normal endocrine function, and how these effects may be passed on to future generations [2].

Strengths and Limitations of Chapter

Although this chapter includes the most recent information, the content is limited to what has been published, which for obvious reasons are not the complete picture.

Knowledge Gaps

There is very little epidemiological evidence to link EDC exposure with adverse pregnancy outcomes, early onset of breast development, obesity or diabetes. There are also data on foetal EDC exposures and adult measures of semen quality. Likewise, no studies explored the potential link between foetal exposure to EDCs and the risk of testicular cancer occurring 20–40 years later.

References

1. IPCS. Global assessment of the state-of-the-science of endocrine disruptors. Geneva: World Health Organization; 2002.
2. Bergman A, Heindel JJ, Jobling S, Kidd KA, Zoeller RT. State of the science of endocrine disrupting chemicals 2012. Geneva: United Nations Environment Programme and the World Health Organization; 2013.
3. Ruenitz PC, Bourne CS, Sullivan KJ, Moore SA. Estrogenic triarylethylene acetic acids: effect of structural variation on estrogen receptor affinity and estrogenic potency and efficacy in MCF-7 cells. J Med Chem. 1996;39(24):4853–9.
4. Clement K, Vaisse C, Lahlou N, Cabrol S, Pelloux V, Cassuto D, et al. A mutation in the human leptin receptor gene causes obesity and pituitary dysfunction. Nature. 1998;392(6674):398–401. Epub 1998/04/16.
5. Tapanainen JS, Aittomaki K, Huhtaniemi IT. New insights into the role of follicle-stimulating hormone in reproduction. Ann Med. 1997;29(4):265–6. Epub 1997/08/01.
6. Itman C, Mendis S, Barakat B, Loveland KL. All in the family: TGF-beta family action in testis development. Reproduction. 2006;132(2):233–46. Epub 2006/08/04.
7. Santen RJ. Is aromatization of testosterone to estradiol required for inhibition of luteinizing hormone secretion in men? J Clin Invest. 1975;56(6):1555–63. Epub 1975/12/01.
8. Hayes FJ, Pitteloud N, DeCruz S, Crowley Jr WF, Boepple PA. Importance of inhibin B in the regulation of FSH secretion in the human male. J Clin Endocrinol Metab. 2001;86(11):5541–6. Epub 2001/11/10.
9. Wennbo H, Kindblom J, Isaksson OG, Tornell J. Transgenic mice overexpressing the prolactin gene develop dramatic enlargement of the prostate gland. Endocrinology. 1997;138(10):4410–5. Epub 1997/10/10.
10. Steger RW, Chandrashekar V, Zhao W, Bartke A, Horseman ND. Neuroendocrine and reproductive functions in male mice with targeted disruption of the prolactin gene. Endocrinology. 1998;139(9): 3691–5. Epub 1998/09/02.
11. Sharpe R. Male reproductive health disorders and the potential role of exposure to environmental chemicals. London: CHEM Trust; 2009.
12. Braw-Tal R. Endocrine disruptors and timing of human exposure. Pediatr Endocrinol Rev. 2010;8(1): 41–6. Epub 2010/11/03.

13. Buck Louis GM, Gray Jr LE, Marcus M, Ojeda SR, Pescovitz OH, Witchel SF, et al. Environmental factors and puberty timing: expert panel research needs. Pediatrics. 2008;121 Suppl 3:S192–207. Epub 2008/02/15.
14. Vandenberg LN, Colborn T, Hayes TB, Heindel JJ, Jacobs Jr DR, Lee DH, et al. Hormones and endocrine-disrupting chemicals: low-dose effects and nonmonotonic dose responses. Endocr Rev. 2012;33(3):378–455. Epub 2012/03/16.
15. Melnick R, Lucier G, Wolfe M, Hall R, Stancel G, Prins G, et al. Summary of the National Toxicology Program's report of the endocrine disruptors low-dose peer review. Environ Health Perspect. 2002;110(4):427–31. Epub 2002/04/10.
16. vom Saal FS, Timms BG, Montano MM, Palanza P, Thayer KA, Nagel SC, et al. Prostate enlargement in mice due to foetal exposure to low doses of estradiol or diethylstilbestrol and opposite effects at high doses. Proc Natl Acad Sci U S A. 1997;94(5):2056–61.
17. Silva E, Rajapakse N, Kortenkamp A. Something from "nothing"—eight weak estrogenic chemicals combined at concentrations below NOECs produce significant mixture effects. Environ Sci Technol. 2002;36(8):1751–6. Epub 2002/05/08.
18. Kortenkamp A, Martin O, Faust M, Evans R, McKinlay R, Orton F, et al. State of the art assessment of endocrine disruptors. Geneva: World Health Organization; 2012.
19. Rajapakse N, Silva E, Kortenkamp A. Combining xenoestrogens at levels below individual no-observed-effect concentrations dramatically enhances steroid hormone action. Environ Health Perspect. 2002;110(9):917–21. Epub 2002/09/03.
20. McKinlay R, Plant JA, Bell JN, Voulvoulis N. Calculating human exposure to endocrine disrupting pesticides via agricultural and non-agricultural exposure routes. Sci Total Environ. 2008;398(1–3):1–12.
21. Bouvier G, Blanchard O, Momas I, Seta N. Environmental and biological monitoring of exposure to organophosphorus pesticides: application to occupationally and non-occupationally exposed adult populations. J Expo Sci Environ Epidemiol. 2006;16(5):417–26.
22. Ambroise D, Moulin JJ, Squinazi F, Protois JC, Fontana JM, Wild P. Cancer mortality among municipal pest-control workers. Int Arch Occup Environ Health. 2005;78(5):387–93.
23. Van Tongeren M, Nieuwenhuijsen MJ, Gardiner K, Armstrong B, Vrijheid M, Dolk H, et al. A job-exposure matrix for potential endocrine-disrupting chemicals developed for a study into the association between maternal occupational exposure and hypospadias. Ann Occup Hyg. 2002;46(5):465–77.
24. Lu C, Fenske RA, Simcox NJ, Kalman D. Pesticide exposure of children in an agricultural community: evidence of household proximity to farmland and take home exposure pathways. Environ Res. 2000;84(3):290–302. Epub 2000/12/01.
25. Grey CN, Nieuwenhuijsen MJ, Golding J. Use and storage of domestic pesticides in the UK. Sci Total Environ. 2006;368(2–3):465–70. Epub 2006/05/16.
26. Menegaux F, Baruchel A, Bertrand Y, Lescoeur B, Leverger G, Nelken B, et al. Household exposure to pesticides and risk of childhood acute leukaemia. Occup Environ Med. 2006;63(2):131–4. Epub 2006/01/20.
27. Whyatt RM, Camann DE, Kinney PL, Reyes A, Ramirez J, Dietrich J, et al. Residential pesticide use during pregnancy among a cohort of urban minority women. Environ Health Perspect. 2002;110(5):507–14. Epub 2002/05/11.
28. Martina CA, Weiss B, Swan SH. Lifestyle behaviors associated with exposures to endocrine disruptors. Neurotoxicology. 2012;33(6):1427–33. Epub 2012/06/29.
29. Rayman RB. Aircraft disinfection. Aviat Space Environ Med. 2006;77(7):733–6. Epub 2006/07/22.
30. van Netten C. Analysis and implications of aircraft disinsectants. Sci Total Environ. 2002;293(1–3):257–62. Epub 2002/07/12.
31. Hahn S, Melching-Kollmuß S, Bitsch A, Schneider K, Oltmans J, Hassauer M, et al. Health risks from biocide-containing products and article of daily use. Hanover: German Federal Environmental Agency; 2005.
32. Steer CD, Grey CN. Socio-demographic characteristics of UK families using pesticides and weed-killers. J Expo Sci Environ Epidemiol. 2006;16(3):251–63. Epub 2005/09/01.
33. Gerhard I, Derner M, Runnebaum B. Prolonged exposure to wood preservatives induces endocrine and immunologic disorders in women. Am J Obstet Gynecol. 1991;165(2):487–8. Epub 1991/08/01.
34. Knopper L, Lean DR. Carcinogenic and genotoxic potential of turf pesticides commonly used on golf courses. J Toxicol Environ Health B Crit Rev. 2004;7(4):267–79. Epub 2004/06/19.
35. Bernard CE, Nuygen H, Truong D, Krieger RI. Environmental residues and biomonitoring estimates of human insecticide exposure from treated residential turf. Arch Environ Contam Toxicol. 2001;41(2):237–40. Epub 2001/07/20.
36. Curl CL, Fenske RA, Elgethun K. Organophosphorus pesticide exposure of urban and suburban preschool children with organic and conventional diets. Environ Health Perspect. 2003;111(3):377–82. Epub 2003/03/04.
37. Lu C, Toepel K, Irish R, Fenske RA, Barr DB, Bravo R. Organic diets significantly lower children's dietary exposure to organophosphorus pesticides. Environ Health Perspect. 2006;114(2):260–3. Epub 2006/02/03.
38. Darnerud PO, Atuma S, Aune M, Bjerselius R, Glynn A, Grawe KP, et al. Dietary intake estimations of organohalogen contaminants (dioxins, PCB,

39. Bro-Rasmussen F. Contamination by persistent chemicals in food chain and human health. Sci Total Environ. 1996;188 Suppl 1:S45–60. Epub 1996/09/01.

40. Givens ML, Lu C, Bartell SM, Pearson MA. Estimating dietary consumption patterns among children: a comparison between cross-sectional and longitudinal study designs. Environ Res. 2007;103(3):325–30. Epub 2006/08/16.

41. United Nations Environment Programme (UNEP). About UNEP chemicals branch. 2013. http://www.chem.unep.ch. Accessed 14 Nov 2013.

42. Woodruff T, Janssen S, Guillette LJ, Giudice L. Environmental impacts on reproductive health and fertility. Cambridge: Cambridge University Press; 2010.

43. Phillips KP, Tanphaichitr N. Human exposure to endocrine disrupters and semen quality. J Toxicol Environ Health B Crit Rev. 2008;11(3–4):188–220.

44. Richthoff J, Rylander L, Jonsson BA, Akesson H, Hagmar L, Nilsson-Ehle P, et al. Serum levels of 2,2',4,4',5,5'-hexachlorobiphenyl (CB-153) in relation to markers of reproductive function in young males from the general Swedish population. Environ Health Perspect. 2003;111(4):409–13.

45. Guo YL, Hsu PC, Hsu CC, Lambert GH. Semen quality after prenatal exposure to polychlorinated biphenyls and dibenzofurans. Lancet. 2000;356(9237):1240–1.

46. Hauser R, Altshul L, Chen Z, Ryan L, Overstreet J, Schiff I, et al. Environmental organochlorines and semen quality: results of a pilot study. Environ Health Perspect. 2002;110(3):229–33.

47. Dallinga JW, Moonen EJ, Dumoulin JC, Evers JL, Geraedts JP, Kleinjans JC. Decreased human semen quality and organochlorine compounds in blood. Hum Reprod. 2002;17(8):1973–9.

48. Toft G, Axmon A, Giwercman A, Thulstrup AM, Rignell-Hydbom A, Pedersen HS, et al. Fertility in four regions spanning large contrasts in serum levels of widespread persistent organochlorines: a cross-sectional study. Environ Health. 2005;4:26. Epub 2005/11/11.

49. Voldner EC, Li YF. Global usage of toxaphene. Chemosphere. 1993;27(10):2073–8.

50. Turusov V, Rakitsky V, Tomatis L. Dichlorodiphenyltrichloroethane (DDT): ubiquity, persistence, and risks. Environ Health Perspect. 2002;110(2):125–8. Epub 2002/02/12.

51. Rogan WJ, Chen A. Health risks and benefits of bis(4-chlorophenyl)-1,1,1-trichloroethane (DDT). Lancet. 2005;366(9487):763–73. Epub 2005/08/30.

52. Kelce WR, Stone CR, Laws SC, Gray LE, Kemppainen JA, Wilson EM. Persistent DDT metabolite p, p'-DDE is a potent androgen receptor antagonist. Nature. 1995;375:581–5.

53. Bhatia R, Shiau R, Paetreas M, Weintraub JM, Farhang L, Eskanazi B. Organochlorine pesticides and male genital anomalies in the child health development studies. Environ Health Perspect. 2005;113:220–4.

54. Danzo BJ. Environmental xenobiotics may disrupt normal endocrine function by interfering with the binding of physiological ligands to steroid receptors and binding proteins. Environ Health Perspect. 1997;105(3):294–301. Epub 1997/03/01.

55. Ying GG, Williams B, Kookana R. Environmental fate of alkylphenols and alkylphenol ethoxylates–a review. Environ Int. 2002;28(3):215–26.

56. Soto AM, Justicia H, Wray JW, Sonnenschein C. p-Nonyl-phenol: an estrogenic xenobiotic released from "modified" polystyrene. Environ Health Perspect. 1991;92:167–73.

57. Jobling S, Sumpter JP. Detergent components in sewage effluent are weakly oestrogenic to fish: An in vitro study using rainbow trout (Oncorhynchus mykiss) hepatocytes. Aquat Toxicol. 1993;27(3–4):361–72.

58. Jobling S, Sumpter JP, Sheahan D, Osborne JA, Matthiessen P. Inhibition of testicular growth in rainbow trout (Oncorhynchus mykiss) exposed to estrogenic alkylphenolic chemicals. Environ Toxicol Chem. 1996;15(2):194–202.

59. Renner R. European bans on surfactant trigger transatlantic debate. Environ Sci Technol. 1997;31(7):316A–20.

60. Bornman R, de Jager C, Worku Z, Farias P, Reif S. DDT and urogenital malformations in newborn boys in a malarial area. BJU Int. 2010;106(3):405–11. Epub 2009/10/24.

61. Inoue K, Kondo S, Yoshie Y, Kato K, Yoshimura Y, Horie M, et al. Migration of 4-nonylphenol from polyvinyl chloride food packaging films into food simulants and foods. Food Addit Contam. 2001;18(2):157–64. Epub 2001/04/06.

62. Soares A, Guieysse B, Jefferson B, Cartmell E, Lester JN. Nonylphenol in the environment: a critical review on occurrence, fate, toxicity and treatment in wastewaters. Environ Int. 2008;34(7):1033–49.

63. Muncke J. Exposure to endocrine disrupting compounds via the food chain: is packaging a relevant source? Sci Total Environ. 2009;407(16):4549–59.

64. Giger W, Brunner PH, Schaffner C. 4-Nonylphenol in sewage sludge: accumulation of toxic metabolites from nonionic surfactants. Science. 1984;225(4662):623–5.

65. Preuss TG, Gehrhardt J, Schirmer K, Coors A, Rubach M, Russ A, et al. Nonylphenol isomers differ in estrogenic activity. Environ Sci Technol. 2006;40(16):5147–53. Epub 2006/09/08.

66. vom Saal FS, Parmigiani S, Palanza PL, Everett LG, Ragaini R. The plastic world: sources, amounts, ecological impacts and effects on development, reproduction, brain and behavior in aquatic and terrestrial animals and humans. Environ Res. 2008;108(2):127–30. Epub 2008/10/25.

67. Wetherill YB, Akingbemi BT, Kanno J, McLachlan JA, Nadal A, Sonnenschein C, et al. In vitro molecular mechanisms of bisphenol A action. Reprod Toxicol. 2007;24(2):178–98.

68. World Health Organization. Toxicological and health aspects of Bisphenol A. Geneva: Joint FAO/WHO Expert Meeting; 2011.
69. Mendiola J, Jorgensen N, Andersson AM, Calafat AM, Ye X, Redmon JB, et al. Are environmental levels of bisphenol A associated with reproductive function in fertile men? Environ Health Perspect. 2010;118(9):1286–91. Epub 2010/05/25.
70. Meeker JD, Ehrlich S, Toth TL, Wright DL, Calafat AM, Trisini AT, et al. Semen quality and sperm DNA damage in relation to urinary bisphenol A among men from an infertility clinic. Reprod Toxicol. 2010;30(4):532–9. Epub 2010/07/27.
71. Li DK, Zhou Z, Miao M, He Y, Wang J, Ferber J, et al. Urine bisphenol-A (BPA) level in relation to semen quality. Fertil Steril. 2011;95(2):625–30. e1–4. Epub 2010/11/03.
72. Department of Health and Human Services, Centers for Disease Control and Prevention (CDC). Third national report on human exposure to environmental chemicals: phtalates. 2005. http://www.cdc.gov/exposurereport/results_06.htm. Accessed 15 Nov 2013.
73. Dehnel LT. The effect of phtalates on the male reproductive system. Maryland: University of Maryland; 2008.
74. NICAS. A summary of physicochemical and human health hazard data for 24 *ortho*-phthalate chemicals existing chemical hazard assessment report. Sydney: National and Industrial Chemicals Notification and Assessment Scheme; 2008.
75. Silva MJ, Barr DB, Reidy JA, Malek NA, Hodge CC, Caudill SP, et al. Urinary levels of seven phthalate metabolites in the U.S. population from the National Health and Nutrition Examination Survey (NHANES) 1999-2000. Environ Health Perspect. 2004;112(3):331–8.
76. Rozati R, Reddy PP, Reddanna P, Mujtaba R. Role of environmental estrogens in the deterioration of male factor fertility. Fertil Steril. 2002;78(6):1187–94. Epub 2002/12/13.
77. Jonsson BA, Richthoff J, Rylander L, Giwercman A, Hagmar L. Urinary phthalate metabolites and biomarkers of reproductive function in young men. Epidemiology. 2005;16(4):487–93. Epub 2005/06/14.
78. Ritter L, Arbuckle TE. Can exposure characterization explain concurrence or discordance between toxicology and epidemiology? Toxicol Sci. 2007;97(2):241–52. Epub 2007/01/20.
79. Diamanti-Kandarakis E, Bourguignon J-P, Giudice L, Hauser R, Prins G, Soto A, Zoeller R, Gore A. Endocrine-disrupting chemicals: an endocrine society scientific statement. Endocr Rev. 2009;30(4): 293–342.
80. Swan SH, Elkin EP, Fenster L. The question of declining sperm density revisited: an analysis of 101 studies published 1934-1996. Environ Health Perspect. 2000;108(10):961–6.
81. Calafat AM, Ye X, Wong L-Y, Reidy JA, Needham LL. Urinary Concentrations of Triclosan in the U.S. Population: 2003–2004. Environ Health Perspect. 2008; 116(3):303–307.

82. Singer H, Muller S, Tixier C, Pillonel L. Triclosan: occurrence and fate of a widely used biocide in the aquatic environment: field measurements in wastewater treatment plants, surface waters, and lake sediments. Environ Sci Technol. 2002;36(23): 4998–5004.
83. Sharpe RM. Pathways of endocrine disruption during male sexual differentiation and masculinization. Best Pract Res Clin Endocrinol Metab. 2006;20(1):91–110. Epub 2006/03/09.
84. Toppari J, Larsen JC, Christiansen P, Giwercman A, Grandjean P, Guillette Jr LJ, et al. Male reproductive health and environmental xenoestrogens. Environ Health Perspect. 1996;104 Suppl 4:741–803. Epub 1996/08/01.
85. Sharpe R, Skakkebaek NE. Male reproductive disorders and the role of endocrine disruption: advances in understanding and identification of areas for future research. Pure Appl Chem. 2003;75(11–12):2023–38.
86. Sharpe RM, Skakkebaek NE. Testicular dysgenesis syndrome: mechanistic insights and potential new downstream effects. Fertil Steril. 2008;89(2 Suppl):e33–8. Epub 2008/03/20.
87. Toppari J, Virtanen HE, Main KM, Skakkebaek NE. Cryptorchidism and hypospadias as a sign of testicular dysgenesis syndrome (TDS): environmental connection. Birth Defects Res A Clin Mol Teratol. 2010;88(10):910–9. Epub 2010/09/25.
88. Toppari J, Kaleva M, Virtanen HE. Trends in the incidence of cryptorchidism and hypospadias, and methodological limitations of registry-based data. Hum Reprod Update. 2001;7(3):282–6. Epub 2001/06/08.
89. Schnack TH, Poulsen G, Myrup C, Wohlfahrt J, Melbye M. Familial coaggregation of cryptorchidism and hypospadias. Epidemiology. 2010;21(1): 109–13. Epub 2009/11/11.
90. Skakkebaek NE, Rajpert-De Meyts E, Main KM. Testicular dysgenesis syndrome: an increasingly common developmental disorder with environmental aspects. Hum Reprod. 2001;16(5):972–8. Epub 2001/05/02.
91. Skakkebaek NE. Endocrine disrupters and testicular dysgenesis syndrome. Horm Res. 2002;57 Suppl 2:43. Epub 2002/06/18.
92. Kalfa N, Cassorla F, Audran F, Oulad Abdennabi I, Philibert P, Beroud C, et al. Polymorphisms of MAMLD1 gene in hypospadias. J Pediatr Urol. 2011;7(6):585–91. Epub 2011/10/28.
93. Nassar N, Bower C, Barker A. Increasing prevalence of hypospadias in Western Australia, 1980-2000. Arch Dis Child. 2007;92(7):580–4. Epub 2007/04/05.
94. Paulozzi LJ. International trends in rates of hypospadias and cryptorchidism. Environ Health Perspect. 1999;107(4):297–302. Epub 1999/03/25.
95. Klip H, Verloop J, van Gool JD, Koster ME, Burger CW, van Leeuwen FE. Hypospadias in sons of women exposed to diethylstilbestrol in utero: a cohort study. Lancet. 2002;359(9312):1102–7. Epub 2002/04/12.

96. Brouwers MM, Feitz WF, Roelofs LA, Kiemeney LA, de Gier RP, Roeleveld N. Hypospadias: a transgenerational effect of diethylstilbestrol? Hum Reprod. 2006;21(3):666–9. Epub 2005/11/19.

97. Kalfa N, Philibert P, Sultan C. Is hypospadias a genetic, endocrine or environmental disease, or still an unexplained malformation? Int J Androl. 2009;32(3):187–97. Epub 2008/07/19.

98. Rocheleau CM, Romitti PA, Dennis LK. Pesticides and hypospadias: a meta-analysis. J Pediatr Urol. 2009;5(1):17–24. Epub 2008/10/14.

99. North K, Golding J. A maternal vegetarian diet in pregnancy is associated with hypospadias. The ALSPAC Study Team. Avon Longitudinal Study of Pregnancy and Childhood. BJU Int. 2000;85(1): 107–13. Epub 2000/01/05.

100. Akre O, Boyd HA, Ahlgren M, Wilbrand K, Westergaard T, Hjalgrim H, et al. Maternal and gestational risk factors for hypospadias. Environ Health Perspect. 2008;116(8):1071–6. Epub 2008/08/19.

101. Christensen JS, Asklund C, Skakkebaek NE, Jorgensen N, Andersen HR, Jorgensen TM, et al. Association between organic dietary choice during pregnancy and hypospadias in offspring: a study of mothers of 306 boys operated on for hypospadias. J Urol. 2013;189(3):1077–82. Epub 2012/10/06.

102. Sweet RA, Schrott HG, Kurland R, Culp OS. Study of the incidence of hypospadias in Rochester, Minnesota, 1940-1970, and a case-control comparison of possible etiologic factors. Mayo Clin Proc. 1974;49(1):52–8. Epub 1974/01/01.

103. Czeizel A. Increasing trends in congenital malformations of male external genitalia. Lancet. 1985;1(8426):462–3. Epub 1985/02/23.

104. Wennerholm UB, Bergh C, Hamberger L, Lundin K, Nilsson L, Wikland M, et al. Incidence of congenital malformations in children born after ICSI. Hum Reprod. 2000;15(4):944–8. Epub 2000/03/31.

105. Klemetti R, Gissler M, Sevon T, Koivurova S, Ritvanen A, Hemminki E. Children born after assisted fertilization have an increased rate of major congenital anomalies. Fertil Steril. 2005;84(5):1300–7. Epub 2005/11/09.

106. Kallen B, Bertollini R, Castilla E, Czeizel A, Knudsen LB, Martinez-Frias ML, et al. A joint international study on the epidemiology of hypospadias. Acta Paediatr Scand Suppl. 1986;324:1–52. Epub 1986/01/01.

107. Czeizel A, Toth J, Erodi E. Aetiological studies of hypospadias in Hungary. Hum Hered. 1979;29(3): 166–71. Epub 1979/01/01.

108. Calzolari E, Contiero MR, Roncarati E, Mattiuz PL, Volpato S. Aetiological factors in hypospadias. J Med Genet. 1986;23(4):333–7. Epub 1986/08/01.

109. Raman-Wilms L, Tseng AL, Wighardt S, Einarson TR, Koren G. Foetal genital effects of first-trimester sex hormone exposure: a meta-analysis. Obstet Gynecol. 1995;85(1):141–9. Epub 1995/01/01.

110. Wahabi HA, Fayed AA, Esmaeil SA, Al Zeidan RA. Progestogen for treating threatened miscarriage. Cochrane Database Syst Rev. 2011;12, CD005943. Epub 2011/12/14.

111. Boisen KA, Kaleva M, Main KM, Virtanen HE, Haavisto AM, Schmidt IM, et al. Difference in prevalence of congenital cryptorchidism in infants between two Nordic countries. Lancet. 2004;363(9417): 1264–9. Epub 2004/04/20.

112. Mathers MJ, Degener S, Roth S. [Cryptorchidism and infertility from the perspective of interdisciplinary guidelines]. Urologe A. 2011;50(1):20–5. Epub 2011/01/06. Hodenhochstand und Infertilitat unter besonderer Berucksichtigung der interdisziplinaren Leitlinie.

113. Lee PA, Coughlin MT. Fertility after bilateral cryptorchidism. Evaluation by paternity, hormone, and semen data. Horm Res. 2001;55(1):28–32.

114. Dieckmann KP, Pichlmeier U. Clinical epidemiology of testicular germ cell tumors. World J Urol. 2004;22(1):2–14. Epub 2004/03/23.

115. Lip SZ, Murchison LE, Cullis PS, Govan L, Carachi R. A meta-analysis of the risk of boys with isolated cryptorchidism developing testicular cancer in later life. Arch Dis Child. 2013;98(1):20–6. Epub 2012/11/30.

116. Rajpert-De Meyts E. Developmental model for the pathogenesis of testicular carcinoma in situ: genetic and environmental aspects. Hum Reprod Update. 2006;12:303–23.

117. Looijenga L, Gillis A, Stoop H, Biermann K, Oosterhuis J. Dissecting the molecular pathways of (testicular) germ cell tumor pathogenesis; from initiation to treatment resistance. Int J Androl. 2011;34:234–51.

118. Carlsen E, Giwercman A, Keiding N, Skakkebaek NE. Evidence for decreasing quality of semen during past 50 years. BMJ. 1992;305(6854):609–13.

119. Mendiola J, Stahlhut RW, Jorgensen N, Liu F, Swan SH. Shorter anogenital distance predicts poorer semen quality in young men in Rochester, New York. Environ Health Perspect. 2011;119(7):958–63. Epub 2011/03/08.

120. Eisenberg ML, Hsieh MH, Walters RC, Krasnow R, Lipshultz LI. The relationship between anogenital distance, fatherhood, and fertility in adult men. PLoS One. 2011;6(5):e18973. Epub 2011/05/19.

121. Irvine DS. Epidemiology and aetiology of male infertility. Hum Reprod. 1998;13 Suppl 1:33–44.

122. Jouannet P, Wang C, Eustache F, Kold-Jensen T, Auger J. Semen quality and male reproductive health: the controversy about human sperm concentration decline. APMIS. 2001;109(5):333–44.

123. Jorgensen N, Carlsen E, Nermoen I, Punab M, Suominen J, Andersen AG, et al. East-West gradient in semen quality in the Nordic-Baltic area: a study of men from the general population in Denmark, Norway, Estonia and Finland. Hum Reprod. 2002;17(8):2199–208. Epub 2002/08/02.

124. Jorgensen N, Asklund C, Carlsen E, Skakkebaek NE. Coordinated European investigations of semen quality: results from studies of Scandinavian young men is a matter of concern. Int J Androl. 2006;29(1): 54–61; discussion 105-8.

125. Jorgensen N, Vierula M, Jacobsen R, Pukkala E, Perheentupa A, Virtanen HE, et al. Recent adverse trends in semen quality and testis cancer incidence among Finnish men. Int J Androl. 2011;34(4 Pt 2):e37–48.

126. Jorgensen N, Joensen UN, Jensen TK, Jensen MB, Almstrup K, Olesen IA, et al. Human semen quality in the new millennium: a prospective cross-sectional population-based study of 4867 men. BMJ Open. 2012;2(4):1–13.

127. Andersson AM, Jorgensen N, Main KM, Toppari J, Rajpert-De Meyts E, Leffers H, et al. Adverse trends in male reproductive health: we may have reached a crucial 'tipping point'. Int J Androl. 2008;31(2): 74–80.

128. Skakkebaek NE, Andersson AM, Juul A, Jensen TK, Almstrup K, Toppari J, et al. Sperm counts, data responsibility, and good scientific practice. Epidemiology. 2011;22(5):620–1.

129. Bonde JP, Giwercman A, Ernst E. Identifying environmental risk to male reproductive function by occupational sperm studies: logistics and design options. Occup Environ Med. 1996;53(8):511–9. Epub 1996/08/01.

130. Tas S, Lauwerys R, Lison D. Occupational hazards for the male reproductive system. Crit Rev Toxicol. 1996;26(3):261–307. Epub 1996/05/01.

131. Abel EL, Moore C, Waselewsky D, Zajac C, Russell LD. Effects of cocaine hydrochloride on reproductive function and sexual behavior of male rats and on the behavior of their offspring. J Androl. 1989;10(1):17–27. Epub 1989/01/01.

132. Torres-Calleja J, Gonzalez-Unzaga M, DeCelis-Carrillo R, Calzada-Sanchez L, Pedron N. Effect of androgenic anabolic steroids on sperm quality and serum hormone levels in adult male bodybuilders. Life Sci. 2001;68(15):1769–74. Epub 2001/03/29.

133. Pasqualotto FF, Lucon AM, Sobreiro BP, Pasqualotto EB, Arap S. Effects of medical therapy, alcohol, smoking, and endocrine disruptors on male infertility. Rev Hosp Clin Fac Med Sao Paulo. 2004;59(6):375–82. Epub 2005/01/18.

134. Verajankorva E, Laato M, Pollanen P. Analysis of 508 infertile male patients in south-western Finland in 1980-2000: hormonal status and factors predisposing to immunological infertility. Eur J Obstet Gynecol Reprod Biol. 2003;111(2):173–8. Epub 2003/11/05.

135. Klaiber EL, Broverman DM. Dynamics of estradiol and testosterone and seminal fluid indexes in smokers and nonsmokers. Fertil Steril. 1988;50(4):630–4. Epub 1988/10/01.

136. Vine MF. Biologic markers of exposure: current status and future research needs. Toxicol Ind Health. 1996;12(2):189–200. Epub 1996/03/01.

137. Mortimer D, Barratt CL, Bjorndahl L, de Jager C, Jequier AM, Muller CH. What should it take to describe a substance or product as 'sperm-safe'. Hum Reprod Update. 2013;19 Suppl 1:i1–45. Epub 2013/04/12.

138. Aneck-Hahn NH, Schulenberg GW, Bornman MS, Farias P, Reif S, De Jager C. Impaired semen quality associated with environmental DDT exposure in young men living in a malaria area in the Limpopo Province, South Africa. J Androl. 2007;28:423–34.

139. Eimers JM, te Velde ER, Gerritse R, Vogelzang ET, Looman CW, Habbema JD. The prediction of the chance to conceive in subfertile couples. Fertil Steril. 1994;61(1):44–52. Epub 1994/01/01.

140. Hirano Y, Shibahara H, Obara H, Suzuki T, Takamizawa S, Yamaguchi C, et al. Relationships between sperm motility characteristics assessed by the computer-aided sperm analysis (CASA) and fertilization rates in vitro. J Assist Reprod Genet. 2001;18(4):213–8. Epub 2001/07/04.

141. Rignell-Hydbom A, Rylander L, Giwercman A, Jonsson BA, Nilsson-Ehle P, Hagmar L. Exposure to CB-153 and p, p′-DDE and male reproductive function. Hum Reprod. 2004;19(9):2066–75. Epub 2004/07/31.

142. De Jager C, Farias P, Barraza-Villarreal A, Avila MH, Ayotte P, Dewailly E, et al. Reduced seminal parameters associated with environmental DDT exposure and p, p′-DDE concentrations in men in Chiapas, Mexico: a cross-sectional study. J Androl. 2006;27(1):16–27. Epub 2006/01/10.

143. Dalvie MA, Myers JE, Thompson ML, Robins TG, Dyer S, Riebow J, et al. The long-term effects of DDT exposure on semen, fertility, and sexual function of malaria vector-control workers in Limpopo Province, South Africa. Environ Res. 2004;96(1):1–8. Epub 2004/07/21.

144. World Health Organization. World Health Organization laboratory manual for the examination of human semen and sperm-cervical mucus interaction. 4th ed. Cambridge: Cambridge University Press; 1999.

145. Parvinen M. Cyclic function of Sertoli cells. In: Russell LD, Griswold MD, editors. The Sertoli cell. Clearwater: Cache River Press; 1998. p. 331–47.

146. Duty SM, Silva MJ, Barr DB, Brock JW, Ryan L, Chen Z, et al. Phthalate exposure and human semen parameters. Epidemiology. 2003;14(3):269–77. Epub 2003/07/16.

147. Aitken RJ, Koopman P, Lewis SE. Seeds of concern. Nature. 2004;432(7013):48–52. Epub 2004/11/05.

148. Aitken RJ, Baker MA. Oxidative stress and male reproductive biology. Reprod Fertil Dev. 2004;16(5):581–8. Epub 2004/09/16.

149. Agarwal A, Sekhon LH. The role of antioxidant therapy in the treatment of male infertility. Hum Fertil (Camb). 2010;13(4):217–25. Epub 2010/12/02.

150. Jacobsen R, Moller H, Thoresen SO, Pukkala E, Kjaer SK, Johansen C. Trends in testicular cancer incidence in the Nordic countries, focusing on the recent decrease in Denmark. Int J Androl. 2006;29(1):199–204. Epub 2005/12/24.

151. Moller H, Skakkebaek NE. Risk of testicular cancer in subfertile men: case-control study. BMJ. 1999;318(7183):559–62. Epub 1999/02/26.

152. Joensen UN, Jorgensen N, Skakkebaek NE. Testicular dysgenesis syndrome and carcinoma in situ of the testes. Nat Clin Pract Urol. 2007;4(8):402–3. Epub 2007/07/12.
153. Gerber GS, Brendler CB. Evaluation of the urologic patient: history, physical examination, and urinalysis. In: Wein AJ, Kavoussi LR, Novick AC, Partin AW, Peters CA, editors. Campbell-Walsh urology. 10th ed. Philadelphia: Elsevier-Saunders; 2012. p. 84.
154. American Cancer Society. Cancer facts and figures 2008. 2008. http://www.cancer.org/acs/groups/content/@nho/documents/document/2008cafffinalsecuredpdf.pdf. Accessed 6 Apr 2011.
155. Karim-Kos HE, de Vries E, Soerjomataram I, Lemmens V, Siesling S, Coebergh JW. Recent trends of cancer in Europe: a combined approach of incidence, survival and mortality for 17 cancer sites since the 1990s. Eur J Cancer. 2008;44(10):1345–89. Epub 2008/02/19.
156. Lichtenstein P, Holm NV, Verkasalo PK, Iliadou A, Kaprio J, Koskenvuo M, et al. Environmental and heritable factors in the causation of cancer–analyses of cohorts of twins from Sweden, Denmark, and Finland. N Engl J Med. 2000;343(2):78–85. Epub 2000/07/13.
157. Bostwick DG, Burke HB, Djakiew D, Euling S, Ho SM, Landolph J, et al. Human prostate cancer risk factors. Cancer. 2004;101(10 Suppl):2371–490. Epub 2004/10/21.
158. Jemal A, Center MM, DeSantis C, Ward EM. Global patterns of cancer incidence and mortality rates and trends. Cancer Epidemiol Biomarkers Prev. 2010;19(8):1893–907. Epub 2010/07/22.
159. Harkonen PL, Makela SI. Role of estrogens in development of prostate cancer. J Steroid Biochem Mol Biol. 2004;92(4):297–305. Epub 2005/01/25.
160. Prins GS, Korach KS. The role of estrogens and estrogen receptors in normal prostate growth and disease. Steroids. 2008;73(3):233–44. Epub 2007/12/21.
161. Ellem SJ, Risbridger GP. The dual, opposing roles of estrogen in the prostate. Ann N Y Acad Sci. 2009;1155:174–86. Epub 2009/03/03.

162. Alavanja MC, Samanic C, Dosemeci M, Lubin J, Tarone R, Lynch CF, et al. Use of agricultural pesticides and prostate cancer risk in the Agricultural Health Study cohort. Am J Epidemiol. 2003;157(9):800–14. Epub 2003/05/03.
163. Koutros S, Alavanja MC, Lubin JH, Sandler DP, Hoppin JA, Lynch CF, et al. An update of cancer incidence in the Agricultural Health Study. J Occup Environ Med. 2010;52(11):1098–105. Epub 2010/11/11.
164. Van Maele-Fabry G, Libotte V, Willems J, Lison D. Review and meta-analysis of risk estimates for prostate cancer in pesticide manufacturing workers. Cancer Causes Control. 2006;17(4):353–73. Epub 2006/04/06.
165. Ritchie JM, Vial SL, Fuortes LJ, Guo H, Reedy VE, Smith EM. Organochlorines and risk of prostate cancer. J Occup Environ Med. 2003;45(7):692–702. Epub 2003/07/12.
166. Ritchie JM, Vial SL, Fuortes LJ, Robertson LW, Guo H, Reedy VE, et al. Comparison of proposed frameworks for grouping polychlorinated biphenyl congener data applied to a case-control pilot study of prostate cancer. Environ Res. 2005;98(1):104–13. Epub 2005/02/22.
167. Parent ME, Siemiatycki J. Occupation and prostate cancer. Epidemiol Rev. 2001;23(1):138–43. Epub 2001/10/09.
168. Verougstraete V, Lison D, Hotz P. Cadmium, lung and prostate cancer: a systematic review of recent epidemiological data. J Toxicol Environ Health B Crit Rev. 2003;6(3):227–55. Epub 2003/05/15.
169. Sahmoun AE, Case LD, Jackson SA, Schwartz GG. Cadmium and prostate cancer: a critical epidemiologic analysis. Cancer Invest. 2005;23(3):256–63. Epub 2005/06/11.
170. Benbrahim-Tallaa L, Waalkes MP. Inorganic arsenic and human prostate cancer. Environ Health Perspect. 2008;116(2):158–64. Epub 2008/02/22.
171. Schuhmacher-Wolz U, Dieter HH, Klein D, Schneider K. Oral exposure to inorganic arsenic: evaluation of its carcinogenic and non-carcinogenic effects. Crit Rev Toxicol. 2009;39(4):271–98. Epub 2009/02/25.

Ionizing Radiation

14

Pieter Johann Maartens, Margot Flint,
and Stefan S. du Plessis

Introduction

Infertility is a term used to describe a couple who cannot achieve pregnancy after attempting to do so for a year without the use of contraceptives. Though technology has progressed at a frightening pace, it is estimated that nearly half of couples seeking infertility treatment unwillingly remain infertile. Unexplained male infertility (UMI) is defined as the reproductive state of a couple who is infertile despite displaying both male and female fertility parameters within the ranges regarded to as normal and able to successfully reproduce [1]. UMI prevalence is estimated between 6 and 27 %. Intensive research has been initiated, by several different sources, attempting to identify the possible causes of UMI. Possible causes such as genetic, molecular and morphologic deficiencies have been identi-

fied and researched. Few theories have, however, successfully provided significant results in proving an identifiable cause or viable treatment strategy. Thus, future hopes of naturally conceiving could remain an elusive ideal for many couples suffering from UMI.

Over the last 50 years, seminal quality has gradually deteriorated, raising concern amongst researchers over the possible connexion between this occurrence and UMI. Intensive research has been launched into the changing environmental and lifestyle conditions to which the human body is exposed over a lifetime. Industrial development and evolving lifestyles cause the reproductive system to be bombarded with toxins, environmental exposures and unhealthy lifestyle choices from initial development (gestational and pre-pubertal) right through to maturity (adulthood). Such external factors can induce morphologic-, genetic- and/ or oxidative impairment of reproductive tissues and functions. A process known as spermatogenesis is very sensitive to external influences and is easily affected, leading to adversely affected semen parameters [2]. One such external factor is ionizing radiation (IR). The effects of IR on reproduction are of growing concern as the number of people exposed to radiation via medical procedures, environmental exposures, air travel and industrial occupations increases.

This chapter aims to address the issue of IR and its effect on male reproduction, briefly discussing some possible sources of IR as well as some biological effects succeeding IR exposure [3, 4].

P.J. Maartens, BSc, BSc (Hons), MSc
S.S. du Plessis, BSc (Hons),
MSc, MBA, PhD (Stell) (✉)
Division of Medical Physiology, Department of Biomedical Sciences, Faculty of Medicine and Health Sciences, Stellenbosch University, PO Box 19063, Tygerberg, Western Cape 7505, South Africa
e-mail: 15076202@sun.ac.za; ssdp@sun.ac.za

M. Flint, BSc, BSc (Hons), MSc
Division of Medical Physiology, Faculty of Medicine and Health Sciences, Stellenbosch University, Tygerberg, Western Cape, South Africa
e-mail: mf@sun.ac.za

S.S. du Plessis et al. (eds.), *Male Infertility: A Complete Guide to Lifestyle and Environmental Factors*,
DOI 10.1007/978-1-4939-1040-3_14, © Springer Science+Business Media New York 2014

Ionizing Radiation

IR is defined as an amount of adequate energy to ionize the medium through which it passes. It comprises either a string of short-wavelength electromagnetic radiation (X-rays, gamma rays, cosmic rays) or a sequence of high energy particles (alpha-particles, electrons, neutrons) [5]. Microwaves, radio waves, ultraviolet rays, infrared rays and radiant heat waves are generally not regarded as IR. Chronic exposures to any of the above can, however, produce enough energy in the form of heat to cause similar effects as caused by IR [6]. IR is produced by any nuclear source (artificial or natural) that can cause the acceleration of particles at high states of energy such as lightning or the supernova reactions of the sun. Typical sources of radiation that are of concern to humans are classified as natural and artificial sources. Natural sources include naturally occurring radionuclides, gamma rays from the decay of uranium in earth, Radon gas decay products in the atmosphere and cosmic rays from outer space. Artificial sources include X-rays from medical procedures, radionuclides found in food and drink, radioactive waste and gamma rays produced as by-products in the nuclear industry and fallout products from atmospheric nuclear testing. IR can be extremely harmful on a molecular level by either transferring energy to the particles of the substance or by causing the release of secondary electrons as a result of the ionizing process. In a biological setting IR can be detrimental to cellular function as it can lead to the secondary emission of an electron from the water (H_2O) molecule leading to the formation of a highly reactive oxygen species, better known as a free radical. Free radicals can have severe effects on biological tissue due to their oxidizing/reducing capabilities [7]. The average radiation which a person is exposed to anywhere on the globe is 2.8 mSv (milliSievert). The maximum amount of IR to which the body can be exposed is dependent on the type of radiation received, the pattern of radiation received and the target tissue in the body. The maximum total uniform radiation which the body can be exposed to, when all the organs receive maximal tissue-specific radiation, with minimal risk of harmful effects is 18.5 mSv. Most Westernized societies have adopted an occupational maximum of 15 mSv [8–10].

Sources of Ionizing Radiation

Natural Sources

IR is present throughout the natural world (see Fig. 14.1). Radioactive cosmic rays constantly reach the earth; radioactive Radon gas is present in the atmosphere; and the earth itself is radioactive. While these sources are the main source of radiation exposure to most people, researchers believe this radiation has been present since the early ages and it would seem that since man and animals have evolved in its presence, it does not present a risk to global health. These exposures are, however, geographically specific and can vary to such an extent as to be of consequence to the health of certain regional inhabitants. Such high exposures should be noted by physicians and inhabitants alike when assessing health of the general population. Natural radiation is responsible for roughly 2.1 mSv of the 2.8 mSv of radiation to which the average person is exposed.

Cosmological

Cosmic rays are radioactive protons and particles from outer space, which come in contact with the earth at a constant rate. Such particles are commonly created by the sun during processes such as solar flares. These protons and other charged particles are affected by the earth's magnetic field and thus occur in higher frequency at higher latitudes. As they enter the atmosphere, they also enter complex reactions and are absorbed by atmospheric particles. Thus, prevalence of these particles also decreases with decreasing altitude. The bulk of the earth's populations live at lower altitudes and experience relatively low doses of radiation. Exceptions are communities living at high altitudes, such as those living in the Andes, Rocky Mountains or the

14 Ionizing Radiation

Fig. 14.1 Sources of ionizing radiation

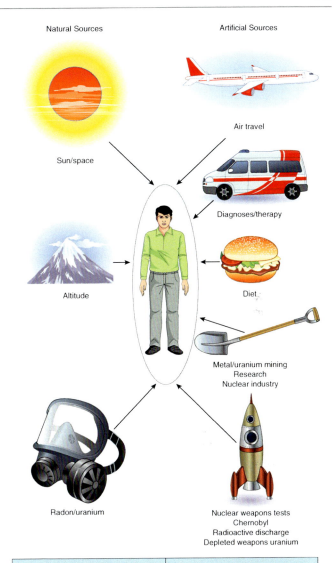

Sources of Ionizing Radiation	Average Global Annual Dose (mSv)
Natural	
Cosmological Exposure	0.4mSv
Environmental Exposure	1.7mSv
Artificial	
Medical Imaging and Therapy	0.4mSv
Occupational Exposure	1.3mSv
Diet	0.3mSv
Environmental Exposure	0.007mSv

Himalayas. These communities may be exposed to radiation levels at several times higher annual doses than those living at lower altitudes. Cosmologic radiation exposure amounts to about 0.4 mSv per person globally [9, 10].

Environmental

All materials from which the earth's crust is constructed contain radionuclides necessary for maintenance of internal temperatures. This energy is harvested mainly from the decay of Uranium and its radio isotopes, which are found in all rocks and soils, to a lesser radioactive form of the element lead. These nuclides radiate people with gamma rays more or less at a constant rate, contributing the greatest fraction of the 2.4 mSv of natural radiation to which the average person is exposed. Building materials, also of course consisting of substances extracted from the earth, are radioactive and expose people to radiation. The dose of such radiation varies remarkably and is influenced by both the style of building and natural geology unique to that region. In places where the earth is naturally abundant in radionuclides, such as India, France and Brazil, people may experience up to 20 times the average global earth-related radiation. Building in such areas would of course be unadvisable but ultimately impossible to prohibit.

One such product of the decay of Uranium is the radioactive gas Radon. Radon is exposed to the atmosphere where it then further decays into more reactive isotopes. The immediate products of the decay of Radon have relatively short half-lives but combine with particles in the air. Radon concentration outdoors are negligibly low due to the dispersion of the particles in the air. However, indoors, the gas enters a building through the floors and concentrates in the building especially if the building is not well ventilated. This problem is an especially notable issue in areas of cold weather, such as Finland, where houses are built to retain heat. When such nuclides are inhaled they expose the lungs to alpha-radiation and increase lung cancer prevalence. Natural environmental radiation exposure amounts to about 1.7 mSv per person globally [9, 10].

Artificial Sources

The Westernized world has expanded at a rapid pace over the last 100 years developing industry and technology and changing lifestyles in terms of diet, medical procedures, waste disposal and occupations. First and third-world country developments have all inevitably led to increased radiation exposure. Artificial radiation is responsible for roughly 0.7 mSv of the 2.8 mSv of radiation to which the average person is exposed.

Medical Imaging and Therapy

IR has two uses in the medical field: diagnosis and therapy. In the field of medical diagnostics, the most common of radiation procedures, X-ray, is used by an expert to diagnose a condition or pathology. X-rays entail radiation from a machine passing through different tissues in the body and being visualized electronically due to the difference in radiation absorption of different tissues. This type of procedure is termed diagnostic radiology and is commonly used to visualize the chest, teeth and limbs. Another less common form of diagnostics entails the administration of radionuclides to a patient and the external imaging of internal bodily processes. Administration takes place in the form of ingestion, injection or inhalation of a pharmaceutical carrying a radionuclide which is then tissue or organ specific for visualization. The radionuclides emit gamma rays which are then observed by a gamma ray detector. This type of procedure is termed nuclear medicine and can also be used as a form of treatment. Nuclear medicine is usually used to visualize the function of a specific tissue or organ or used to treat conditions such as hyperthyroidism. Radiation levels in such diagnostic procedures are relatively low, but can be increased substantially to treat malignant cells.

In cases where radiation beams are used to treat a medical condition or pathology, by irradiating the affected tissue, the procedure is termed radiotherapy. Radiotherapy is of cardinal importance to modern day medical practitioners, as it is used to treat certain forms of cancer and alleviate associated stress. Radiation beams consisting of

X-rays, electrons or gamma rays are directed at a malignant tissue, from several directions to minimize peripheral tissue damage, in an attempt to kill the compromised cells. Radiotherapy is however a slightly ambiguous treatment as it can often cause tissue malignancy in other tissues after treating a specific tissue. Radiotherapy also utilizes high levels of radiation and can affect the hereditary status of an individual resulting in adverse effects for subsequent generations. Most people that undergo radiotherapy, therefore, are usually past reproductive age and past the age where secondary delayed cancers are a viable risk. Radiotherapy is also only used when the chances of a cure or symptom relief are good, the side effects are minimal and other treatments would not be as effective. Medical radiation exposure amounts to approximately 0.4 mSv per person globally, but will of course increase exponentially for a person undergoing a radiation procedure [9–14].

Occupational Exposure

Occupational exposure to IR occurs in two settings: occupational exposure to naturally occurring IR and occupational exposure to artificially induced IR. Artificial sources of occupational IR are commonly found in industry, research, power-generating plants and medical care [15]. Natural sources of occupational IR are commonly found in the mining industry and air travel. In the artificially induced IR industries, there are about 800,000 workers in the nuclear industry and over 2,000,000 workers in the medical radiology industry globally. These workers are at highest risk of IR exposure. As mentioned earlier in the chapter, the earth contains significant amounts of decomposing Uranium. Geological sites that contain more than 1,000 parts per million of Uranium are regarded to be economic mining prospects for nuclear uses, thus exposing the workers to significant amounts of IR. The average annual dose of IR exposure to people in the uranium mining industry is 4.5 mSv. Other occupations also exposing workers to high annual levels of IR are medical isotope production, 1.9 mSv, radiography, 1.6 mSv and nuclear reactor occupations

with 1.4 mSv average annual exposure. Most occupations involving such an active IR risk require personnel to monitor their particular IR exposure by way of some form of electronic- or thermoluminescent device. This helps industry and government officials manage the overall annual average of personnel that are occupationally exposed to IR so they may attempt to restrict it to less than 2 mSv per worker globally. The average in the nuclear industry is still slightly higher than this average, but global doses have declined remarkably in the last decade due to these precautions [8–10, 16, 17].

In the naturally induced IR industries, some of the workers at highest risk are metal mining personnel. This occurrence is caused by insufficient ventilation and Radon gas build-up in the metal mines rather than exposure to metals. As mentioned earlier in the chapter, IR exposure is affected by altitude. Thus aircraft travel increases exposure to cosmic rays and subsequent IR at a dramatic rate. A passenger on an intercontinental flight may experience up to 100 times the dose of radiation than a person on the ground, posing a significant risk for frequent flying business individuals and regular flight crew. The annual average exposure for flight personnel is around 3 mSv but it could increase to twice that amount if regularly involved with long flights at high altitude [18, 19]. Occupational radiation exposure is negligible to the average person not working with radiation on a day-to-day basis but is of concern to workers in the nuclear industry and flight industry and amounts to an annual average of about 1.3 mSv per worker globally.

Diet

Radionuclides are also present in food and drink. Lead, polonium and potassium are all present in the environment and the natural diet and are thus a source of radiation. On average, the human body is exposed to 0.3 mSv annually from dietary sources. This figure varies immensely, however, between individuals. A young man, for example, is exposed to twice as much radiation than an elderly lady due to dietary absorption. This is due to the fact that more than half of the dietary radiation source is made up of potassium and thus is biologically controlled and dependent on amount of muscle mass. Diet-associated radiation exposure amounts to about 0.3 mSv per person globally [9, 10].

Environmental

There are also sources of radiation present in the earth's atmosphere which are artificially created. Nuclides originating from nuclear tests, the Chernobyl accident and discharge of nuclear waste into the atmosphere by nuclear plants and military installations disperse into the atmosphere, the water, the ground and food and drink and thus are a source of radiation. The testing of nuclear weapons causes several nuclides to be exposed to the atmosphere. There were about 500 tests conducted before the limited test treaty was signed in 1963. Since then environmental concentrations of nuclides have decreased substantially. The average annual dose has decreased from 0.1 to 0.005 mSv.

The Chernobyl nuclear accident on 26 April 1986 at the Chernobyl nuclear plant in Ukraine caused the exposure of an enormous amount of radiation to the atmosphere over a period of 10 days. This radioactive material dispersed throughout Europe and exposure was exacerbated in certain areas by heavy rainfall. Radiation exposure led to the deaths of 31 people, primarily emergency workers, who were exposed to external doses of between 3 and 16 Sv. Over 200 people were hospitalized, of which 109 were diagnosed with acute radiation sickness. Over 100,000 people were relocated from communities in Ukraine, Belarus and Russia and serious restrictions were implemented to prohibit people from living in areas where fallout exposure was highest [20–25].

Radionuclides discharged by nuclear power plants and military installations are exposed to the atmosphere in significant quantities to be regarded a source of radioactive materials to the general public. Nuclear power plants contribute about 20 % of the world's electricity. During each stage of the nuclear fuel cycle, several nuclides in the form of matter are released to the environment. These doses are normally low, about 1 μSv,

but have to be constantly measured and regulated. Many military installations in the past and present have worked with ammunition utilizing depleted uranium. Depleted uranium occurs in a concentrated metallic form when found in munitions. Radiation exposure could take place when handling such spent munitions or inhaling such vapours and dust after the detonation of such munitions. Exposure doses can be as high as 2.5 mSv/h. There is active concern amongst researchers and the public over the possible adverse health effects both to military personnel and people living in recent war zones [26–30]. Artificial environmental annual radiation amounts to about 0.007 mSv per person globally.

Effects of Ionizing Radiation on the Male Reproductive System

Ionizing Radiation-Induced Oxidative Stress

The human body consists of a finely balanced interaction between pro- and antioxidants. Intracellular homeostasis is achieved when prooxidants, which consist of free radicals and antioxidants, the body's natural scavenging capability, are maintained in balance. Free radicals are short-lived atoms or molecules that contain one or more electrons with unpaired spin [31, 32]. Within the context of reproductive biology, the following chemical intermediates have been recognized as the predominant reactive oxidizing agents: peroxyl radical (ROO^-), hydrogen peroxide (H_2O_2), superoxide anion (O_2^-) and the hydroxyl radical (OH^-) [33], all of which are natural by-products of normal physiological processes [34–36]. ROS elicits a bio positive influence when maintained at low concentrations; however, excessive concentrations that overwhelm the natural defence mechanisms can result in damage to biomolecules and a state of oxidative stress (OS) [31, 34]. All cellular components, including nucleic acids, lipids and proteins are potentially OS targets as a result of supraphysiological concentrations of ROS [32]. Due to the fact that free radicals predominantly attack

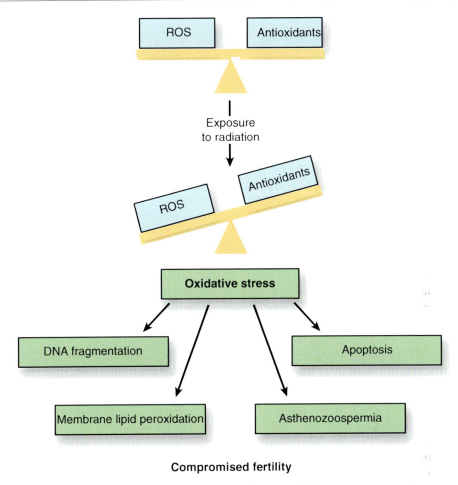

Fig. 14.2 Effects of radiation exposure on the male reproductive status. *ROS* reactive oxygen species

the closest stable molecule, which subsequently turns that specific particle into a free radical; ROS can be involved in a cascade of reactions which can damage a wide variety of biomolecules [35, 37].

Exposure of the body to external influences such as IR can cause the onset of a state of OS, which can result in a variety of damaging cellular effects (See Fig. 14.2). OS results from an excessive generation of reactive oxidizing species (ROS) accompanied by a lack of inactivation of these free radicals. IR causes results in the formation of HO and H atoms as a result of the decomposition of H_2O, which leads to an imbalance in the antioxidant capability of the cells [38]. Studies have also demonstrated that high concentrations of ROS can negatively impact crucial steps in the steroidogenic pathway [39]. Human spermatozoa are uniquely sensitive to OS, which targets these cells vulnerable to states such as IR. The natural defence system of scavenging antioxidants can be overwhelmed and basic semen parameters are negatively affected. A state of OS can induce nucleic acid damage, oxidation of proteins, lipid peroxidation and ultimately cell death [40].

Mechanism of Cell Injury Due to IR

Developmental Injury (Spermatogenesis)

The damaging effect of exposure to IR can be attributed to the high radio-sensitivity of the male reproductive tissue. Data collected from American research projects conducted in the 1970s, which included prisoners who volunteered to have exposure of their testicles to X-ray radiation, showed the damaging effect on male fertility [12]. In 1986, Martin et al., reported the first findings from a study to demonstrate that an increase in chromosomal abnormalities may be a result of exposure to radiation [41]. The male testes are identified as one of the most radiosensitive organs, and the germinal epithelium, as well as the spermatogonia known to be incredibly sensitive to radiation exposure [24, 42]. IR is responsible for the apoptotic and mitotic death of spermatocyte cells and spermatogonia [24]. Spermatogenesis can be described as "a well-organized and sequential developmental and differentiation process" [7]. This particular biological feature is the only process in mammals whereby meiosis happens in the adult state [43]. The pachytene stage of meiosis, whereby chromosomal cross over occurs, is recognized to be incredibly sensitive to xenobiotic influences which includes IR [41]. Low doses such as 0.15–0.5 Gy can cause suppression of the spermatogenesis process and a significant decrease in the sperm count, whereas long-lasting or permanent azoospermia can result from 2 Gy or more [42, 44].

Molecular Injury

DNA damage from IR can be a result of the following two mechanisms: firstly, the direct interaction of DNA with ionizing particles and secondly, through the indirect reaction which occurs in the area encircling the DNA whereby the particle generates an increase in free radicals [45]. The result can include an excessive occurrence of single- and double strand DNA breaks [46, 47], chromosomal rearrangements [48, 49], chromatin cross-linkage and DNA base oxidation [50]. DNA integrity can be termed as "the absence of both single strand and double strand and break absence of nucleotide modifications in the DNA" [51]. Despite spermatozoa DNA being remarkably resilient against denaturation from chemical or physical influences, strand breaks within the doughnut-shaped DNA is indicative of a decline in the functional capacity [52].

When assessing the reproductive potential of the male partner, the analysis of sperm DNA integrity offers a comprehensive insight beyond the parameters established by the WHO [51]. With the burden of infertility increasing, it has been estimated that amongst the couples experiencing idiopathic infertility, sperm DNA fragmentation was a causative factor behind 20 % of the cases [53]. The sperm plasma membrane, made up of redox-sensitive polyunsaturated fatty acids (PUFA), is particularity vulnerable to OS as it can cause peroxidation of the lipids [32, 54, 55]. The predominant PUFA is docosahexaenoic acid and peroxidation induced by IR-induced OS can result in permeability of the plasma membrane [31, 34, 56] which causes decreased fluidity [36]. This peroxidation process results in a loss of motility, which compromises successful oocyte fertilization.

Hypothalamic-Anterior Pituitary-Testicular Axis

In addition to the high sensitivity of the testes to irradiation and the subsequent damaging effects that exposure may cause on the male fertility status, the production of the sex steroids are also under influence. Exposure of the body to radiation may compromise the male's fertility status as a result cranial irradiation damaging the central nervous system, which includes the hypothalamic–pituitary–gonadal system [57]. Spermatogenesis is a system under endocrine feedback regulation by the hypothalamus (See Fig. 14.3). The hypothalamus is responsible for the increased neuron activity that causes the secretion of the gonadotropin releasing hormone (GnRH) [58]. The GnRH acts upon the anterior pituitary (also termed the adenohypophysis) which contains the cells that secrete the following two gonadotropins: the luteinizing hormone (LH), also known as the interstitial cell stimulating hormone, and the follicle stimulating hormone (FSH) [58]. The hormones are glycopeptides consisting of two peptide chains (alpha and beta) and are required for the completion of the process to yield motile spermatozoa capable of successful oocyte fertilization [57]. FSH is a pituitary hormone essential for the final

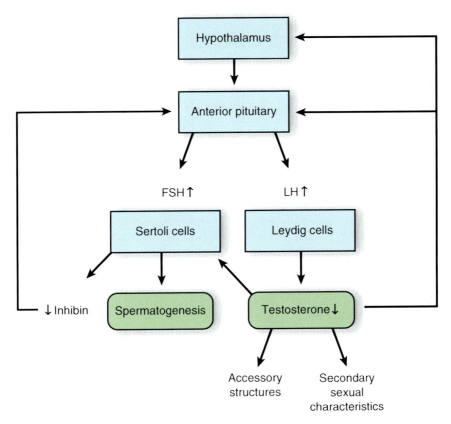

Fig. 14.3 Effect of ionizing radiation on the hypothalamus-anterior pituitary gonadal-axis. *FSH* follicle stimulating hormone, *LH* luteinizing hormone

phase of the transformation of the haploid spermatids to spermatozoa. The hormone acts on the Sertoli cells of the testis and the release of FSH is controlled through a negative feedback system. The system is controlled by the hormone inhibin, which is peptide growth factor that is secreted from the Sertoli cells and regulates the anterior pituitary's secretion of the gonadotropin [58]. Upon exposure of the Sertoli cells to radiation, spermatogenesis is impaired and the concentration of FSH released by the anterior pituitary increases [59].

The second hormone involved in the feedback regulation of spermatogenesis is the LH. This pituitary hormone promotes the secretion of testosterone by the Leydig cells, which are the interstitial cells situated between the seminiferous tubules [58]. The release of sex steroid testosterone acts on the Sertoli cells to stimulate spermatogenesis, as well as maintaining the hormone-dependent secondary sexual characteristics. Exposure to radiation at concentrations as low as 0.78 Gy may elicit temporary azoospermia, and doses exceeding 2 Gy can cause irreversible azoospermia [8]. Comparatively, the Leydig cells have been shown to have a higher resistance to radiation [60]. As testosterone is responsible for feedback control on the secretion of LH at both the hypothalamus and pituitary gland, IR-induced damage will result in compromised testosterone release as well as compensatory increase in the level of LH [59].

Future Research

Treatment for patients undergoing radiation or a combination of chemotherapy and radiation protocols have been identified as being vulnerable to conditions such as renal failure, cardiovascular disease, as well as infertility [60]. With the use of IR in medical scenarios, there has been a

Table 14.1 Recovery period of spermatogenesis following exposure of the testes to ionizing radiation

Radiation dose	Time to recovery (return of the patient's sperm concentration prior to radiation)
<1 Gy	9–18 months
2–3 Gy	30 months
≥4 Gy	>5 years

heightened concern of azoospermia and temporary or permanent infertility [44]. Despite advancements in cancer treatments that offer increased survival rates for individuals diagnosed with the condition of malignancy, it has been approximated that up to two-thirds will experience long-term adverse health consequences [56, 60, 61]. The testes are protected during the time that the male patient is exposed to radiation for medical treatment. However, certain cases of IR therapy can result in substantial damage to the reproductive system such as whole body irradiation prior to bone marrow transplantation and IR of malignant cells in the testes [60]. Men undergoing radiation therapy for rectal, prostate and testicular cancer are treated with high-dose pelvic irradiation. This form of site-specific treatment can cause permanent damage to the function of the testes as well as erectile dysfunction [52]. Patients with testicular cancer and Hodgkin's lymphoma were shown to have sperm DNA damage for up to a period of 2 years following IR therapy [44, 62].

The dose and duration of radiation therapy predict the cytotoxic effects that may be elicited. With studies focusing on the effects of cancer treatment on the fertility status of male patients, it was shown that the dosage and sperm production were directly proportional with decreased sperm production starting approximately 60–80 days following IR exposure [63]. A study which examined the effects of graded doses of IR on the recovery of spermatogenesis, which was considered as the period taken for the individuals sperm to return to the concentration it was before IR exposure, is represented in Table 14.1. From the collection of data focusing on infertility as a result of IR exposure, the risk for sterility was localized to doses in excess of 40 Gy [63]. Men undergoing radiation therapy

are advised to abstain from impregnating their partner for 12–18 months following the exposure to IR as the effects that gonadotoxic agents may have on spermatozoa are not fully understood [64]. Advances in assisted reproductive technology (ART) have offered the hope of preserving the fertility status of male patients undergoing radiation treatment through the cryopreservation of semen samples [64]. ART has progressed significantly over the years and advancements such as in vitro fertilization (IVF) and intracytoplasmic sperm injection (ICSI) allow for a degree of assurance to male partners. This is due to the fact that even if the sperm removed from a semen sample and prepared for ICSI have parameters such as poor motility can be implanted into the ovum to fertilize the oocyte upon reaching the cytoplasm [64]. With the introduction of cryopreservation, it has been shown that sperm can maintain functional capacity for successful oocyte fertilization for up to a period of 28 years [65].

With the threat of compromised spermatogenesis as a result of cytotoxic therapy, research has been initiated to protect and preserve germ cells in the testes exposed to IR. One such approach has been the retrieval and harvesting of spermatogonial stem cells from testicular tissue prior to treatment. This stem cell transplantation method has been shown to be effective in restoring spermatogenesis in studies utilizing rodent models [60]. The second example of preserving fertility has been the approach of testicular allografting whereby cloned donor mice testicular tissue was extracted and transplanted into recipient mice's testes. After a period, the donor germ cells were shown to have colonized the donor mouse's seminiferous tubules and in some rodents, spermatogenesis had been induced [66]. At present, cryopreservation is the only viable option available to men undergoing radiation therapy [60]. The challenging aspect of studying the effects of IR exposure on the male reproductive profile is the obvious ethical considerations. There remains a limited amount of experimental data that has investigated the potential toxic effects of IR on the male fertility status [12] and the vast majority of the studies have been conducted on experimental animal models. The monkey and rodent spermatogenesis process and molecular response of testicular tissue to IR has been found to be significantly similar to humans; therefore, the investigation into long-term exposure to IR on the fertility status has been conducted in primates and rodents [64].

Conclusion

Compromised fertility can be attributed to a range of causative factors contributed by both partners. The male's fertility status has been estimated to play a crucial role in the observed failed fertilization rates, with up to a third of the cases of reported sub-fertility being solely contributed by the male partner [2]. With the past 50 years having displayed the deterioration of seminal quality, it is crucial to isolate the impacting factors responsible for this phenomenon. With the twenty-first lifestyle, humans are exposed to a range of lifestyle, environmental and industrial factors that can insult the reproductive profile, for example obesity, smoking, and exposure to IR. The effects that exposure to radiation can elicit on spermatogenesis through the generation of OS and hormonal impacts, the risk for transient or permanent infertility is possible.

References

1. Hamada A, Esteves S, Agarwal A. Unexplained male infertility—looking beyond routine semen analysis. Euro Urol Rev. 2012;7(1):90–6.
2. World Health Organization. WHO manual for the standardized investigation and diagnosis of the infertile couple. Cambridge: Cambridge University Press; 2000.
3. Wilson JW, Goldhagen P, Rafnsson V, Clem JM, De Angelis G, Friedberg W. Overview of atmospheric ionizing radiation (AIR) research: SST-present. Adv Space Res. 2003;32(1):3–16.
4. Lipshultz L, Sigman M. Office evaluation of the subfertile male. In: Howards S, Lipshultz L, Niederberger C, editors. Infertility in the male. Cambridge: Cambridge University Press; 2009. p. 153–76.
5. Bullock J, Boyle J, Wang MB, Ajello RR. Physiology. Pennsylvania: Harwal Publishing Company; 1984.
6. Lancranjan I, Maicanescu M, Rafaila E, Klepsch I, Popescu HI. Gonadic function in workmen with long-term exposure to microwaves. Health Phys. 1975; 29(3):381–3.

7. Rowley MJ, Leach DR, Warner GA, Heller CG. Effect of graded doses of ionizing radiation on the human testis. Radiat Res. 1974;59(3):665–78.
8. Doyle P, Roman E, Maconochie N, Davies G, Smith PG, Beral V. Primary infertility in nuclear industry employees: report from the nuclear industry family study. Occup Environ Med. 2001;58(8):4.
9. International Atomic Energy Agency (IAEA). Radiation, people and the environment. Vienna: IAEA; 2004.
10. United Nations Scientific Committee on the Effects of Atomic Radiation. Sources and effects of ionizing radiation: sources (Vol 1). Vienna: United Nations Publications; 2000.
11. Clifton DK, Bremner WJ. The effect of testicular x-irradiation on spermatogenesis in man. A comparison with the mouse. J Androl. 1983;4(6):387–92.
12. Sharma OP, Oswanski MF, Sidhu R, Krugh K, Culler AS, Spangler M, et al. Analysis of radiation exposure in trauma patients at a level I trauma center. J Emerg Med. 2011;41(6):640–8.
13. Fleurian G, Perrin J, Ecochard R, Dantony E, Lanteaume A, Achard V, Sari-Minodier I. Occupational exposures obtained by questionnaire in clinical practice and their association with semen quality. J Androl. 2009;30(5):566–79.
14. Naysmith TE, Blake DA, Harvey VJ, Johnson NP. Do men undergoing sterilizing cancer treatments have a fertile future? Hum Reprod. 1998;13(11):3250–5.
15. Dias FL, Antunes LM, Rezende PA, Carvalho FE, Silva C, Matheus JM, Balarin MA. Cytogenetic analysis in lymphocytes from workers occupationally exposed to low levels of ionizing radiation. Environ Toxicol Pharmacol. 2007;23(2):228–33.
16. Sahin A, Tatar A, Oztas S, Seven B, Varoglu E, Yesilyurt A, et al. Evaluation of the genotoxic effects of chronic low-dose ionizing radiation exposure on nuclear medicine workers. Nucl Med Biol. 2009; 36(5):575–8.
17. Cardis E, Gilbert ES, Carpenter L, Howe G, Kato I, Armstrong BK, et al. Effects of low doses and low dose rates of external ionizing radiation: cancer mortality among nuclear industry workers in three countries. Radiat Res. 1995;142(2):117–32.
18. De Angelis G, Caldora M, Santaquilani M, Scipione R, Verdecchia A. Radiation exposure of civilian airline crew members and associated biological effects due to the atmospheric ionizing radiation environment. Phys Med. 2001;17:258–60.
19. Iulu C, Cheburakova OP. Disorders of spermatogenesis in people working at the clean-up of the Chernobyl nuclear power plant accident. Radiats Biol Radioecol. 1993;33(6):1.
20. Moller AP, Mousseau TA. Biological consequences of Chernobyl: 20 years on. Trends Ecol Evol. 2006; 21(4):200–7.
21. Belyakov OV, Steinhäusler F, Trott KR. Chernobyl liquidators. The people and the doses. Tenth International Congress of the International Radiation Protection Association: Hiroshima; 2000.

22. Fairlie I. Chernobyl: consequences of the catastrophe for people and the environment. Radiat Protect Dosim. 2010;141(1):97–101.
23. Moller AP, Mousseau TA, Lynn C, Ostermiller S, Rudolfsen G. Impaired swimming behaviour and morphology of sperm from barn swallows Hirundo rustica in Chernobyl. Mutat Res. 2008;650(2):210–6.
24. Fischbein A, Zabludovsky N, Eltes F, Grischenko V, Bartoov B. Ultramorphological sperm characteristics in the risk assessment of health effects after radiation exposure among salvage workers in Chernobyl. Environ Health Perspect. 1997;105(6):1445–9.
25. Ferguson CD, Kazi T, Perera J. Commercial radioactive sources: surveying the security risks. Monterey: Monterey Institute of International Studies, Center for Nonproliferation Studies; 2003.
26. De la Calle JFV, Rachou E, le Martelot MT, Ducot B, Multigner L, Thonneau PF. Male infertility risk factors in a French military population. Hum Reprod. 2001;16(3):481–6.
27. Schrader SM, Langford RE, Turner TW, Breitenstein MJ, Clark JC, Jenkins BL, et al. Reproductive function in relation to duty assignments among military personnel. Reprod Toxicol. 1998;12(4):3.
28. Weyandt TB, Schrader SM, Turner TW, Simon SD. Semen analysis of military personnel associated with military duty assignments. Reprod Toxicol. 1996;10(6):521–8.
29. Saleh RA, Agarwal A, Kandirali E, Sharma RK, Thomas AJ, Nada EA, et al. Leukocytospermia is associated with increased reactive oxygen species production by human spermatozoa. Fertil Steril. 2002;78(6):1215–24.
30. Ochsendorf FR. Infections in the male genital tract and reactive oxygen species. Hum Reprod Update. 1999;5(5):399–420.
31. Maneesh M, Jayalekshmi H. Role of reactive oxygen species and antioxidants on pathophysiology of male reproduction. Indian J Clin Biochem. 2006; 21(2):80–9.
32. Aitken RJ, Buckingham D, Harkiss D. Use of a xanthine oxidase free radical generating system to investigate the cytotoxic effects of reactive oxygen species on human spermatozoa. J Reprod Fertil. 1993;97(2): 441–50.
33. Cocuzza M, Sikka SC, Athayde KS, Agarwal A. Clinical relevance of oxidative stress and sperm chromatin damage in male infertility: an evidence based analysis. Int Braz J Urol. 2007;33(5):603–21.
34. Makker K, Agarwal A, Sharma R. Oxidative stress & male infertility. Indian J Med Res. 2009;129(4): 357–67.
35. Sanocka D, Kurpisz M. Reactive oxygen species and sperm cells. Reprod Biol Endocrinol. 2004;2:12.
36. Gorczyca W, Gong J, Darzynkiewicz Z. Detection of DNA strand breaks in individual apoptotic cells by the in situ terminal deoxynucleotidyl transferase and nick translation assays. Cancer Res. 1993;53(8):1945–51.
37. Sharma RK, Agarwal A. Role of reactive oxygen species in male infertility. Urology. 1996;48(6):835–50.

38. Martin RH, Hildebrand K, Yamamoto J, Rademaker A. An increased frequency of human sperm chromosomal abnormalities after radiotherapy. Mutat Res. 1986;174(3):6.
39. Jennet S. Human physiology. 1st ed. London: Churchill Livingstone; 1989.
40. Hyer S, Vini L, O'Connell M, Pratt B, Harmer C. Testicular dose and fertility in men following I(131) therapy for thyroid cancer. Clin Endocrinol. 2002;56(6):755–8.
41. Moghbeli-Nejad S, Mozdarani H, Behmanesh M, Rezaiean Z, Fallahi P. Genome instability in AZFc region on Y chromosome in leukocytes of fertile and infertile individuals following exposure to gamma radiation. J Assist Reprod Genet. 2012;29(1):53–61.
42. Xu G, Intano GW, McCarrey JR, Walter RB, McMahan CA, Walter CA. Recovery of a low mutant frequency after ionizing radiation-induced mutagenesis during spermatogenesis. Mutat Res. 2008;654(2): 150–7.
43. Nikjoo H, O'Neill P, Wilson WE, Goodhead DT. Computational approach for determining the spectrum of DNA damage induced by ionizing radiation. Radiat Res. 2001;156:577–83.
44. Twigg J, Fulton N, Gomez E, Irvine DS, Aitken RJ. Analysis of the impact of intracellular reactive oxygen species generation on the structural and functional integrity of human spermatozoa: lipid peroxidation, DNA fragmentation and effectiveness of antioxidants. Hum Reprod. 1998;13(6):1429–36.
45. Aitken RJ, Krausz C. Oxidative stress, DNA damage and the Y chromosome. Reproduction. 2001;122(4): 497–506.
46. Duru NK, Morshedi M, Schuffner A, Oehninger S. Semen treatment with progesterone and/or acetyl-L-carnitine does not improve sperm motility or membrane damage after cryopreservation-thawing. Fertil Steril. 2000;74(4):715–20.
47. Ramos L, Wetzels AM. Low rates of DNA fragmentation in selected motile human spermatozoa assessed by the TUNEL assay. Hum Reprod. 2001;16(8): 1703–7.
48. Kullisaar T, Turk S, Punab M, Korrovits P, Kisand K, Rehema A, Zilmer M, Mandar R. Oxidative stress in leucocytospermic prostatitis patients: preliminary results. Andrologia. 2007;40:11.
49. Shamsi MB, Venkatesh S, Tanwar M, Talwar P, Sharma RK, Dhawan A, et al. DNA integrity and semen quality in men with low seminal antioxidant levels. Mutat Res. 2009;665(1–2):29–36.
50. Philpott A, Leno GH. Nucleoplasmin remodels sperm chromatin in Xenopus egg extracts. Cell. 1992; 69(5):759–67.
51. Nakayama K, Milbourne A, Schover LR, Champlin RE, Ueno NT. Gonadal failure after treatment of hematologic malignancies: from recognition to management for health-care providers. Nat Clin Pract Oncol. 2008;2:78–89.
52. Aydemir B, Onaran I, Kiziler AR, Alici B, Akyolcu MC. The influence of oxidative damage on viscosity

of seminal fluid in infertile men. J Androl. 2008; 29(1):41–6.

53. Agarwal A, Prabakaran SA. Mechanism, measurement, and prevention of oxidative stress in male reproductive physiology. Indian J Exp Biol. 2005;43(11):963–74.

54. de Lamirande E, Gagnon C. Human sperm hyperactivation in whole semen and its association with low superoxide scavenging capacity in seminal plasma. Fertil Steril. 1993;59(6):1291–5.

55. Agarwal A, Ranganathan P, Kattal N, Pasqualotto F, Hallak J, Khayal S, et al. Fertility after cancer: a prospective review of assisted reproductive outcome with banked semen specimens. Fertil Steril. 2004;81(2): 342–8.

56. Ogilvy-Stuart AL, Shalet SM. Effect of radiation on the human reproductive system. Environ Health Perspect. 1993;101 Suppl 2:109–16.

57. Yau I, Vuong T, Garant A, Ducruet T, Doran P, Faria S, et al. Risk of hypogonadism from scatter radiation during pelvic radiation in male patients with rectal cancer. Int J Radiat Oncol Biol Phys. 2009;74(5): 1481–6.

58. Dohle GR. Male infertility in cancer patients: review of the literature. Int J Urol. 2010;17(4):327–31.

59. Lass A, Akagbosu F, Brinsden P. Sperm banking and assisted reproduction treatment for couples following

cancer treatment of the male partner. Hum Reprod Update. 2001;7(4):370–7.

60. Tempest HG, Ko E, Chan P, Robaire B, Rademaker A, Martin RH. Sperm aneuploidy frequencies analysed before and after chemotherapy in testicular cancer and Hodgkin's lymphoma patients. Hum Reprod. 2008; 23(2):251–8.

61. Barber HR. The effect of cancer and its therapy upon fertility. Int J Fertil Steril. 1981;26(4):250–9.

62. Shin D, Lo KC, Lipshultz LI. Treatment options for the infertile male with cancer. J Natl Cancer Inst Monogr. 2005;34:48–50.

63. Feldschuh J, Brassel J, Durso N, Levine A. Successful sperm storage for 28 years. Fertil Steril. 2005; 84(4):1017.

64. Ohta H, Wakayama T. Generation of normal progeny by intracytoplasmic sperm injection following grafting of testicular tissue from cloned mice that died postnatally. Biol Reprod. 2005;73(3):390–5.

65. de Rooij DG, van de Kant HJ, Dol R, Wagemaker G, van Buul PP, van Duijn-Goedhart A, et al. Long-term effects of irradiation before adulthood on reproductive function in the male rhesus monkey. Biol Reprod. 2002;66(2):486–94.

66. Saalu LC. The incriminating role of reactive oxygen species in idiopathic male infertility: an evidence based evaluation. Pak J Biol Sci. 2010;13(9):413–22.

Part III

Other Factors Affecting Male Fertility

Risks from Medical and Therapeutic Treatments

15

Yagil Barazani and Edmund S. Sabanegh Jr.

Introduction

Despite modern advances in the understanding and treatment of male infertility, almost a quarter of men with infertility still have an idiopathic cause [1]. In part, the etiology of male factor infertility is so challenging to define because it is a polygenic multifactorial disease with a heterogeneous phenotype. Moreover, it is probable that many cases of gonadal dysfunction result from a combination of genetic susceptibility to subfertility and certain environmental factors [2].

While a number of epigenetic factors have been implicated as potential causes of male infertility such as environmental pollutants and social habits [3], infertility can also be an unintended consequence of medical treatment. This includes both pharmacologically mediated male infertility and spermatogenic impairment resulting from treatment with ionizing radiation. Knowledge of these reproductive effects is crucial in the management of male patients trying to conceive because it allows for identification of modifiable risk factors and selection of agents less likely to adversely affect male fertility.

This chapter is designed to highlight the iatrogenic causes of male infertility, including the untoward reproductive consequences of both medical and radiation therapies. In doing so, our goal is threefold: (1) to help prevent treatment-related infertility in patients with a desire to conceive, (2) to help diagnose iatrogenic causes as part of a comprehensive male infertility evaluation, and (3) to help clinicians identify patients at high risk for infertility due to essential treatments with whom options for fertility preservation such as cryopreservation should be discussed prior to initiating treatment.

Complications of Medical Therapy

Multiple drug classes adversely affect male fertility, their effects generally being dependent on the specific drug, dose, and length of exposure. Detailed information about the known human reproductive risks of various agents is available in the *Physicians' Desk Reference* and in a number of databases including the REPRORISK® System.

While a wide variety of medications are known to negatively impact male fertility, these agents all exert their effects through one of several basic mechanisms [4–6]. The first of these (pre-testicular) consists of alterations to the hypothalamic-pituitary-gonadal (HPG) axis. For example, HPG axis feedback mechanisms can be interrupted by

---

Y. Barazani, MD
Department of Urology, Cleveland Clinic,
Cleveland Clinic Main Campus, Mail Code Q10-1,
9500 Euclid Avenue, Cleveland, OH 44195, USA
e-mail: yagilb@gmail.com

E.S. Sabanegh Jr., MD (✉)
Glickman Urological and Kidney Institute,
Cleveland Clinic, Cleveland, OH, USA
e-mail: sabanee@ccf.org

S.S. du Plessis et al. (eds.), *Male Infertility: A Complete Guide to Lifestyle and Environmental Factors*,
DOI 10.1007/978-1-4939-1040-3_15, © Springer Science+Business Media New York 2014

Table 15.1 Medications That Negatively Impact Male Fertility

Medication	Altered HPG axis	Gonadotoxic	Post-testicular		
			Decreased libido	Erectile dysfunction	Fertilization potential
Antihypertensives					
Thiazide diuretics	–	–	–	+	–
Spironolactone	+	–	+	+	–
Beta-blockers	–	–	+	+	–
Calcium channel blockers	–	–	–	–	+
Alpha-adrenergic blockers	–	–	–	+	–
Psychotherapeutic agents					
Antipsychotics	+	–	+	+	–
Tricyclic antidepressants	+	–	+	+	–
MAOIs	–	–	–	+	–
Phenothiazines	+	–	–	–	–
Lithium	–	–	+	+	–
Chemotherapeutic agents	–	+	–	–	–
Hormones					
Anabolic steroids	+	–	–	+	–
Testosterone	+	–	–	+	–
Antiandrogens	+	–	+	–	–
Progesterone derivatives	+	–	+	+	–
Estrogens	+	–	+	+	–
Antibiotics					
Nitrofurantoin	+	+	–	–	–
Erythromycin	–	+	–	–	–
Tetracyclines	–	–	–	–	+
Gentamicin	–	+	–	–	–
Miscellaneous medications					
Marijuana	+	+	–	–	–
Opiates	+	–	+	–	–
Cimetidine	+	–	–	–	–
Cyclosporine	+	–	–	–	–
Colchicine	–	–	–	–	+
Finasteride/dutasteride	–	–	+	+	–
Treatments for IBD					
Sulfasalazine	+	+	–	–	–
Methotrexate	–	+	–	–	–
Infliximab	–	+	–	–	–

MAOIs monoamine oxidase inhibitors, *IBD* inflammatory bowel disease, + effect present, – effect not present
[Adapted from Nudell DM, et al. Common medications and drugs: how they affect male fertility. Urol Clin North Am. 2002;29:965-973. With permission from Elsevier]

hormonal therapies, administration of exogenous hormones, and various psychotherapeutic agents that alter concentrations of gonadotropins or testosterone [4]. The second basic mechanism (testicular) refers to direct gonadotoxic effects. Medications that damage germ cells, supporting Sertoli cells and/or Leydig cells, invariably impair spermatogenesis [4]. Finally, post-testicular mechanisms describe agents that exert effects on libido, erectile function, and/or ejaculation, thereby interfering with the deposition of semen in the female reproductive tract [4, 5].

Table 15.1 summarizes the various classes of drugs known to adversely affect male reproduction; it would be prudent for clinicians to consider a patient's desire for future fertility prior to prescribing any agent listed. This table classifies each medication according to the mechanism(s) by which it exerts its effects (pre-testicular, testicular, or post-testicular) and will serve as a framework to organize the detailed review that follows.

Pre-testicular (Endocrine Disturbances)

Spermatogenesis requires feedback-controlled, pulsatile secretion of gonadotropin-releasing hormone (GnRH), gonadotropins (FSH/LH), and testosterone by the hypothalamus, pituitary, and testes, respectively. Any medication that perturbs the reproductive axis at one or more of these levels has the potential to compromise gonadal function. While only 3–20 % of infertile men are found to have an underlying endocrinopathy [1, 7–9], multiple classes of medications interfere with the HPG axis and contribute to endocrine-derived subfertility.

Exogenous Hormones, Antiandrogens, and GnRH Agonists

Exogenous hormonal steroids (e.g., testosterone, progesterone derivatives, and estrogens), antiandrogens, and constitutive GnRH agonists all adversely affect male fertility by directly targeting the HPG axis, as illustrated in Fig. 15.1 [4, 6]. Some of these agents are prescribed specifically to produce a castrate state (as in the treatment of prostate cancer or hormone replacement therapy for transsexuals), and therefore impaired gonadal function is the goal. Other medications like exogenous androgens, however, suppress gonadal function inadvertently.

Exogenous testosterone supplementation, whether medically prescribed or used recreationally, paradoxically inhibits spermatogenesis [1]. This effect results directly from negative feedback by testosterone on the HPG axis, reducing FSH/LH and subsequently intratesticular testosterone levels. Drops in intratesticular testosterone can lead to oligospermia/azoospermia,

testicular atrophy, and an increased percentage of morphologically abnormal sperm [10]. This hypogonadism is usually reversible within 3–6 months of discontinuation but occasionally may be irreversible [4]. Thus, testosterone replacement therapy should be avoided in hypogonadal men attempting to conceive, and alternative agents like clomiphene or tamoxifen may be considered instead [1].

Antiepileptics

Epilepsy itself may directly influence the HPG axis, leading to decreased testosterone and increased estrogen levels [4, 11]. However, a number of antiepileptic drugs such as valproate, oxcarbazepine, and carbamazepine may exacerbate these hormonal effects and affect semen quality as well [4, 12]. A study of men with epilepsy taking valproate or carbamazepine as monotherapy revealed significantly lower FSH values than age-matched controls. Moreover, valproate-treated patients had significantly higher dehydroepiandrosterone levels and lower FSH/LH concentrations compared with the controls [13]. In addition to these effects, anticonvulsants are known to increase sex hormone-binding globulin (SHBG) levels and decrease the testosterone/SHBG ratio, thereby influencing levels of bioavailable testosterone [1, 13].

Animal studies have demonstrated impaired semen quality with the use of various anticonvulsants [14], and these effects have been mirrored in human studies as well. For example, men taking carbamazepine, oxcarbazepine, and valproic acid are more likely to demonstrate morphologically abnormal sperm (e.g., sperm-head abnormalities), poor sperm motility, and/or low sperm concentration compared to controls [12, 14].

Psychotherapeutic Medications

Many psychotherapeutic agents including selective serotonin reuptake inhibitors (SSRIs), monoamine oxidase (MAO) inhibitors, antipsychotics, phenothiazines, tricyclic antidepressants (TCAs), and lithium can affect male fertility by reducing libido and impairing erectile function and/or ejaculation [1, 4]. These will be discussed further under "Post-testicular Causes."

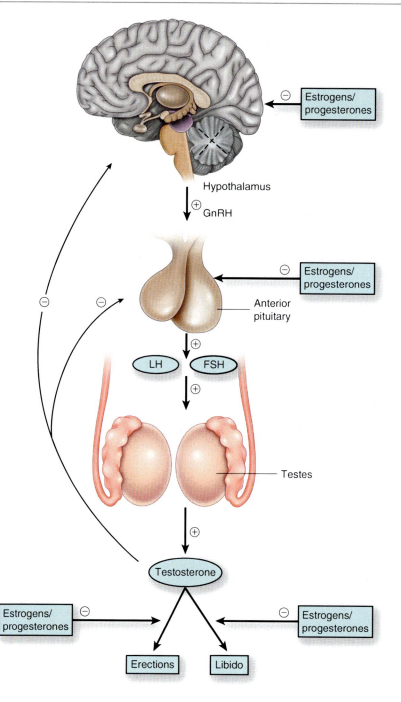

Fig. 15.1 Adverse effects of estrogens and progesterone derivatives on the hypothalamic-pituitary-gonadal axis. *Abbreviations*: *GnRH* gonadotropin-releasing hormone, *FSH* follicle-stimulating hormone, *LH* luteinizing hormone

However, several classes of psychotherapeutic agents can also impair fertility more directly by significantly suppressing the HPG axis; this section will highlight these pre-testicular effects.

Antipsychotics

Infertility secondary to hyperprolactinemia is a well-known side effect of traditional antipsychotic agents [15, 16]. Neuroleptics have in common the ability to block dopamine receptors, thereby reducing dopamine transmission. Reduction of dopamine results in greater circulating levels of prolactin in nearly half of patients taking antipsychotics [17], which in turn inhibits GnRH production. Reduced secretion of GnRH leads to reduced secretion of FSH and therefore decreased gonadal steroidogenesis [15, 16]. As many as 28 % of patients receiving antipsychotic treatment experience hypotestosteronism [18], and the degree of hypogonadism is usually proportional to the degree of prolactin elevation [16]. Effects include reduced libido, erectile dysfunction, gynecomastia, galactorrhea, decreased sperm production, and infertility, though the exact effect of neuroleptics on male fertility has not been investigated or reported systematically [16, 17].

Selective Serotonin Reuptake Inhibitors

Like antipsychotics, SSRI antidepressants are associated with elevation of prolactin levels and subsequent suppression of spermatogenesis [4]. It has been suggested that serotonin increases prolactin by stimulating the activity of prolactin-releasing factors and inhibiting dopamine and that the resulting hyperprolactinemia suppresses the HPG axis as described above [19]. One study comparing semen samples from men treated with SSRIs against untreated controls revealed lower mean total sperm counts, motility rates, and rates of normal sperm morphology. Moreover, each of these parameters significantly correlated with treatment duration, such that further detrimental effects by SSRIs on count, motility, and morphology were observed with extended treatment duration [20]. Another study evaluating the effect of escitalopram treatment on semen parameters in men with lifelong premature ejaculation demonstrated that at the third month of treatment, there was a significant decrease in mean sperm concentration (from 68 to 26 million/mL), motility (from 58 to 23 %), and morphology (19–7 % normal-shaped spermatozoa) when compared with the baseline semen measures [21]. Fortunately, the prolactin-mediated effects on semen parameters appear to be reversible within only a few weeks of SSRI discontinuation [19].

Tricyclic Antidepressants

Like SSRIs, TCAs adversely affect male fertility by altering the HPG axis [4]. Clomipramine and imipramine, for example, are known to have negative effects on sperm viability, motility, count, morphology, and volume [22]. One comparison of men taking clomipramine with age-matched controls not taking this medication demonstrated a significantly higher incidence of abnormal ejaculate parameters, especially with regard to volume, sperm motility, and sperm morphology [23]. Elsewhere, it has been reported that 3 weeks of continuous therapy with the TCA desmethylimipramine resulted in a significant decrease in sperm viability but no significant change in sperm count or motility [24]. While the reported effects of tricyclics vary depending on the specific agent and dose utilized, these studies nevertheless indicate that there is a negative association between sperm quality and exposure to TCAs [25].

Opiates

Long-acting narcotics suppress the HPG axis by inhibiting GnRH pulse patterns, which leads to suppression of LH release, androgen deficiency, and impaired spermatogenesis [10, 26]. Moreover, SHBG is elevated in men taking opioids, which further reduces the levels of bioavailable testosterone [10].

Numerous studies of men chronically using intrathecal, oral, and transdermal opioids for nonmalignant pain have demonstrated significantly reduced testosterone and LH levels compared to men not receiving opioids. While androgen deficiency is particularly profound in men treated with methadone maintenance therapy because of its long duration of action, hypogonadotropic hypogonadism results from the other narcotics in comparable doses [10, 26]. In fact, the high prevalence of hypogonadism in men taking any long-term narcotics has led the 2010 Endocrine Society Clinical Practice Guideline Committee to list men receiving chronic opioids as a candidate group in whom there is a high prevalence of low testosterone levels and in whom serum testosterone levels should be measured [26].

Clinically, hypogonadism in men taking narcotics presents with decreased libido, impotence, and impaired gonadal function. Semen analyses from men taking narcotics reveal significantly higher rates of asthenospermia, teratospermia, and oligospermia than those observed in the general population [27].

Glucocorticoids

Glucocorticoids affect gonadal function at multiple levels in the HPG axis, including the hypothalamus (suppressing the release of GnRH), the pituitary (inhibiting the release of LH/FSH), and the testes (modulating steroidogenesis and/or gametogenesis directly) [26, 28]. Moreover, glucocorticoids interfere with normal levels of bioavailable testosterone by decreasing SHBG levels [1].

Clinically, suppression of the HPG axis at all levels results in a combined primary and secondary hypogonadism [26]. Testosterone levels are lower in glucocorticoid-treated men than in age-matched controls, and the administration of greater than 5–7.5 mg/day of prednisone or its equivalent increases the risk of gonadotropin and testosterone suppression [26]. The propensity of this class of agents to cause hypogonadism is also reflected in the 2010 Endocrine Society Clinical Practice Guideline, which lists men receiving chronic glucocorticoids as a candidate group in whom there is a high prevalence of low testosterone levels and for whom measurement of serum testosterone is recommended [26].

Miscellaneous Drugs That Cause Endocrine Disturbances

Like the aforementioned drug classes, a number of individual agents also interfere with the HPG axis at various levels, producing endocrine disturbances that negatively impact male reproductive potential.

Spironolactone

The aldosterone antagonist spironolactone is widely used to treat chronic illnesses including cardiovascular and liver diseases. In addition to its actions on the mineralocorticoid receptor, spironolactone also acts as an antiandrogen by blocking testosterone synthesis and competing with testosterone for the androgen receptor. These effects interrupt hypothalamic and pituitary components of the testosterone negative feedback loop [1, 29], resulting in gynecomastia and impotence especially at doses exceeding 100 mg daily [30].

Interruption of the HPG feedback axis also negatively impacts semen parameters. In a study by Caminos-Torres et al., administration of spironolactone daily to healthy young men for up to 24 weeks produced decreased sperm density and motility in 22 % of subjects. Semen analysis in affected individuals had been normal prior to spironolactone administration, decreased markedly to subnormal levels within 4 weeks of initiating spironolactone, remained subnormal throughout the course of treatment, and returned to normal after spironolactone was discontinued [30].

Ketoconazole

Ketoconazole, an imidazole derivative, is widely used throughout the world as an antifungal agent [31]. In addition to its antimycotic properties, ketoconazole also inhibits both adrenal and testicular steroidogeneses [1, 31, 32]. While these antiandrogenic effects are useful in the treatment of prostate cancer, hirsutism, and Cushing's syndrome [31], they have a deleterious impact on male reproduction.

When administered at therapeutic doses of 200–600 mg/day, ketoconazole transiently reduces serum testosterone levels in men. In fact, the decline in testosterone concentration is substantial after even a single dose, with testosterone levels returning to normal over 8–24 h. Conventional antifungal doses of ketoconazole temporarily block testosterone synthesis and the adrenal response to corticotropin but rarely lead to endocrine complications [31]. However, higher therapeutic doses (800–1,200 mg/day) cause a more prolonged and profound hormone inhibition associated with oligo- or azoospermia, impotence, impaired libido, and gynecomastia. Fortunately, even the substantial inhibitory effects of high-dose ketoconazole regimens on testicular and adrenal steroidogenesis appear to be reversible with discontinuation of therapy [31, 33].

Cimetidine

Cimetidine, a histamine H_2-receptor antagonist, inhibits testosterone production and functions as a weak antiandrogen by competing for androgen receptors. Like other antiandrogens, it leads to elevated gonadotropin levels by antagonizing the negative feedback control of gonadotropin secretion by testosterone [1, 34]. Cimetidine has been reported to have antiandrogenic effects ranging from gynecomastia to oligospermia [4]. In one clinical study, men administered cimetidine exhibited a significant reduction in sperm concentration compared to placebo-treated controls [35]. In another study of men receiving cimetidine for chronic duodenal ulcers, testosterone and FSH were elevated during treatment with cimetidine compared to both pre- and posttreatment levels. Moreover, these hormonal effects were associated with a reduction in mean sperm count compared to the period after drug withdrawal [34].

Cyclosporine

The long-term use of the immunosuppressant cyclosporine is known to cause hirsutism and gynecomastia in male transplant recipients as a result of hormonal alterations. While the exact mechanism of these effects is still unknown, proposed mechanisms include action on fibroblasts and glandular cells, humoral and/or immunologic pathways [36], and effects on the hypothalamus and/or the pituitary [4, 37].

Gonadal effects resulting from hormonal alterations have been documented in animal models. In one experiment, administration of cyclosporine to rats led to significant reductions in serum testosterone levels, testicular weight, sperm count, haploid testicular cell population, and fertility compared to untreated controls [38]. In another rat study, cyclosporine administration produced hypo-androgenism associated with reduced reproductive organ weights, testicular and epididymal sperm counts, sperm motility, and fertilizing ability [39].

While human studies are limited in number and confounded by concurrent illness, cyclosporine has been shown to exert effects in men that are similar to those described in rats. For example, transplant patients taking cyclosporine demonstrate lower baseline levels of plasma prolactin and low or normal LH/FSH levels despite low testosterone levels. Moreover, cyclosporine appears to directly antagonize gonadal function, manifested as lower testosterone levels that are refractory to the administration of HCG [37].

Medical Marijuana

Marijuana contains the psychoactive cannabinoid delta-9-tetrahydrocannabinol (THC), which has repeatedly been shown to negatively affect male reproductive physiology. Specifically, cannabinoids block LHRH release from the hypothalamus which in turn reduces secretion of LH by the anterior pituitary. THC also increases the release of hypothalamic dopamine (the major physiological inhibitory factor of prolactin), reducing prolactin release from the adenohypophysis and further deregulating the reproductive axis [40]. Moreover, THC may activate endocannabinoid receptors on sperm, reducing motility in a dose-dependent manner and inhibiting the acrosomal reaction [10].

In men, THC decreases serum LH and subsequently plasma testosterone levels [41]. While patients experience variable sensitivities to marijuana, the resulting hypo-androgenism is dose dependent and may take as long as 2–3 months to resolve after cessation [4, 10]. Clinically, this manifests as gynecomastia, loss of libido, impotence, and ejaculatory dysfunction, as well as elevated seminal leukocytes [1, 4, 42].

With respect to gonadal function, marijuana reduces testosterone production by the testis and negatively influences the spermatogenetic process, reducing germ cell proliferation and sperm concentrations [41]. In mice, chronic administration of THC and other cannabinoids has been shown to impair spermatogenesis at both mitotic and meiotic stages, with mature spermatozoa characterized by severe morphological abnormalities [43]. Similarly, more than one-third of men who chronically smoke marijuana are characterized by oligospermia [10]. While human studies are observational and include subjects using marijuana in different formulations and doses and at varying frequencies, it is clear that consumption of this agent—be it illicit or prescribed—has a clear negative impact on male reproductive potential.

Testicular (Direct Toxic Effect on Gonadocytes)

Various medications have been shown to impair spermatogenesis by exerting direct gonadotoxic effects. These agents are listed in Table 15.1 and include antineoplastic drugs, medications frequently used to treat inflammatory bowel disease (IBD) and gout, and several common classes of antibiotics [4]. While these agents exert their effects through a variety of pathophysiologic mechanisms, they all have in common the ability to interfere with spermatogenesis. This section will review these gonadotoxic drug classes in detail, focusing on the impact that each has on male reproductive potential.

Chemotherapy

Approximately 1.5 million men and women were diagnosed with cancer in the United States in 2010, with approximately 1 % of these individuals under the age of 20 years at diagnosis [44]. While advances in cancer therapies have vastly improved disease-specific survival in these patients, many of them will face late treatment-related morbidities. Iatrogenic reproductive failure resulting from chemotherapy is a frequently encountered late effect and one which is of particular concern for younger patients undergoing cancer treatments [45]. Chemotherapy can have devastating effects on male fertility secondary to direct germ cell toxicity, with potential long-term spermatogenic impairment lasting years if recovery occurs at all [1].

Low-dose chemotherapy can deplete differentiating spermatogonia, resulting in temporary oligo- or azoospermia. The less sensitive mitotically quiescent spermatogonial stem cell lines survive the cytotoxic insult and recolonize the seminiferous tubules with differentiating spermatogonia, ultimately restoring spermatogenesis. However, when the spermatogonial stem cell pool is entirely depleted by high-dose treatment, a Sertoli cell-only pattern results and leads to permanent infertility [44, 46].

The germinal epithelium is particularly sensitive to several classes of chemotherapeutic agents (Table 15.2). Alkylating agents (notably chlorambucil, procarbazine, melphalan, cyclophosphamide, and busulfan) and platinum-based drugs, which cause direct DNA and RNA damage and induce apoptosis, are especially gonadotoxic and pose a greater risk of prolonged azoospermia [46, 47]. Antimetabolites, vinca alkaloids, podophyllotoxins, and antitumor antibiotics, on the other hand, depress germ cell function to a lesser extent [46].

The adverse effects of gonadotoxic chemotherapeutic agents largely depend on the type and dose of medication used. For example, the alkylating agent cyclophosphamide has a threshold dose of approximately 10 g/m^2 in postpubertal patients for impairing fertility. However, gradual recovery of spermatogenesis may occur even at this dose, with permanent sterility only occurring at 19–20 g/m^2 or higher doses [46]. Moreover, multiple low-dose insults with cyclophosphamide appear to cause more damage than a single high-dose insult as a result of repeated injury to reserve stem cells that become mitotically active following the initial injury to the seminiferous epithelium. Similar threshold cumulative doses required for prolonged azoospermia have been reported for other alkylating and platinum agents [46]. Cisplatin-based chemotherapy, for example, results in azoospermia immediately after therapy in most patients, with subsequent reversal of this effect in at least 50 % of patients receiving standard-dose chemotherapy up to four cycles [48]. At doses of 500–600 mg/m^2 however, cisplatin is associated with prolonged azoospermia [46, 47]. Table 15.2 lists the threshold cumulative doses associated with various alkylating and platinum agents.

While it was earlier suggested that germ cells of younger males are less susceptible to the toxic effects of chemotherapy compared to older boys and young adults, more recent studies have demonstrated that boys receiving gonadotoxic treatment prior to puberty are not protected from posttreatment gonadal dysfunction [49, 50]. In fact, some chemotherapeutic agents that exhibit reversible spermatogenic effects in postpubertal males result in permanent azoospermia when given to prepubertal boys [47]. The prepubertal testis appears particularly vulnerable due to its

Table 15.2 Gonadotoxic chemotherapeutic medications

High or moderate risk		Low risk	
Non-cell cycle-specific drugs		Cell cycle-specific drugs	Non-cell cycle-specific drugs
Drug	Cumulative dose for prolonged azoospermia	Drug	Drug
Alkylating agents		Antimetabolites	Antitumor antibiotics
Cyclophosphamide	19 g/m^2	Methotrexate	Bleomycin
Busulfan	600 mg/kg	Mercaptopurine	Dactinomycin
Melphalan	140 mg/m^2	Vinca alkaloids	
BCNU		Vincristine	
CCNU		Vinblastine	
Chlorambucil	1.4 g/m^2	Podophyllotoxins	
Ifosfamide	42 g/m^2	Asparaginase	
Procarbazine	4 g/m^2		
Platinum agents			
Cic-platinum	600 mg/m^2		
Mechanism of action		Mechanism of action	Mechanism of action
– DNA/RNA damage		– DNA/RNA synthesis inhibition	– Induction of DNA strand breaks
– Induction of apoptosis		– Inhibition of mitosis	
		– Deamination of proteins	

[Reprinted from Jahnukainen K, Ehmcke J, Hou M, Schlatt S. Testicular function and fertility preservation in male cancer patients. *Best Pract Res Clin Endocrinol Metab*. 2011 Apr;25(2):287-302. With permission from Elsevier]

constant turnover of early germ cells [46]. Thomson et al. reported that only 33 % of male survivors of childhood cancer have normal semen quality [51]. In a review of 6,224 male childhood cancer survivors (all younger than 21 years at diagnosis and not surgically sterile), Green et al. demonstrated that survivors were nearly half as likely to sire a pregnancy compared to their siblings. Specifically, the hazard ratio of siring a pregnancy was decreased by treatment with cyclophosphamide or procarbazine and inversely related to the cumulative alkylating agent dose (AAD) score. Importantly, participants without a summed AAD score ≥ 2, treatment with procarbazine, or treatment with higher doses of cyclophosphamide were as likely as their siblings to sire a pregnancy [52]. In another large study of 565 childhood cancer survivors, Tromp et al. showed that one-third of male childhood cancer survivors have elevated FSH levels (a surrogate for spermatogenic dysfunction) after a median follow-up of 15 years. Among the various antineoplastic agents, the authors identified the use of procarbazine, cyclophosphamide, vinca alkaloids, or alkylating agents as independent treatment-related risk factors for elevated FSH levels [45].

In contrast to the testicular germinal epithelium, Leydig cells are characterized by a slow rate of turnover which makes them much less vulnerable to damage from antineoplastic agents. Chemotherapy-induced Leydig cell failure leading to androgen insufficiency that requires testosterone supplementation is extremely rare. Some studies have suggested that Leydig cell dysfunction may be observed following treatment with alkylating agents, with anywhere from 10 to 88 % of male subjects developing elevated serum concentrations of LH. However, most males undergo a normal puberty and produce normal adult levels of testosterone. Thus, Leydig cell dysfunction is generally subclinical when present [44, 46, 53].

Treatment of Inflammatory Bowel Disease

Numerous studies have shown that treatments for IBD are associated with reversible impairment of male reproductive function, including reductions in sperm concentration and motility

[1]. The reproductive impact of these treatments is particularly important given that half of patients are under the age of 35 years when diagnosed with IBD and a quarter of them conceive for the first time after being diagnosed [54]. Specific agents believed to impair male fertility include sulfasalazine, methotrexate, and infliximab.

Sulfasalazine

Commonly used to treat ulcerative colitis, Crohn's disease, and rheumatoid arthritis, sulfasalazine is composed of sulfapyridine linked to 5-aminosalicylic acid (5-ASA) by an azo bond. While 5-ASA is the active therapeutic moiety of sulfasalazine, most of the drug's adverse effects are attributed to the nontherapeutic sulfapyridine constituent [55]. Male infertility resulting from sulfasalazine was first reported in 1979 by Levi et al. in patients treated for ulcerative colitis [56]. Since then, numerous clinical studies have demonstrated sulfasalazine's gonadotoxic effects, including oligospermia, impaired sperm motility, and alterations in sperm morphology [54]. Moreover, multiple studies have demonstrated restoration of semen quality (improvement in sperm count, morphology, and motility) and successful conception when other 5-ASA preparations not containing a sulfapyridine moiety are substituted for sulfasalazine [54, 57, 58]. While the exact mechanism for this spermatogenic toxicity remains poorly elucidated, research using rat models has suggested that sulfasalazine-induced oxidative stress may play an important role [55].

Methotrexate

The immunosuppressive drug methotrexate is a folic acid antagonist that binds to the enzyme dihydrofolate reductase, disrupting synthesis of DNA, RNA, and protein [59]. In men, methotrexate is used in higher doses to treat malignancy and in lower doses to treat a number of autoimmune conditions including rheumatoid arthritis, psoriasis, psoriatic arthritis, lupus, and IBD. Concerns about the effect of methotrexate on male fertility and pregnancy outcomes stem from the fact that methotrexate damages or kills cells undergoing division, a process continually occurring during spermatogenesis [59].

Studies in animals have shown altered spermatogenesis, cytotoxicity, and degeneration of spermatocytes, Sertoli cells, and Leydig cells resulting from methotrexate use; however, conflicting data exists regarding the reproductive effects of methotrexate in men [57, 59, 60]. While some studies have failed to demonstrate suppression of spermatogenesis or impairment of semen quality with methotrexate use [60, 61], others have documented reversible oligospermia and/or sterility in men taking this immunosuppressant [57, 59]. Additional concern has focused on the known teratogenic effects of methotrexate in women, for whom the FDA has classified this medication as a Pregnancy Category X [54, 57]. However, there are no reports to date describing adverse pregnancy outcomes in the female partners of men who were treated with methotrexate [54, 59, 60].

Although the gonadotoxic effects of low-dose methotrexate are unclear and there are no reports of methotrexate-induced congenital abnormalities in infants born to men taking this medication, authorities nonetheless recommend that methotrexate be stopped prior to conception. Some have advocated that this agent be discontinued at least 3–4 months before attempts at conception due to its prolonged tissue-binding characteristics [54, 57, 60].

Infliximab

The tumor necrosis factor (TNF) antagonist infliximab is commonly used for treatment of reproductive-age men with IBD, and some studies have reported adverse gonadal effects with this agent. In one prospective study comparing pre- and posttreatment semen parameters of men with IBD receiving infliximab, the authors found that infliximab therapy decreased sperm motility and the number of normal oval forms [62]. Moreover, case reports have described reduced sperm motility in patients with ankylosing spondylitis who were treated with infliximab [63]. However, in a study of men with spondyloarthritis taking TNF blockers (infliximab, etanercept, or adalimumab), the authors concluded that the sperm quality of patients receiving long-term TNF inhibition was comparable to that of healthy controls [64]. Given the conflicting reports regarding its effect on semen parameters and the fact that no studies have specifically evaluated the effects of infliximab on fertility, experts agree that infliximab need not be stopped before attempts at conception for men with IBD [57].

Antibiotics

Antibiotics are routinely prescribed to men for a variety of everyday conditions, oftentimes without regard for fertility. Unfortunately, adverse effects on male fertility have been well established for individual agents from all the major classes of antibiotics, including impairment of both spermatogenesis and spermatozoal function [1, 3, 4, 65].

A number of animal studies have documented adverse reproductive effects related to antibiotic exposures. Research using DNA flow cytometry of testicular aspirate to quantitatively evaluate testicular function in rats receiving various antibiotics demonstrates that Bactrim, nitrofurantoin, ofloxacin, and doxycycline significantly alter spermatogenesis [66]. Hargreaves et al. cultured sperm with increasing concentrations of various antibiotics to investigate their effects on sperm movement characteristics and viability. In this in vitro experiment, tetracycline was the most potent drug tested, exerting significant effects on sperm movement at concentrations as low as 2.5 µg/mL, well within the levels seen with therapeutic doses of this antibiotic. On the other hand, erythromycin did not exert effects on sperm movement at concentrations <100 µg/mL, and amoxicillin had no effect on sperm movement characteristics over the dose range used. Because tetracyclines penetrate into semen with concentrations about 60 % of those found in serum, the effects that tetracycline exerts on sperm movement in vitro would be expected to occur in vivo during a course of tetracycline treatment [3].

While in vitro and animal data suggest that multiple classes of antibiotics have the potential to adversely affect fertility, documentation of an in vivo effect in humans is lacking [4]. Nonetheless, a number of antibiotics have been well established to impair spermatogenesis and/or sperm function in men. For example, significant alterations in semen parameters have been documented following treatment with nitrofurans [65], with high doses of nitrofurantoin reported to cause early maturation arrest at the primary spermatocyte stage [4]. Other antibiotics known to be gonadotoxic include erythromycin and gentamicin [4]. Tetracyclines, on the other hand, are relatively nontoxic to spermatogenesis, exerting their effect on mature sperm function and motility as illustrated by the aforementioned in vitro experiments [3].

While additional research is needed to define the relative toxicity of antibiotics and the exact mechanisms by which they exert their effects, clinicians must be aware that a number of antibiotics may impair the reproductive potential of men.

Colchicine

Colchicine, an alkaloid used to treat gouty arthritis, familial Mediterranean fever, and Behçet's disease, is a modulator of microtubules at the cytoskeleton level [67]. In vitro, high-dose colchicine arrests mitotic division at metaphase, raising concern that it might arrest meiosis as well [68]. However, controversial results have been published regarding the adverse effect of colchicine on sperm production in vivo. Sporadic reports have described negative impacts on sperm production and function ranging from oligo- and azoospermia to normospermia with disturbances in sperm motility [69]. Others have reported that colchicine induces oligospermia and impacts fertilization potential in patients with Behçet's disease with long-term exposure; however, short-term exposure in healthy males has failed to reproduce these effects [4]. On the basis of inconsistent sperm pathologies, the general consensus is that treatment with typical doses of colchicine (<2 mg daily) does not have a significant adverse effect on sperm production and function [67, 68]. However, it may be possible that underlying factors make some men particularly sensitive to a cytotoxic effect of colchicine on germinal epithelium, accounting for rare cases of reversible infertility associated with its use [68].

Calcium Channel Blockers (Functional Sperm Defects)

Calcium channel blockers have been scrutinized for their potential to inhibit the sperm fertilization process. Two mechanisms have been proposed: (1) these agents may directly block calcium influx, a necessary component of the acrosome reaction, and (2) lipophilic calcium ion antagonists may insert into the lipid bilayer of the sperm plasma membrane, altering surface molecules required for normal fertilization [70, 71].

A number of case reports and human experiments have demonstrated that therapeutic administration of calcium antagonists leads to reversible male infertility and IVF failure associated with normal semen analysis parameters. Moreover, discontinuation of these agents has been shown to restore parameters associated with sperm fertilizing potential, including recovery of spontaneous acrosome reactions and increases in surface mannose-ligand binding in vitro [70, 72]. However, other clinical studies have failed to demonstrate an adverse effect of calcium channel blockers on fertility [71]. Given these conflicting data, it may nevertheless be prudent for clinicians to select alternative antihypertensive agents in men pursuing fertility.

Post-testicular (Impaired Libido/Erection/Emission/ Ejaculation)

While a number of medications act at the pre-testicular or testicular levels to inhibit sperm production, other classes of medications act at the post-testicular level, interfering with delivery of sperm into the female reproductive tract. These include effects on libido, erectile function, emission, and ejaculation. A number of drugs disrupt male libido by acting on the central nervous system, affecting fertility indirectly by decreasing sexual drive. Other agents interfere with the neurologic or vascular-mediated events necessary for normal erectile function. Finally, some medications interfere with intra-vaginal sperm deposition by inhibiting ejaculate emission and/or causing retrograde ejaculation [4]. This section will address the drug classes most commonly implicated in post-testicular causes of male subfertility, including a detailed review of the specific impairments associated with each of these.

Medications Used to Treat Lower Urinary Tract Symptoms

Lower urinary tract symptoms (LUTS) and male sexual dysfunction are both common in older men, and the link between these two conditions has been well established. In large part, this link results from the adverse sexual effects associated with 5-α reductase inhibitors and alpha blockers, both of which are used in the treatment of benign prostatic hyperplasia (BPH) [73].

5-α Reductase Inhibitors

The 5-α reductase inhibitors finasteride and dutasteride, which inhibit conversion of testosterone to the metabolically active dihydrotestosterone, are commonly used in the treatment of BPH and male pattern baldness [1, 4]. While randomized, placebo-controlled trials have demonstrated that each of these medications has a clinically insignificant effect on spermatogenesis [74], the use of these agents is strongly associated with sexual dysfunction. 5-α reductase inhibitors have been shown to adversely affect libido and erectile function as well as to increase the incidence of low-volume ejaculate [1, 4, 73], with finasteride and dutasteride exhibiting a similar profile and incidence of adverse sexual events [75].

A number of studies have demonstrated reductions in libido associated with both finasteride and dutasteride. Dutasteride has been reported to produce a 4.2 % incidence of reduced libido compared to approximately 2 % in placebo [75, 76]. In another trial, approximately 2.8 % of patients taking dutasteride reported a decreased libido, with 1.3 % of the patients in this group reporting a complete loss of libido [76]. Similarly, finasteride is associated with a 6.4 % rate of diminished libido compared to 3.4 % for placebo [75].

Effects on erectile function are also comparable for these two agents, dutasteride being associated with a 7.3 % rate of ED (compared to 4.0 % for placebo) and finasteride causing an 8.1 % rate of ED compared to 3.7 % for placebo [75]. Several other trials have documented ED in approximately 6–8 % of patients taking 5-α reductase inhibitors, and this side effect is often the most common adverse event leading to withdrawal [76].

Ejaculatory dysfunction is also adversely affected in patients taking 5-α reductase inhibitors, with dutasteride causing a 2.2 % rate of ejaculatory dysfunction (compared to 0.8 % for placebo) and finasteride causing a 4.5 % rate of ejaculatory dysfunction compared to 0.9 % for placebo [75]. Symptoms of ejaculatory dysfunction were subdivided in the CombAT study, which reported a 0.6 % rate of retrograde ejaculations, 0.5 % rate of ejaculation failure, and 0.3 % rate of semen volume decrease in patients taking dutasteride [77].

Alpha-Blockers

Alpha-1-adrenoceptor antagonists (α1-blockers) are widely utilized as a first-line treatment for LUTS and, less commonly, to treat hypertension. However, their use has been clearly shown to cause varying degrees of ejaculatory dysfunction, ranging from decreased ejaculate volume to complete anejaculation. These effects are mediated by loss of seminal emission as well as relaxation of the bladder neck resulting in retrograde ejaculation [78].

Multiple alpha-blockers are available (alfuzosin, doxazosin, tamsulosin, terazosin, and silodosin), and each of these differs in its degree of uroselectivity and therefore in its associated risk of adverse sexual events. While the reported incidence of ejaculatory dysfunction with nonselective alpha-blockers such as doxazosin and terazosin is generally less than 1.5 %, adverse ejaculatory effects occur more commonly with tamsulosin and silodosin because these medications exhibit the highest degree of uroselectivity for the α1-adrenoceptor subtype A receptor [75]. Tamsulosin is reportedly associated with a 4–26 % rate of ejaculatory dysfunction, depending on its dose and duration of use [75]. In a randomized, placebo-controlled study, administration of tamsulosin 0.8 mg once daily to healthy volunteers markedly decreased mean ejaculate volume in almost 90 % of subjects, with 35 % having no ejaculation [73]. Silodosin, approved by the FDA in 2008, is the newest and most highly selective α1A-blocker. The selectivity of silodosin toward the α1A-adrenoceptor subtype has been reported to be 38 times greater than that of tamsulosin [78]. This uroselectivity translates into the highest reported rates of ejaculatory dysfunction among the alpha-blockers, ranging from 28 to 100 % [75, 78]. In one double-blind, placebo-controlled, randomized trial randomizing men to silodosin vs. placebo, every participant receiving silodosin had a complete lack of emission and expulsion of semen from the urethra despite there being a normal average semen volume at baseline [78].

Antihypertensives

Increasing emphasis on blood pressure control has led to greater numbers of younger patients taking antihypertensives, a category of agents commonly associated with impaired libido and erectile dysfunction. A review of hypertensive men taking selected antihypertensive therapy (thiazide diuretics, beta-blockers, spironolactone, methyldopa, and clonidine) demonstrated complete ED prevalence rates in this group that were threefold greater than normotensive men and 2.4-fold greater than hypertensive men who did not use these agents [79].

Among the classes of antihypertensive drugs most commonly utilized, diuretics and β-adrenoceptor antagonists stand out as the two groups most often implicated in causing sexual dysfunction, and these will be covered in greater detail below [80, 81]. While older-generation antihypertensive drugs (central-acting beta-blockers and diuretics) negatively impact erectile function, the newer-generation agents (calcium antagonists, angiotensin-converting enzyme inhibitors, and angiotensin receptor blockers) have neutral or even beneficial effects on erectile function [82]. Alpha-adrenergic blockers, though used more frequently nowadays for the treatment of BPH than to treat hypertension, demonstrate negative effects on ejaculatory function as described in the previous section. While the aforementioned antihypertensive agents do not directly affect fertility, the antihypertensive spironolactone acts as an antiandrogen, altering the HPG axis and leading to impaired semen quality in addition to decreased libido and erectile dysfunction (refer to the section entitled "Miscellaneous Drugs That Cause Endocrine Disturbances" [4].

Beta-Blockers

Beta-blockers have traditionally been considered a major cause of erectile dysfunction, with effects that are dose dependent but more prevalent with older-generation beta-blockers such as propranolol than with newer ones like celiprolol and carvedilol [81, 82]. A recent observational study of more than 1,000 hypertensive men taking beta-blockers demonstrated a 71 % incidence of erectile dysfunction in this group. In this study, metoprolol and carvedilol were associated with the highest rates and degrees of erectile dysfunction, atenolol and bisoprolol with intermediate rates, and nebivolol with the lowest rates and degrees of erectile dysfunction [83]. Studies have also demonstrated that the prevalence of erectile dysfunction seen with this class of drugs translates clinically into a reduction in the number of sexual intercourse events per month [81, 82]. Atenolol significantly reduced the number of intercourse events per month from 7.8 to 4.2 in one randomized, double-blinded study and from 6.0 to 4.2 in another. Similarly, carvedilol has been shown to reduce sexual intercourse episodes per month from 8.2 to 3.7 [82]. Thus, while beta-blockers do not prohibit most men from being able to deposit sperm in the female reproductive tract, they may nonetheless contribute to subfertility by posing a barrier to sexual intercourse.

Diuretics

Thiazide diuretics are the most commonly prescribed antihypertensive drugs for the treatment of hypertension and are the most implicated class of antihypertensives with respect to erectile function [82, 84]. Multiple randomized, placebo-controlled trials have reported that patients taking thiazide diuretics experience significantly greater sexual dysfunction than control subjects, including decreased libido, difficulty obtaining and maintaining an erection, and difficulty with ejaculation [38, 84]. In the Trial of Antihypertensive Interventions and Management study, erectile function worsened in 28 % of men receiving chlorthalidone (a thiazide), compared with 11 % of men receiving atenolol and only 3 % of men receiving placebo [38]. Similarly, in the Treatment of Mild Hypertension Study, participants randomized to chlorthalidone experienced a 17.1 % incidence of erectile dysfunction at 2 years compared to 8.1 % of patients randomized to placebo [38]. Like beta-blockers, consideration should therefore be given to discontinuing thiazide diuretics in men trying to conceive who report adverse sexual effects.

Psychotherapeutic Medications

This drug category as a whole, including antipsychotics, TCAs, SSRIs, selective norepinephrine reuptake inhibitors (SNRI), monoamine oxidase inhibitors (MAOIs), phenothiazines, and lithium, has been implicated in suppressing the HPG axis and adversely affecting libido, erectile function, and ejaculation [1, 4, 85]. While disruption of the HPG axis leads to impaired spermatogenesis as discussed earlier (see "Pre-testicular Causes, Psychotherapeutic Medications"), the adverse sexual effects also contribute to subfertility at the post-testicular level.

Antipsychotics produce a rise in circulating levels of prolactin, which in turn inhibits GnRH release and gonadal steroidogenesis [15, 16]. Hyperprolactinemia (>25 ng/mL) and secondary hypogonadism are highly prevalent among treated schizophrenics, affecting 51 % and 28 % of men, respectively [16, 86]. These endocrine abnormalities manifest clinically as reduced libido and erectile dysfunction [16]. Cross-sectional, comparative studies of male schizophrenics taking neuroleptics have reported a high incidence of sexual dysfunction, ranging from 50 to 70 % [86]. In particular, drugs that induce hyperprolactinemia such as risperidone are associated with significantly higher rates of sexual problems (40–60 %) compared to prolactin-sparing drugs like quetiapine, ziprasidone, and aripiprazole (<30 %) [86].

Antidepressants, especially selective SSRIs, venlafaxine (an SNRI), and clomipramine (a TCA), are also frequently associated with sexual dysfunction [85]. These agents all have in common the ability to raise serotonin levels, which increases prolactin and leads to sexual side effects. Montejo et al. analyzed the incidence of antidepressant-related sexual dysfunction in a multicenter, prospective study carried out by the Spanish Working Group for the Study of

Psychotropic-Related Sexual Dysfunction. In this review of 412 men with previously normal sexual function who were being treated with antidepressants, the authors reported a 62.4 % overall incidence of sexual dysfunction in men. Rates of sexual dysfunction were highest for citalopram (73 %), followed by paroxetine (71 %), venlafaxine (67 %), sertraline (63 %), fluvoxamine (62 %), fluoxetine (58 %), and mirtazapine (24 %) [85].

While the effects of psychotherapeutic medications on sexual function are not absolute barriers to reproduction, they may contribute to subfertility in patients undergoing treatment for psychiatric disease. Thus, clinicians should consider modifying these regimens in affected men being evaluated for infertility when it is clinically safe to do so.

Exogenous Hormones, Antiandrogens, and GnRH Agonists

Exogenous hormonal steroids (e.g., progesterone derivatives and estrogens), antiandrogens (e.g., flutamide, nilutamide, bicalutamide), and constitutive GnRH agonists (e.g., leuprolide) all directly target the HPG axis [4, 6]. While the resulting hypogonadotropic hypogonadism can impair spermatogenesis (see "Pre-testicular Causes"), the endocrine changes may also profoundly reduce libido and erectile function [4]. The magnitude and quality of this effect vary according to the specific medication, dose, and duration of use, but clinicians should be aware that this broad category of agents may exert substantial post-testicular barriers to reproduction in addition to the aforementioned spermatogenic effects.

Complications of Radiation Therapy

Men diagnosed with cancer must often face the long-term reproductive consequences of treatment with intensive, multimodal therapies [53]. As with chemotherapy, the testis is exquisitely sensitive to ionizing radiation, exhibiting significant functional impairment after exposure to even low doses [87]. Such exposures can be from radiation directed specifically at the testis (as in the treatment of testicular CIS) or from collateral scatter during treatment directed at adjacent tissues such as the pelvis or abdomen. Regardless of the target, gonadal irradiation can cause damage to germinal epithelium and to a lesser extent Leydig cells, impairing spermatogenesis and testosterone production, respectively [88]. Moreover, radiation-mediated reproductive insults take an altogether different form: hypothalamic-pituitary dysfunction secondary to cranial irradiation, resulting in central hypogonadism and disruption of spermatogenesis. This section will provide a detailed review of the reproductive effects observed following treatment with radiation, including spermatogenic and endocrine impairments that result from testis exposure as well as hypogonadotropic hypogonadism resulting from irradiation damage to the hypothalamus and/or pituitary.

Radiation-Induced Injury to Germinal Epithelium

The seminiferous epithelium is quite sensitive to the effects of irradiation at all stages of life, with the degree of functional impairment depending on the radiation dose and ranging from mild oligospermia to complete azoospermia [45, 87, 89]. Like chemotherapy, low-dose radiation may destroy differentiating spermatogonia, resulting in temporary oligo- or azoospermia. The less sensitive spermatogonial stem cells survive and must repopulate the pool of differentiating spermatogonia to restore sperm production. However, at higher doses of radiation, spermatogonial stem cells are lost, leading to a Sertoli cell-only pattern and permanent infertility [46].

The timing of spermatogonial recovery depends on the radiation dose received, with recolonization of surviving spermatogonia detected 6 months after a dose of 0.2 Gy, 9–18 months after a dose of 1 Gy, and more than 4 years after a dose of 10 Gy [46]. Whether recovery happens at all also depends on the radiation dose received. While scatter doses as low as 0.1 Gy lead to temporary azoospermia, doses of

2–3 Gy are associated with long-term azoospermia, and doses of 6 Gy or more (as with direct testis radiation for testicular CIS) can result in permanent sterility [44, 46]. It is important to note that fractionated radiation is more toxic than single-dose exposure because the repeated insults do damage to reserve stem cell lines as they repopulate the germinal epithelium [52, 88].

While the effects of scatter radiation depend largely on dose and fractionation, they also vary greatly according to the specific field utilized. For example, in a study of long-term survivors of acute lymphoblastic leukemia, the authors reported that the incidence of germ cell dysfunction was significantly greater following craniospinal + abdominal RT including the gonads than following craniospinal RT, which in turn was associated with a higher incidence of germ cell dysfunction than with cranial RT alone [90]. Pelvic irradiation poses a particular reproductive risk given the proximity of this region to the testes. In one study measuring the radiation doses delivered to the testicles in male patients receiving radiotherapy for rectal cancer, the authors demonstrated that on average, 7.1 % of the prescribed dose is scattered to the testis depending on the distance between the testis and the lower field margin. In this study, the testes received an average of 3.6 Gy during the course of pelvic radiotherapy, and in 73 % of patients the testes received more than 2 Gy, a dose associated with long-term azoospermia. The scattered dose to the testes occurring during pelvic irradiation has also been measured for prostate cancer. During a conventional course of irradiation for prostate cancer, the testes receive between 2 and 8 % of the target dose, corresponding to an approximately 1.8–2.4 Gy testicular dose in patients receiving 60–66 Gy external beam irradiation of the prostate [88, 91].

Radiation-Induced Injury to Leydig Cells

Leydig cells are far less vulnerable than germ cells to damage from radiotherapy because of their relatively slow rate of turnover. Nevertheless, Leydig cells are susceptible at higher doses, with the likelihood of sustaining radiation-induced injury being directly related to the dose delivered and inversely related to patient age at treatment. Doses greater than 20 Gy cause Leydig cell failure in most prepubertal males, whereas doses greater than 30 Gy are generally required to cause failure in adolescent boys and young adults [53]. Thus, high-dose irradiation during childhood does more harm to adult Leydig cell function than irradiation to the adult testis does [44].

At lower doses, Leydig cell injury leads to compensatory subclinical hypogonadism. For example, LH levels are elevated in about 20 % of patients receiving just 1 Gy of fractionated irradiation to their testes. However, the majority of men who receive 20 Gy or less as a fractionated testicular dose continue to produce normal amounts of testosterone and therefore do not experience any symptoms of hypogonadism [88].

When high-dose testicular radiation is utilized, particularly in younger patients, Leydig cell failure may result. In one study of boys undergoing testicular irradiation at 24 Gy for acute lymphoblastic leukemia, 83 % of patients demonstrated Leydig cell dysfunction at a median of 5 years after therapy [44]. When it occurs, Leydig cell failure leads to hypogonadism, manifested as loss of libido and erectile function. Moreover, because the germinal epithelium is much more sensitive to the effects of ionizing radiation than Leydig cells, doses that lead to Leydig cell dysfunction are invariably associated with spermatogenic failure and semen abnormalities as well (see "Radiation-Induced Injury to Germinal Epithelium").

Pituitary Radiation Causing Hypopituitarism

Patients treated with cranial irradiation for malignancy have benefited from greater survival in recent years; however, these advances have been hampered by long-term effects including radiation-induced hypopituitarism [46, 92]. The hypothalamus and to a lesser extent the pituitary [93] are inadvertently affected in patients receiving total body radiotherapy, prophylactic cranial irradiation for leukemia, and radiotherapy for intracranial, skull base, sinonasal, and nasopharyngeal tumors [94]. While radiation affects multiple hypothalamic-pituitary-end organ axes, the growth hormone axis is the most radiosensitive followed by the gonadal axis. Thus, irradiation may lead to hypopituitarism in the form of growth hormone deficiency in addition to hypogonadotropic hypogonadism [93].

The *timing* of radiation-induced empty sella or pituitary atrophy varies depending on the dose, fractionation, and age at treatment, though the effect is usually insidious, progressive, and irreversible [93, 94]. Hypopituitarism is known to increase up to 10 years after radiation exposure [95]. For example, the prevalence of pituitary failure in patients treated for nasopharyngeal tumors is reportedly 6 % after 1 year, 35 % after 2 years, 56 % after 3 years, and 62 % after 4–5 years. Moreover, individual pituitary axes fail in a predictable sequential order, with growth hormone insufficiency manifesting after an average of 2.6 years, followed by failure of the HPG axis after 3.8 years, ACTH deficiency after 6 years, and finally TSH insufficiency after 11 years [92].

The *incidence* and *degree* of radiation-induced pituitary injury also depend on the dose, fractionation, and patient age [93, 94]. The clinical manifestations of hypopituitarism are more severe in children and young adults, though effects are increasingly being observed in older adults as well [94]. The reported incidence of side effects varies considerably between studies in part because of the long follow-up interval required to observe them. Hypopituitarism is present in approximately half to two-thirds of adult patients previously treated with cranial radiation, and hypogonadotropic hypogonadism has been reported in 30 % of patients radiated for non-pituitary tumors, including 30–82 % of patients treated for nasopharyngeal cancer, and in 38–61 % of patients treated for intracerebral tumors [92]. Similarly, two-thirds of leukemia patients who receive prophylactic cranial irradiation or total body irradiation in preparation for bone marrow transplantation suffer from pituitary atrophy 10 to 20 years after irradiation [93]. These findings are reflected in the 2010 Endocrine Society Clinical Practice Guideline, which identifies men with a history of radiation to the sellar region as a candidate group in whom there is a high prevalence of low testosterone levels [26].

Given the prevalence of radiation-induced sellar injury, an infertility evaluation for any patient with a history of cranial or total body radiotherapy should include an assessment of pituitary function. Specifically, low LH and FSH levels in the setting of abnormal semen parameters would be suggestive of hypothalamic and/or pituitary dysfunction causing central suppression of spermatogenesis [5].

Conclusion

Approximately 15 % of couples fail to conceive a child after 1 year of unprotected intercourse, with male factor infertility solely present in 20 % of these cases and contributing to female factor infertility in another 30–40 % of cases [4]. While 23 % of men found to be infertile or subfertile will have no known etiology [1], a significant number of infertile men have impaired fertility attributable to prior or ongoing pharmaco- and radiotherapies. Attention by clinicians to their male patients' desire for future fertility and awareness of the impact that these treatments have on subsequent reproductive potential are critical in order to avoid iatrogenic causes of male infertility. In cases where therapy takes priority over future reproductive ability (as in the treatment of malignancy), a discussion of anticipated reproductive effects is critical and should include options for male fertility preservation such as cryopreservation of semen or testicular tissue before initiating therapy when possible.

References

1. Sabanegh Jr E, Agarwal A. Male infertility. In: Wein AJ, Kavoussi LR, Novick AC, Partin AW, Peters CA, editors. Campbell-Walsh urology. 10th ed. Philadelphia, PA: Saunders; 2011.
2. Krausz C. Male infertility: pathogenesis and clinical diagnosis. Best Pract Res Clin Endocrinol Metab. 2011;25(2):271–85.

3. Hargreaves CA, Rogers S, Hills F, Rahman F, Howell RJ, Homa ST. Effects of co-trimoxazole, erythromycin, amoxycillin, tetracycline and chloroquine on sperm function in vitro. Hum Reprod. 1998;13(7): 1878–86.
4. Sigman M. Medications that impair male fertility. A clinical publication of the American Society for Reproductive Medicine 2007;5(2). http://www.srmejournal.com/article.asp?AID=7104. Accessed 29 Oct 2013.
5. Shindel AW, Smith JF. Evaluation of male factor infertility. AUA Update Series 2011;30. Lesson 16.
6. Buchanan JF, Davis LJ. Drug-induced infertility. Drug Intell Clin Pharm. 1984;18(2):122–32.
7. Baker HWG, et al. Relative incidence of etiologic disorders in male infertility. In: Santen RJ, Swerdloff RS, editors. Male reproductive dysfunctions. NY: Marcel Dekker; 1986. p. 341–72.
8. Jequier AM, Holmes SC. Primary testicular disease presenting as azoospermia or oligozoospermia in an infertility clinic. Br J Urol. 1993;71(6):731–5.
9. de Kretser DM. Male infertility. Lancet. 1997; 349(9054):787–90.
10. Fronczak CM, Kim ED, Barqawi AB. The insults of illicit drug use on male fertility. J Androl. 2012;33(4): 515–28.
11. Hamed SA. Neuroendocrine hormonal conditions in epilepsy: relationship to reproductive and sexual functions. Neurologist. 2008;14(3):157–69.
12. Isojärvi JI, Löfgren E, Juntunen KS, Pakarinen AJ, Päivänsalo M, Rautakorpi I, Tuomivaara L. Effect of epilepsy and antiepileptic drugs on male reproductive health. Neurology. 2004;62(2):247–53.
13. Røste LS, Taubøll E, Mørkrid L, Bjørnenak T, Saetre ER, Mørland T, Gjerstad L. Antiepileptic drugs alter reproductive endocrine hormones in men with epilepsy. Eur J Neurol. 2005;12(2):118–24.
14. Røste LS, Taubøll E, Haugen TB, Bjørnenak T, Saetre ER, Gjerstad L. Alterations in semen parameters in men with epilepsy treated with valproate or carbamazepine monotherapy. Eur J Neurol. 2003;10(5):501–6.
15. Currier GW, Simpson GM. Antipsychotic medications and fertility. Psychiatr Serv. 1998;49(2):175–6.
16. Cookson J, Hodgson R, Wildgust HJ. Prolactin, hyperprolactinaemia and antipsychotic treatment: a review and lessons for treatment of early psychosis. J Psychopharmacol. 2012;26(5 Suppl):42–51.
17. Haddad PM, Wieck A. Antipsychotic-induced hyperprolactinaemia: mechanisms, clinical features and management. Drugs. 2004;64(20):2291–314.
18. Howes OD, Wheeler MJ, Pilowsky LS, Landau S, Murray RM, Smith S. Sexual function and gonadal hormones in patients taking antipsychotic treatment for schizophrenia or schizoaffective disorder. J Clin Psychiatry. 2007;68(3):361–7.
19. Koyuncu H, Serefoglu EC, Ozdemir AT, Hellstrom WJ. Deleterious effects of selective serotonin reuptake inhibitor treatment on semen parameters in patients with lifelong premature ejaculation. Int J Impot Res. 2012;24(5):171–3.

20. Safarinejad MR. Sperm DNA, damage and semen quality impairment after treatment with selective serotonin reuptake inhibitors detected using semen analysis and sperm chromatin structure assay. J Urol. 2008;180(5):2124–8.
21. Koyuncu H, Serefoglu EC, Yencilek E, Atalay H, Akbas NB, Sarıca K. Escitalopram treatment for premature ejaculation has a negative effect on semen parameters. Int J Impot Res. 2011;23(6):257–61.
22. Relwani R, Berger D, Santoro N, Hickmon C, Nihsen M, Zapantis A, Werner M, Polotsky AJ, Jindal S. Semen parameters are unrelated to BMI but vary with SSRI use and prior urological surgery. Reprod Sci. 2011;18(4):391–7. Epub 2010 Oct 19.
23. Maier U, Koinig G. Andrological findings in young patients under long-term antidepressive therapy with clomipramine. Psychopharmacology (Berl). 1994; 116(3):357–9.
24. Levin RM, Amsterdam JD, Winokur A, Wein AJ. Effects of psychotropic drugs on human sperm motility. Fertil Steril. 1981;36(4):503–6.
25. Hall E, Burt VK. Male fertility: psychiatric considerations. Fertil Steril. 2012;97(2):434–9.
26. Bhasin S, Cunningham GR, Hayes FJ, Matsumoto AM, Snyder PJ, Swerdloff RS, Montori VM. Testosterone therapy in men with androgen deficiency syndromes: an Endocrine Society clinical practice guideline. J Clin Endocrinol Metab. 2010;95(6):2536–59.
27. Ragni G, De Lauretis L, Bestetti O, Sghedoni D, Gambaro V. Gonadal function in male heroin and methadone addicts. Int J Androl. 1988;11(2):93–100.
28. Whirledge S, Cidlowski JA. Glucocorticoids, stress, and fertility. Minerva Endocrinol. 2010;35(2):109–25.
29. Santen RJ, Kulin HE, Loriaux DL, Friend J. Spironolactone stimulation of gonadotropin secretion in boys with delayed adolescence. J Clin Endocrinol Metab. 1976;43(6):1386–90.
30. Caminos-Torres R, Ma L, Snyder PJ. Gynecomastia and semen abnormalities induced by spironolactone in normal men. J Clin Endocrinol Metab. 1977;45(2): 255–60.
31. Feldman D. Ketoconazole and other imidazole derivatives as inhibitors of steroidogenesis. Endocr Rev. 1986;7(4):409–20.
32. Soriano-Guillén L, Lahlou N, Chauvet G, Roger M, Chaussain JL, Carel JC. Adult height after ketoconazole treatment in patients with familial male-limited precocious puberty. J Clin Endocrinol Metab. 2005; 90(1):147–51.
33. Pont A, Graybill JR, Craven PC, Galgiani JN, Dismukes WE, Reitz RE, Stevens DA. High-dose ketoconazole therapy and adrenal and testicular function in humans. Arch Intern Med. 1984;144(11):2150–3.
34. Wang C, Lai CL, Lam KC, Yeung KK. Effect of cimetidine on gonadal function in man. Br J Clin Pharmacol. 1982;13(6):791–4.
35. Van Thiel DH, Gavaler JS, Heyl A, Susen B. An evaluation of the anti-androgen effects associated with H2 antagonist therapy. Scand J Gastroenterol Suppl. 1987;136:24–8.

36. Iaria G, Urbani L, Catalano G, De Simone P, Carrai P, Petruccelli S, Morelli L, Coletti L, Garcia C, Liermann R, Mosca F, Filipponi F. Switch to tacrolimus for cyclosporine-induced gynecomastia in liver transplant recipients. Transplant Proc. 2005;37(6):2632–3.
37. Ramirez G, Narvarte J, Bittle PA, Ayers-Chastain C, Dean SE. Cyclosporine-induced alterations in the hypothalamic hypophyseal gonadal axis in transplant patients. Nephron. 1991;58(1):27–32.
38. Srinivas M, Agarwala S, Datta Gupta S, Das SN, Jha P, Misro MM, Mitra DK. Effect of cyclosporine on fertility in male rats. Pediatr Surg Int. 1998;13(5–6): 388–91.
39. Seethalakshmi L, Flores C, Diamond DA, Menon M. Reversal of the toxic effects of cyclosporine on male reproduction and kidney function of rats by simultaneous administration of hCG + FSH. J Urol. 1990;144(6):1489–92.
40. Rettori V, De Laurentiis A, Fernandez-Solari J. Alcohol and endocannabinoids: neuroendocrine interactions in the reproductive axis. Exp Neurol. 2010;224(1):15–22.
41. Park B, McPartland JM, Glass M. Cannabis, cannabinoids and reproduction. Prostaglandins Leukot Essent Fatty Acids. 2004;70(2):189–97.
42. Bari M, Battista N, Pirazzi V, Maccarrone M. The manifold actions of endocannabinoids on female and male reproductive events. Front Biosci. 2011;16:498–516.
43. Patra PB, Wadsworth RM. Quantitative evaluation of spermatogenesis in mice following chronic exposure to cannabinoids. Andrologia. 1991;23(2):151–6.
44. Holoch P, Wald M. Current options for preservation of fertility in the male. Fertil Steril. 2011;96(2):286–90.
45. Tromp K, Claessens JJ, Knijnenburg SL, van der Pal HJ, van Leeuwen FE, Caron HN, Beerendonk CC, Kremer LC. Reproductive status in adult male long-term survivors of childhood cancer. Hum Reprod. 2011;26(7):1775–83.
46. Jahnukainen K, Ehmcke J, Hou M, Schlatt S. Testicular function and fertility preservation in male cancer patients. Best Pract Res Clin Endocrinol Metab. 2011;25(2):287–302.
47. Meistrich ML. Male gonadal toxicity. Pediatr Blood Cancer. 2009;53(2):261–6.
48. Abouassaly R, Fossa SD, Giwercman A, Kollmannsberger C, Motzer RJ, Schmoll HJ, Sternberg CN. Sequelae of treatment in long-term survivors of testis cancer. Eur Urol. 2011;60(3):516–26.
49. Kenney LB, Laufer MR, Grant FK, Grier H, Diller L. High risk of infertility and long term gonadal damage in males treated with high dose cyclophosphamide for sarcoma during childhood. Cancer. 2001; 91(3):613–21.
50. van Casteren NJ, van der Linden GH, Hakvoort-Cammel FG, Hählen K, Dohle GR, van den Heuvel-Eibrink MM. Effect of childhood cancer treatment on fertility markers in adult male long-term survivors. Pediatr Blood Cancer. 2009;52(1):108–12.
51. Thomson AB, Campbell AJ, Irvine DC, Anderson RA, Kelnar CJ, Wallace WH. Semen quality and spermatozoal DNA integrity in survivors of childhood

cancer: a case-control study. Lancet. 2002;360(9330): 361–7.
52. Green DM, Kawashima T, Stovall M, Leisenring W, Sklar CA, Mertens AC, Donaldson SS, Byrne J, Robison LL. Fertility of male survivors of childhood cancer: a report from the childhood cancer survivor study. J Clin Oncol. 2010;28:332–9.
53. Sklar C. Reproductive physiology and treatment-related loss of sex hormone production. Med Pediatr Oncol. 1999;33(1):2–8.
54. Heetun ZS, Byrnes C, Neary P, O'Morain C. Review article: reproduction in the patient with inflammatory bowel disease. Aliment Pharmacol Ther. 2007;26(4): 513–33.
55. Alonso V, Linares V, Bellés M, Albina ML, Sirvent JJ, Domingo JL, Sánchez DJ. Sulfasalazine induced oxidative stress: a possible mechanism of male infertility. Reprod Toxicol. 2009;27(1):35–40.
56. Levi AJ, Fisher AM, Hughes L, Hendry WF. Male infertility due to sulphasalazine. Lancet. 1979;2: 276–8.
57. Feagins LA, Kane SV. Sexual and reproductive issues for men with inflammatory bowel disease. Am J Gastroenterol. 2009;104(3):768–73.
58. Zelissen PM, van Hattum J, Poen H, Scholten P, Gerritse R, te Velde ER. Influence of salazosulphapyridine and 5-aminosalicylic acid on seminal qualities and male sex hormones. Scand J Gastroenterol. 1988;23(9):1100–4.
59. French AE, Koren G. Effect of methotrexate on male fertility. Can Fam Physician. 2003;49:577–8.
60. Kalb RE, Strober B, Weinstein G, Lebwohl M. Methotrexate and psoriasis: 2009 National Psoriasis Foundation Consensus Conference. J Am Acad Dermatol. 2009;60(5):824–37.
61. Grunnet E, Nyfors A, Hansen KB. Studies of human semen in topical corticosteroid—treated and in methotrexate-treated psoriatics. Dermatologica. 1977; 154:78–84.
62. Mahadevan U, Terdiman JP, Aron J, Jacobsohn S, Turek P. Infliximab and semen quality in men with inflammatory bowel disease. Inflamm Bowel Dis. 2005;11(4):395–9.
63. Montagna GL, Malesci D, Buono R, Valentini G. Asthenoazoospermia in patients receiving anti-tumour necrosis factor {alpha} agents. Ann Rheum Dis. 2005;64(11):1667.
64. Villiger PM, Caliezi G, Cottin V, Förger F, Senn A, Østensen M. Effects of TNF antagonists on sperm characteristics in patients with spondyloarthritis. Ann Rheum Dis. 2010;69(10):1842–4.
65. Schlegel PN, Chang TS, Marshall FF. Antibiotics: potential hazards to male fertility. Fertil Steril. 1991;55(2):235–42.
66. Crotty KL, May R, Kulvicki A, Kumar D, Neal Jr DE. The effect of antimicrobial therapy on testicular aspirate flow cytometry. J Urol. 1995;153(3 Pt 1): 835–8.
67. Haimov-Kochman R, Ben-Chetrit E. The effect of colchicine treatment on sperm production and function: a review. Hum Reprod. 1998;13(2):360–2.

68. Kastrop P, Kimmel I, Bancsi L, Weima S, Giltay J. The effect of colchicine treatment on spermatozoa: a cytogenetic approach. J Assist Reprod Genet. 1999;16(9):504–7.
69. Kirchin VS, Southgate HJ, Beard RC. Colchicine: an unusual cause of reversible azoospermia. BJU Int. 1999;83(1):156.
70. Benoff S, Cooper GW, Hurley I, Mandel FS, Rosenfeld DL, Scholl GM, Gilbert BR, Hershlag A. The effect of calcium ion channel blockers on sperm fertilization potential. Fertil Steril. 1994;62(3):606–17.
71. Pasqualotto FF, Lucon AM, Sobreiro BP, Pasqualotto EB, Arap S. Effects of medical therapy, alcohol, smoking, and endocrine disruptors on male infertility. Rev Hosp Clin Fac Med Sao Paulo. 2004;59(6):375–82.
72. Hershlag A, Cooper GW, Benoff S. Pregnancy following discontinuation of a calcium channel blocker in the male partner. Hum Reprod. 1995;10(3):599–606.
73. Giuliano F. Impact of medical treatments for benign prostatic hyperplasia on sexual function. BJU Int. 2006;97 Suppl 2:34–8; discussion 44–5.
74. Amory JK, Wang C, Swerdloff RS, Anawalt BD, Matsumoto AM, Bremner WJ, Walker SE, Haberer LJ, Clark RV. The effect of 5alpha-reductase inhibition with dutasteride and finasteride on semen parameters and serum hormones in healthy men. J Clin Endocrinol Metab. 2007;92(5):1659–65.
75. Mirone V, Sessa A, Giuliano F, Berges R, Kirby M, Moncada I. Current benign prostatic hyperplasia treatment: impact on sexual function and management of related sexual adverse events. Int J Clin Pract. 2011;65(9):1005–13.
76. Traish AM, Hassani J, Guay AT, Zitzmann M, Hansen ML. Adverse side effects of 5α-reductase inhibitors therapy: persistent diminished libido and erectile dysfunction and depression in a subset of patients. J Sex Med. 2011;8(3):872–84.
77. Roehrborn CG, Siami P, Barkin J, Damião R, Major-Walker K, Morrill B, Montorsi F. The effects of dutasteride, tamsulosin and combination therapy on lower urinary tract symptoms in men with benign prostatic hyperplasia and prostatic enlargement: 2-year results from the CombAT study. J Urol. 2008;179(2):616–21.
78. Kobayashi K, Masumori N, Kato R, Hisasue S, Furuya R, Tsukamoto T. Orgasm is preserved regardless of ejaculatory dysfunction with selective alpha1A-blocker administration. Int J Impot Res. 2009;21(5):306–10.
79. Francis ME, Kusek JW, Nyberg LM, Eggers PW. The contribution of common medical conditions and drug exposures to erectile dysfunction in adult males. J Urol. 2007;178(2):591–6; discussion 596. Epub 2007 Jun 13.
80. Düsing R. Sexual dysfunction in male patients with hypertension: influence of antihypertensive drugs. Drugs. 2005;65(6):773–86.
81. Manolis A, Doumas M. Antihypertensive treatment and sexual dysfunction. Curr Hypertens Rep. 2012; 14(4):285–92.
82. Doumas M, Douma S. The effect of antihypertensive drugs on erectile function: a proposed management algorithm. J Clin Hypertens (Greenwich). 2006;8(5): 359–64.
83. Cordero A, Bertomeu-Martínez V, Mazón P, Fácila L, Bertomeu-González V, Conthe P, González-Juanatey JR. Erectile dysfunction in high-risk hypertensive patients treated with beta-blockade agents. Cardiovasc Ther. 2010;28(1):15–22.
84. Chang SW, Fine R, Siegel D, Chesney M, Black D, Hulley SB. The impact of diuretic therapy on reported sexual function. Arch Intern Med. 1991;151(12): 2402–8.
85. Montejo AL, Llorca G, Izquierdo JA, Rico-Villademoros F. Incidence of sexual dysfunction associated with antidepressant agents: a prospective multicenter study of 1022 outpatients. Spanish Working Group for the Study of Psychotropic-Related Sexual Dysfunction. J Clin Psychiatry. 2001;62 Suppl 3:10–21.
86. Kikuchi T, Iwamoto K, Sasada K, Aleksic B, Yoshida K, Ozaki N. Sexual dysfunction and hyperprolactinemia in Japanese schizophrenic patients taking antipsychotics. Prog Neuropsychopharmacol Biol Psychiatry. 2012;37(1):26–32.
87. Kim JS, Heo K, Yi JM, Gong EJ, Yang K, Moon C, et al. Genistein mitigates radiation-induced testicular injury. Phytother Res. 2012;26(8):1119–25.
88. Hermann RM, Henkel K, Christiansen H, Vorwerk H, Hille A, Hess CF, Schmidberger H. Testicular dose and hormonal changes after radiotherapy of rectal cancer. Radiother Oncol. 2005;75(1):83–8.
89. Lavranos G, Balla M, Tzortzopoulou A, Syriou V, Angelopoulou R. Investigating ROS sources in male infertility: a common end for numerous pathways. Reprod Toxicol. 2012;34(3):298–307.
90. Sklar CA, Robison LL, Nesbit ME, Sather HN, Meadows AT, Ortega JA, Kim TH, Hammond GD. Effects of radiation on testicular function in long-term survivors of childhood acute lymphoblastic leukemia: a report from the Children Cancer Study Group. J Clin Oncol. 1990;8(12):1981–7.
91. King CR, Lo A, Kapp DS. Testicular dose from prostate cyberknife: a cautionary note. Int J Radiat Oncol Biol Phys. 2009;73(2):636–7.
92. Appelman-Dijkstra NM, Kokshoorn NE, Dekkers OM, Neelis KJ, Biermasz NR, Romijn JA, Smit JW, Pereira AM. Pituitary dysfunction in adult patients after cranial radiotherapy: systematic review and meta-analysis. J Clin Endocrinol Metab. 2011;96(8): 2330–40.
93. Nishi Y, Hamamoto K, Fujita N, Okada S. Empty sella/pituitary atrophy and endocrine impairments as a consequence of radiation and chemotherapy in long-term survivors of childhood leukemia. Int J Hematol. 2011;94(4):399–402.
94. Sathyapalan T, Dixit S. Radiotherapy-induced hypopituitarism: a review. Expert Rev Anticancer Ther. 2012;12(5):669–83.
95. Livesey EA, Brook CG. Gonadal dysfunction after treatment of intracranial tumours. Arch Dis Child. 1988;63(5):495–500.

The Aging Male: Longevity and Subsequent Implications

16

Sonja Grunewald and Uwe Paasch

Introduction

The effects of aging on fertility are complex, as is aging itself. In women, the loss of functional oocytes contributes to sub-/infertility by their late 30s. In men, however, spermatogenesis continues well into advanced ages, thereby allowing men to reproduce until senescence. In recent decades, a social trend of late parenthood has developed, particularly in Western countries. For this reason, many studies have investigated the age-related effects on female fertility issues and the health risks to children. Consequently, methods such as oocyte freezing were developed to maintain female fertility beyond that time frame. Although the impact of age on male fertility is less obvious, in recent years, more data have been published on the age-related ceasing of male reproductive function and the impact to the offspring.

The objective of this chapter is to focus on the implications of advanced age on male fertility. It furthermore aims to support evidence-based counseling of older fathers-to-be with regard to the risks and benefits to reproduction and their offspring.

S. Grunewald, MD (✉) • U. Paasch, MD, PhD
Department of Dermatology, University of Leipzig,
European Training Centre of Andrology,
Philipp-Rosenthal-Straße 23, Leipzig,
Saxony 04103, Germany
e-mail: sonja_grunewald@medizin.uni-leipzig.de

Effect of Age on Male Fertility

Age-Related Effect on Semen Parameters

Many studies have investigated the effect of male aging on standard semen parameters. Not all of these studies have been adjusted for confounding factors, such as abstinence time and smoking habits, amongst others, while some have investigated healthy donors and infertile patients as well. Overall, spermiogram changes are rather minor [1, 2]; in donor populations, the changes are often still within normal limits [3]. Table 16.1 provides an overview.

Apart from the standard spermiogram [3], subcellular markers of sperm quality have also been studied with regard to male aging; most importantly these included sperm DNA damage, apoptosis signaling, and oxidative stress.

Nuclear sperm DNA damage is associated with failed oocyte fertilization, impaired preimplantation development, and poor pregnancy outcomes, whether the insemination is natural or artificial [8]. Multiple large studies have evaluated sperm DNA fragmentation rates with respect to male aging [9]. In a group of 508 male partners of couples attending infertility investigation, Vagnini et al. clearly demonstrated a significant increase in sperm DNA damage by TUNEL assay in men were older than 35 years of age [10]. Similarly, Wyrobek et al. reported a fivefold increase in the percentage of sperm DNA fragmentation in men

---

S.S. du Plessis et al. (eds.), *Male Infertility: A Complete Guide to Lifestyle and Environmental Factors*,
DOI 10.1007/978-1-4939-1040-3_16, © Springer Science+Business Media New York 2014

Table 16.1 Literature overview on age-related effect on standard spermiogram parameters

Spermiogram parameter	Age-related change	Reference	Comment
Semen volume	↓	[4]	Effect is more pronounced in studies adjusted for abstinence time [5]
Sperm concentration	↔/↑	[1, 4, 6]	Slight but significant increase of sperm concentration in large study adjusted for abstinence time [1]
Total sperm count	↔/↓	[1, 4, 6]	
Sperm motility	↔/↓	[1, 7]	In some studies, the age effect on sperm motility appears to be slightly more pronounced in infertile patients; other studies deny such an effect in infertile patients [6]
Sperm morphology	↔/↓	[4, 6, 7]	Study results vary because of different staining protocols and reference values; however, the majority has observed degenerative changes in the germinal epithelium resulting in decreasing amounts of normal-shaped sperm
Sperm vitality	↓	[4]	

Arrows indicate decrease (↓), no change (↔), and increase (↑) of spermiogram parameters, respectively

between 20 and 80 years of age, and Moskovtsev et al. set the threshold for significantly increased sperm DNA damage in a cohort of 1,125 men presenting for fertility evaluations at age 45 (15.2 % DNA fragmentation index in men <30 years vs. 32.0 % in men ≥45 years) [11, 12]. However, the results may depend on the method used for the DNA fragmentation test [13].

Oxidative stress appears to be the most likely culprit for age-related increases in sperm DNA fragmentation. Small amounts of reactive oxygen species (ROS) are necessary for physiological processes, such as capacitation, hyperactivation, and acrosome reaction [14]. However, because of the high content of polyunsaturated fatty acids in their membranes, sperm are particularly susceptible to high oxidative stress levels. Seminal ROS levels are significantly elevated in men older than 40 years [15]. Increased mitochondrial ROS production is associated with cell senescence and a causative factor of aging. Unfortunately, although demonstrated in principal [16], there is a lack of data on sperm mitochondrial ROS production with regard to male age.

Activated sperm apoptosis signaling contributes significantly to male subfertility [17]. In 2010, a small study on 25 healthy volunteers with proven fertility ranging in age from 20 to 68 years showed that advancing male age was associated with increased plasma membrane translocation of phosphatidylserine, as well as with higher DNA fragmentation rates [18]. These findings are supported by data from our own laboratory which proved stronger activation of apoptosis signaling with increasing male age [19].

Age-Related Effect on Reproductive Hormones

Follicle-stimulating hormone (FSH) and inhibin B are important serum markers of spermatogenesis. A recent investigation of a large unselected infertility patient group that included 2,448 men revealed a U-shaped dependence of FSH on age with an optimum at 20–40 years. The same result (inverse U-shaped dependence on age) was found for inhibin B and the inhibin B/FSH ratio (IFR). However, in men with normal spermiogram, there was only a slight increase of serum FSH and a slight decrease of serum inhibin B concentrations ($p > 0.05$) in men older than 40 years [20]. The effects of age on reproductive hormones are rather mild but more prominent in infertility patients with altered spermiogram. The figure displays inhibin B serum levels in regard to age in an unselected population of 2,263 men seeking infertility treatment in our department (Fig. 16.1).

Age-Related Effect on Testosterone and Sexual Function

It is well known from several studies that testosterone levels gradually decline during the male aging process [21]. Sexual dysfunction is

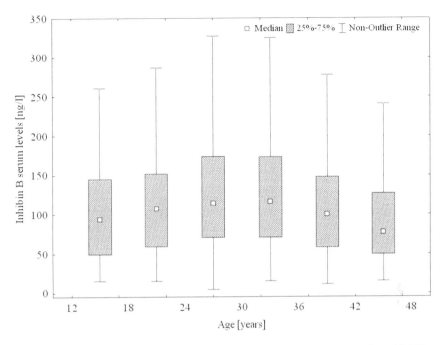

Fig. 16.1 Age-related inhibin B profile: change of inhibin B levels with age in a population of 2,263 non-selected consecutive andrological patients from our clinic

associated with low testosterone levels, and it is also an important determinant of late-onset male hypogonadism [22].

Weight gain in particularly is associated with decreased testosterone levels in middle-aged and older men. Obesity-associated changes in hypothalamic-pituitary-testicular axis hormones are shown to be reversible following weight reduction. For this reason, weight management appears to be important in maintaining circulating testosterone levels in aging men [23].

Although normal testosterone levels are required to regulate spermatogenesis, high testosterone levels suppress spermatogenesis, which is only partially reversible. Testosterone replacement therapy may not be considered in men with milder cases of late-onset male hypogonadism who are still seeking to father a child.

Population-Based Studies and Results from Assisted Reproduction Programs

Numerous studies of natural conceiving couples have suggested an influence of paternal age on pregnancy rates. A data analysis of 8,515 fertile couples from the Avon Longitudinal Study of Pregnancy and Childhood (ALSPAC) revealed that the time to conception was significantly greater in men older than 40 years [5]. Similarly, Hassan et al. documented longer conception times in males older than 45 years in a cohort study of 2,112 consecutive pregnancies. Relative to men younger than 25 years, men older than 45 years were 4.6 times more likely to have had a time to conception of greater than 1 year and 12.5 times more likely to have had a time to pregnancy of more than 2 years [24]. The results of a smaller study of 782 couples underlined the negative impact of advanced paternal age on pregnancy rates but set the critical point of male age as early as 35 years [25].

Although all of the before-mentioned studies have been adjusted for maternal age, other female confounders, such as obesity, diabetes, etc., might have influenced the data. For this reason, the data from assisted reproduction procedures, particularly from oocyte donation programs, might provide more insight.

As expected, the majority of studies from couples undergoing intrauterine insemination (IUI) or in vitro fertilization (IVF)/intracytoplasmic (ICSI) cycles with autologous oocytes (in total over 20,000 cycles) confirmed the data derived from couples with spontaneous conception. Pregnancy rates decreased with advanced paternal age. However, the threshold of age varied between 35 and 50 years [26–30]. Studies from IUI or IVF/ICSI cycles with autologous oocytes have shown different results. No influence of paternal age was detected in one study analyzing 2,204 IUI cycles [31]. Spandorfer et al. analyzed 398 couples undergoing ICSI in which the female partner was younger than 35 years; the authors reported that pregnancy outcomes were not influenced by the age of the male partner [32]. However, this cohort only included nine men younger than 40 years. Another case-control study of 1,024 couples in an ICSI setting did not observe any influence of paternal age in normo-zoospermic patients. In contrast, the same study found that for couples in which the men were oligozoospermic, the chance of pregnancy decreased by 5 % for each year of advanced paternal age [33].

Until now, there have been six studies on the effect of advanced paternal age in oocyte donation programs with >5,000 cycles. Because donor oocytes are generally obtained from young healthy women, age and other maternal confounding factors are reduced to a minimum. Only one of the six studies, which included 1,023 donor oocyte cycles, revealed a significantly decreased live birth rate of approximately −15 % in men older than 50 years [34]. These findings are supported by a study that included 672 cycles and showed lower fertilization as well as implantation rates in men older than 60 years of age [35]. However, both studies did not adjust for the oocyte recipient's age. The other four studies of donor oocyte programs could not show any influence of the paternal age [31, 36, 37]. The most recent investigation included 1,083 couples and adjusted the data for the oocyte recipient's age, but did not observe any effects from the advanced age of the male partner [38].

Paternal Age: Effects in the Offspring?

Paternal Age Effect Disorders

Advanced paternal age has been linked with a higher risk for a small group of rare spontaneous congenital disorders, such as Apert syndrome, achondroplasia, thanatophoric dysplasia, and Costello syndrome—the so-called paternal age effect (PAE) disorders [39, 40]. Recent systematic investigations of mutations in sperm and testes in cases of the PAE disorders revealed that the PAE is mediated through the growth factor receptor-RAS signal transduction pathway. Although the tested PAE mutations rarely arise, they are positively selected and expand clonally in the normal testes of all men. This expansion leads to the relative enrichment of mutant sperm over time and could explain the observed PAE that is associated with these disorders.

The regulation of RAS and other mediators of cellular proliferation and survival is important in many different biological contexts; for example, during tumorigenesis, organ homeostasis, and neurogenesis, the consequences of selfish mutations that hijack this process within the testes might extend far beyond congenital skeletal disorders to include complex diseases, such as neuro-cognitive disorders and cancer predisposition [41]. Although this hypothesis remains highly speculative, there are population-based data suggesting that common complex diseases might be more frequent in the progeny of older fathers. Examples described in the literature include schizophrenia [42], bipolar disorder [43], autism [44], and some cancers [45]. However, the association is not consistent and critically discussed [46–48].

Telomere Hypothesis

We tend to assume that advanced paternal age has rather negative effects on fertility, but as the American Association of Physical Anthropologists has stated: "Older dads have healthier kids than you think" [49].

With every round of cell division, the process of DNA synthesis fails to replicate a small amount of DNA at the chromosome end. Telomeres serve as disposable caps that protect the gene-rich DNA on the interior of the chromosome from this end-replication problem. An insufficient number of telomere repeats leads to chromosome uncapping, cell senescence, and death. The length of telomeres is considered a highly heritable trait; it decreases with age and provides a surrogate marker for biological age [50]. Surprisingly, several large reports have described a positive correlation between paternal age at birth and leukocyte telomere length in the offspring [51, 52].

Conditions in the Aging Male Affecting Reproductive Function

Several specific comorbidities in elderly men influence the reproductive function, most do so by affecting sexual function.

Prostate: Benign Prostatic Hyperplasia and Prostate Cancer

Benign prostatic hyperplasia (BPH) is common in older men, and epidemiological studies have confirmed an association with sexual dysfunction. Moreover, current treatment includes alpha-blockers and 5-alpha reductase inhibitors, which cause the loss of libido, erectile dysfunction, and ejaculatory disorders [53].

Prostate cancer surgery frequently leads to sexual dysfunction. Treatment is difficult although oral phosphodiesterase-5 (PDE5) inhibitors are routinely applied, particularly after nerve-sparing radical prostatectomy [54]. Some studies have shown the beneficial motility effects of sildenafil [55], but the side effects of PDE5 inhibitors are indicative of an acrosome reaction to sildenafil [56] and decreased sperm motility

from tadalafil [57]. However, the fertilization rates in ICSI cycles were not influenced by vardenafil treatment [58]. Published studies have shown that prostatic brachytherapy significantly damages spermatogenesis. Specific semen parameters, such as semen volume, total sperm concentration, and percent sperm motility, were significantly lower than the normal reference values, and high DNA fragmentation (mean 46.4 %) rates occurred [59]. For this reason, semen analysis with sperm cryopreservation should be routinely offered to men with prostate cancer before any therapy, particularly if there is a desire for parenthood.

Hypertension and Atherosclerosis

Hypertension and the resulting pelvic organ atherosclerosis directly impair sexual function [60]. Moreover, erectile dysfunction is a common side effect of antihypertensive drugs, such as thiazide diuretics, beta blockers, spironolactone, and angiotensin-converting enzyme inhibitors, but not loop diuretics [61]. Angiotensin II receptor type-1 blockers are exceptions that may even improve sexual function in hypertensive men [62].

Apart from sexual function, antihypertensive treatment can also impair sperm function. There are several studies demonstrating that calcium channel blockers profoundly affect sperm fertilizing abilities [63]. The effect is reversible. Nifedipine analogues are still discussed as potential nonhormonal male contraceptives [64]. Hypertension itself also may alter sperm quality. A recent pilot study showed significant higher DNA fragmentation rates and clusterin immunolabeling in 25 men with high blood pressure compared to controls [65].

Overweight and Diabetes

On a subcellular level, the ejaculates of diabetic males contain significantly higher levels of sperm with disrupted transmembrane mitochondrial potential, activated caspase-3, ROS, and fragmented DNA when compared to healthy, fertile donors. The effect is particularly pronounced in males with diabetes type-II, a group of patients with increased age and BMI. All measured parameters (activated apoptosis signaling, oxidative stress, and DNA fragmentation) were inversely correlated with the sperm fertilizing potential, indicating a possible mechanism of subfertility in these patients [19]. Furthermore, significantly positive correlations between the spermatozoa exhibiting signs of apoptosis (e.g., sperm with disrupted transmembrane mitochondrial potential and activated caspase-3) or between DNA fragmentations and the clinical parameters of age, abdominal girth, BMI, and HbA1c have been detected [66–68]. In addition to sperm quality, overweight, diabetes, and metabolic syndrome appear to be strongly related to erectile dysfunction as well as hypogonadism [60, 69].

Mental Diseases

The frequency of depressive disorders rises with age. Selective serotonin reuptake inhibitors (SSRI) are the treatment of choice. They adversely affect orgasm, and escitalopram also significantly decreases sperm concentration, motility, and morphology when compared with the baseline semen measures [70]. The same result was found for the tricyclic antidepressant clomipramine [71]. Paroxetine induced abnormal sperm DNA fragmentation without any measurable effect on semen parameters [72]. The fertility potential of a substantial number of men on antidepressants may be adversely affected by these changes.

Discussion and Conclusion

Key Points

In contrast to the relatively abrupt hormonal changes that occur during female menopause, male reproductive function gradually declines during the aging process. Spermiogram changes appear to be rather mild; however, it might be advantageous to check additional parameters, such as the DNA fragmentation rate, for age-related changes. PAE genetic disorders are limited to rare cases. The results of studies on the supposed higher frequency of mental disorders in the offspring of older fathers have been inconsistent, but several diseases that negatively impact fertility and sexual function are frequently seen in aging males, including obesity, diabetes mellitus, hypertension, and prostate disorders. It is important to analyze co-medications and change them accordingly to avoid side effects on male fertility. Recently, studies have also shown the positive effects of late fatherhood (i.e., telomere length increases in the offspring, thereby potentially leading to a higher life expectancy in the next generation).

Strengths and Limitations of This Chapter

Guidelines for evaluating older potential fathers have not been developed, and few studies have evaluated the specific fertility treatment options in men at advanced ages. Moreover, it is difficult to advise couples on the magnitude of the potential risk of abnormalities in the offspring of older men. There is some risk, but the age at which this risk develops is still poorly defined [73].

However, the absolute degree of increased risk appears to be small, and based on current knowledge, this chapter offers a variety of approaches to investigate the older father-to-be more specifically (e.g., sperm DNA fragmentation, monitor ROS levels, apoptosis signaling, optimize co-medication, and counsel the couple with regard to the current scientific literature).

5-Year View

Future Directions for Research

Because of the strong social trend of late childbirth in developed countries and the potential of assisted reproductive techniques to maintain female reproductive function (e.g., egg freezing), future research on age-related male fertility and the effects in the offspring is urgently needed. Such research, including if and how age-related effects can be minimized, is currently under investigation.

The clinical aspects of further research could include the development of specialized embryo testing for PAE disorders as an option in the ART setting. Another approach would be to expand the indications for sperm cryopreservation. Moreover, with regard to the intense discussion in the past, further studies are needed to clarify effects of advanced paternal age on mental health in the offspring (e.g., using larger sibling groups with long time intervals between their births).

One example to minimize age-related effects on male fertility might be the treatment of elevated oxidative stress levels to reduce sperm DNA fragmentation levels. While the benefits of antioxidant supplementation are still under debate [74], better life choices during many years of delay may be one of the keys to fertility preservation. A healthy lifestyle, including healthy food, sports, and avoidance of exposure to toxic pollutants, might protect male fertility [75]. Although this advice to patients improves their health and well-being, more studies are necessary to show the effects on reproductive functions. Another approach is to deplete sperm with high DNA fragmentation (e.g., using an electrophoretic approach) [76]. Sperm with activated apoptosis signaling can be specifically depleted using Annexin V-based techniques, such as the MACS® GMP Annexin V kit (Miltenyi Biotec, Bergisch Gladbach, Germany), which enhances the pregnancy rates in IVF/ICSI programs [77, 78]. This method must be tested to determine whether it also improves pregnancy rates in couples with older male partners.

References

1. Fisch H, Goluboff ET, Olson JH, Feldshuh J, Broder SJ, Barad DH. Semen analyses in 1,283 men from the United States over a 25-year period: no decline in quality. Fertil Steril. 1996;65:1009–14.
2. Rolf C, Behre HM, Nieschlag E. Reproductive parameters of older compared to younger men of infertile couples. Int J Androl. 1996;19:135–42.
3. World Health Organization (WHO). WHO laboratory manual for the examination and processing of human semen. 5th ed. Geneva, Switzerland: WHO; 2010.
4. Ng KK, Donat R, Chan L, Lalak A, Di Pierro I, Handelsman DJ. Sperm output of older men. Hum Reprod. 2004;19:1811–5.
5. Ford WC, North K, Taylor H, Farrow A, Hull MG, Golding J. Increasing paternal age is associated with delayed conception in a large population of fertile couples: evidence for declining fecundity in older men. Hum Reprod. 2000;15:1703–8.
6. Berling S, Wolner-Hanssen P. No evidence of deteriorating semen quality among men in infertile relationships during the last decade: a study of males from Southern Sweden. Hum Reprod. 1997;12:1002–5.
7. Pasqualotto FF, Sobreiro BP, Hallak J, Pasqualotto EB, Lucon AM. Sperm concentration and normal sperm morphology decrease and follicle-stimulating hormone level increases with age. BJU Int. 2005;96: 1087–91.
8. Aitken RJ, De Iuliis GN. Value of DNA integrity assays for fertility evaluation. Soc Reprod Fertil Suppl. 2007;65:81–92.
9. Humm KC, Sakkas D. Role of increased male age in IVF and egg donation: is sperm DNA fragmentation responsible? Fertil Steril. 2013;99:30–6.
10. Vagnini L, Baruffi RL, Mauri AL, Petersen CG, Massaro FC, Pontes A, Oliveira JB, Franco Jr JG. The effects of male age on sperm DNA damage in an infertile population. Reprod Biomed Online. 2007;15:514–9.
11. Wyrobek AJ, Eskenazi B, Young S, Arnheim N, Tiemann-Boege I, Jabs EW, Glaser RL, Pearson FS, Evenson D. Advancing age has differential effects on DNA damage, chromatin integrity, gene mutations, and aneuploidies in sperm. Proc Natl Acad Sci U S A. 2006;103:9601–6.
12. Moskovtsev SI, Willis J, Mullen JB. Age-related decline in sperm deoxyribonucleic acid integrity in patients evaluated for male infertility. Fertil Steril. 2006;85:496–9.
13. Schmid TE, Eskenazi B, Baumgartner A, Marchetti F, Young S, Weldon R, Anderson D, Wyrobek AJ. The effects of male age on sperm DNA damage in healthy non-smokers. Hum Reprod. 2007;22:180–7.
14. de Lamirande E, O'Flaherty C. Sperm activation: role of reactive oxygen species and kinases. Biochim Biophys Acta. 2008;1784:106–15.
15. Cocuzza M, Athayde KS, Agarwal A, Sharma R, Pagani R, Lucon AM, Srougi M, Hallak J. Age-related increase of reactive oxygen species in neat semen in healthy fertile men. Urology. 2008;71:490–4.
16. Koppers AJ, De Iuliis GN, Finnie JM, McLaughlin EA, Aitken RJ. Significance of mitochondrial reactive oxygen species in the generation of oxidative stress in spermatozoa. J Clin Endocrinol Metab. 2008;93:3199–207.
17. Grunewald S, Said TM, Paasch U, Glander HJ, Agarwal A. Relationship between sperm apoptosis signalling and oocyte penetration capacity. Int J Androl. 2008;31:325–30.

18. Colin A, Barroso G, Gomez-Lopez N, Duran EH, Oehninger S. The effect of age on the expression of apoptosis biomarkers in human spermatozoa. Fertil Steril. 2010;94(7):2609–14.
19. Roessner C, Paasch U, Kratzsch J, Glander HJ, Grunewald S. Sperm apoptosis signalling in diabetic men. Reprod Biomed Online. 2012;25:292–9.
20. Grunewald S, Glander HJ, Paasch U, Kratzsch J. Age-dependent inhibin B concentration in relation to FSH and semen sample qualities: a study in 2448 men. Reproduction. 2013;145:237–44.
21. Wang C, Nieschlag E, Swerdloff R, Behre HM, Hellstrom WJ, Gooren LJ, Kaufman JM, Legros JJ, Lunenfeld B, Morales A, Morley JE, Schulman C, Thompson IM, Weidner W, Wu FC. ISA, ISSAM, EAU, EAA and ASA recommendations: investigation, treatment and monitoring of late-onset hypogonadism in males. Int J Impot Res. 2009;21:1–8.
22. Corona G, Rastrelli G, Vignozzi L, Mannucci E, Maggi M. How to recognize late-onset hypogonadism in men with sexual dysfunction. Asian J Androl. 2012;14:251–9.
23. Camacho EM, Huhtaniemi IT, O'Neill TW, Finn JD, Pye SR, Lee DM, Tajar A, Bartfai G, Boonen S, Casanueva FF, Forti G, Giwercman A, Han TS, Kula K, Keevil B, Lean ME, Pendleton N, Punab M, Vanderschueren D, Wu FC. Age-associated changes in hypothalamic-pituitary-testicular function in middle-aged and older men are modified by weight change and lifestyle factors: longitudinal results from the European Male Ageing Study. Eur J Endocrinol. 2013;168:445–55.
24. Hassan MA, Killick SR. Effect of male age on fertility: evidence for the decline in male fertility with increasing age. Fertil Steril. 2003;79 Suppl 3:1520–7.
25. Dunson DB, Colombo B, Baird DD. Changes with age in the level and duration of fertility in the menstrual cycle. Hum Reprod. 2002;17:1399–403.
26. Mathieu C, Ecochard R, Bied V, Lornage J, Czyba JC. Cumulative conception rate following intrauterine artificial insemination with husband's spermatozoa: influence of husband's age. Hum Reprod. 1995;10:1090–7.
27. Belloc S, Cohen-Bacrie P, Benkhalifa M, Cohen-Bacrie M, De MJ, Hazout A, Menezo Y. Effect of maternal and paternal age on pregnancy and miscarriage rates after intrauterine insemination. Reprod Biomed Online. 2008;17:392–7.
28. Klonoff-Cohen HS, Natarajan L. The effect of advancing paternal age on pregnancy and live birth rates in couples undergoing in vitro fertilization or gamete intrafallopian transfer. Am J Obstet Gynecol. 2004;191:507–14.
29. de la Rochebrochard E, de Mouzon J, Thepot F, Thonneau P. Fathers over 40 and increased failure to conceive: the lessons of in vitro fertilization in France. Fertil Steril. 2006;85:1420–4.
30. Aboulghar M, Mansour R, Al-Inany H, Abou-Setta AM, Aboulghar M, Mourad L, Serour G. Paternal age and outcome of intracytoplasmic sperm injection. Reprod Biomed Online. 2007;14:588–92.
31. Bellver J, Garrido N, Remohi J, Pellicer A, Meseguer M. Influence of paternal age on assisted reproduction outcome. Reprod Biomed Online. 2008;17:595–604.
32. Spandorfer SD, Avrech OM, Colombero LT, Palermo GD, Rosenwaks Z. Effect of parental age on fertilization and pregnancy characteristics in couples treated by intracytoplasmic sperm injection. Hum Reprod. 1998;13:334–8.
33. Ferreira RC, Braga DP, Bonetti TC, Pasqualotto FF, Iaconelli Jr A, Borges Jr E. Negative influence of paternal age on clinical intracytoplasmic sperm injection cycle outcomes in oligozoospermic patients. Fertil Steril. 2010;93:1870–4.
34. Frattarelli JL, Miller KA, Miller BT, Elkind-Hirsch K, Scott Jr RT. Male age negatively impacts embryo development and reproductive outcome in donor oocyte assisted reproductive technology cycles. Fertil Steril. 2008;90:97–103.
35. Luna M, Finkler E, Barritt J, Bar-Chama N, Sandler B, Copperman AB, Grunfeld L. Paternal age and assisted reproductive technology outcome in ovum recipients. Fertil Steril. 2009;92:1772–5.
36. Paulson RJ, Milligan RC, Sokol RZ. The lack of influence of age on male fertility. Am J Obstet Gynecol. 2001;184:818–22.
37. Gallardo E, Simon C, Levy M, Guanes PP, Remohi J, Pellicer A. Effect of age on sperm fertility potential: oocyte donation as a model. Fertil Steril. 1996;66:260–4.
38. Whitcomb BW, Turzanski-Fortner R, Richter KS, Kipersztok S, Stillman RJ, Levy MJ, Levens ED. Contribution of male age to outcomes in assisted reproductive technologies. Fertil Steril. 2011;95:147–51.
39. Orioli IM, Castilla EE, Scarano G, Mastroiacovo P. Effect of paternal age in achondroplasia, thanatophoric dysplasia, and osteogenesis imperfecta. Am J Med Genet. 1995;59:209–17.
40. Tolarova MM, Harris JA, Ordway DE, Vargervik K. Birth prevalence, mutation rate, sex ratio, parents' age, and ethnicity in Apert syndrome. Am J Med Genet. 1997;72:394–8.
41. Goriely A, Wilkie AO. Paternal age effect mutations and selfish spermatogonial selection: causes and consequences for human disease. Am J Hum Genet. 2012;90:175–200.
42. Malaspina D. Paternal factors and schizophrenia risk: de novo mutations and imprinting. Schizophr Bull. 2001;27:379–93.
43. Frans EM, Sandin S, Reichenberg A, Lichtenstein P, Langstrom N, Hultman CM. Advancing paternal age and bipolar disorder. Arch Gen Psychiatry. 2008;65:1034–40.
44. Grether JK, Anderson MC, Croen LA, Smith D, Windham GC. Risk of autism and increasing maternal and paternal age in a large north American population. Am J Epidemiol. 2009;170:1118–26.

45. Yip BH, Pawitan Y, Czene K. Parental age and risk of childhood cancers: a population-based cohort study from Sweden. Int J Epidemiol. 2006;35:1495–503.
46. Chen XK, Wen SW, Krewski D, Fleming N, Yang Q, Walker MC. Paternal age and adverse birth outcomes: teenager or 40+, who is at risk? Hum Reprod. 2008;23:1290–6.
47. Petersen L, Mortensen PB, Pedersen CB. Paternal age at birth of first child and risk of schizophrenia. Am J Psychiatry. 2011;168:82–8.
48. Grigoroiu-Serbanescu M, Wickramaratne PJ, Mihailescu R, Prelipceanu D, Sima D, Codreanu M, Grimberg M, Elston RC. Paternal age effect on age of onset in bipolar I disorder is mediated by sex and family history. Am J Med Genet B Neuropsychiatr Genet. 2012;159B:567–79.
49. Gibbons A. American Association of Physical Anthropologists. Older dads have healthier kids than you think. Science. 2012;336:539.
50. Kalmbach KH, Fontes Antunes DM, Dracxler RC, Knier TW, Seth-Smith ML, Wang F, Liu L, Keefe DL. Telomeres and human reproduction. Fertil Steril. 2013;99:23–9.
51. Kimura M, Cherkas LF, Kato BS, Demissie S, Hjelmborg JB, Brimacombe M, Cupples A, Hunkin JL, Gardner JP, Lu X, Cao X, Sastrasinh M, Province MA, Hunt SC, Christensen K, Levy D, Spector TD, Aviv A. Offspring's leukocyte telomere length, paternal age, and telomere elongation in sperm. PLoS Genet. 2008;4:e37.
52. Eisenberg DT, Hayes MG, Kuzawa CW. Delayed paternal age of reproduction in humans is associated with longer telomeres across two generations of descendants. Proc Natl Acad Sci U S A. 2012; 109:10251–6.
53. Mirone V, Sessa A, Giuliano F, Berges R, Kirby M, Moncada I. Current benign prostatic hyperplasia treatment: impact on sexual function and management of related sexual adverse events. Int J Clin Pract. 2011;65:1005–13.
54. Chung E, Brock G. Sexual rehabilitation and cancer survivorship: a state of art review of current literature and management strategies in male sexual dysfunction among prostate cancer survivors. J Sex Med. 2013;10 Suppl 1:102–11.
55. Dimitriadis F, Giannakis D, Pardalidis N, Zikopoulos K, Paraskevaidis E, Giotitsas N, Kalaboki V, Tsounapi P, Baltogiannis D, Georgiou I, Saito M, Watanabe T, Miyagawa I, Sofikitis N. Effects of phosphodiesterase-5 inhibitors on sperm parameters and fertilizing capacity. Asian J Androl. 2008;10:115–33.
56. Glenn DR, McVicar CM, McClure N, Lewis SE. Sildenafil citrate improves sperm motility but causes a premature acrosome reaction in vitro. Fertil Steril. 2007;87:1064–70.
57. Pomara G, Morelli G, Canale D, Turchi P, Caglieresi C, Moschini C, Liguori G, Selli C, Macchia E, Martino E, Francesca F. Alterations in sperm motility after acute oral administration of sildenafil or tadalafil in young, infertile men. Fertil Steril. 2007;88:860–5.
58. Dimitriadis F, Tsampalas S, Tsounapi P, Giannakis D, Chaliasos N, Baltogiannis D, Miyagawa I, Saito M, Takenaka A, Sofikitis N. Effects of phosphodiesterase-5 inhibitor vardenafil on testicular androgen-binding protein secretion, the maintenance of foci of advanced spermatogenesis and the sperm fertilising capacity in azoospermic men. Andrologia. 2012;44 Suppl 1:144–53.
59. Singh DK, Hersey K, Perlis N, Crook J, Jarvi K, Fleshner N. The effect of radiation on semen quality and fertility in men treated with brachytherapy for early stage prostate cancer. J Urol. 2012;187:987–9.
60. Ryan JG, Gajraj J. Erectile dysfunction and its association with metabolic syndrome and endothelial function among patients with type 2 diabetes mellitus. J Diabetes Complications. 2012;26:141–7.
61. Reffelmann T, Kloner RA. Sexual function in hypertensive patients receiving treatment. Vasc Health Risk Manag. 2006;2:447–55.
62. Ferrario CM, Levy P. Sexual dysfunction in patients with hypertension: implications for therapy. J Clin Hypertens (Greenwich). 2002;4:424–32.
63. Enders G. Clinical approaches to male infertility with a case report of possible nifedipine-induced sperm dysfunction. J Am Board Fam Pract. 1997;10:131–6.
64. Waghmare A, Kanyalkar M, Joshi M, Srivastava S. In-vitro metabolic inhibition and antifertility effect facilitated by membrane alteration: search for novel antifertility agent using nifedipine analogues. Eur J Med Chem. 2011;46:3581–9.
65. Muciaccia B, Pensini S, Culasso F, Padula F, Paoli D, Gandini L, Di VC, Bianchini G, Stefanini M, D'Agostino A. Higher clusterin immunolabeling and sperm DNA damage levels in hypertensive men compared with controls. Hum Reprod. 2012;27:2267–76.
66. Amiri I, Karimi J, Piri H, Goodarzi MT, Tavilani H, Khodadadi I, Ghorbani M. Association between nitric oxide and 8-hydroxydeoxyguanosine levels in semen of diabetic men. Syst Biol Reprod Med. 2011; 57:292–5.
67. La Vignera S, Condorelli R, Vicari E, Calogero AE. Negative impact of increased body weight on sperm conventional and non-conventional flow cytometric sperm parameters. J Androl. 2012;33(1):53–8.
68. Karimi J, Goodarzi MT, Tavilani H, Khodadadi I, Amiri I. Relationship between advanced glycation end products and increased lipid peroxidation in semen of diabetic men. Diabetes Res Clin Pract. 2011;91:61–6.
69. Lee RK, Chughtai B, Te AE, Kaplan SA. Sexual function in men with metabolic syndrome. Urol Clin North Am. 2012;39:53–62.
70. Koyuncu H, Serefoglu EC, Yencilek E, Atalay H, Akbas NB, Sarica K. Escitalopram treatment for premature ejaculation has a negative effect on semen parameters. Int J Impot Res. 2011;23:257–61.
71. Maier U, Koinig G. Andrological findings in young patients under long-term antidepressive therapy with clomipramine. Psychopharmacology (Berl). 1994; 116:357–9.

72. Tanrikut C, Feldman AS, Altemus M, Paduch DA, Schlegel PN. Adverse effect of paroxetine on sperm. Fertil Steril. 2010;94:1021–6.
73. Stewart AF, Kim ED. Fertility concerns for the aging male. Urology. 2011;78:496–9.
74. Hamada AJ, Montgomery B, Agarwal A. Male infertility: a critical review of pharmacologic management. Expert Opin Pharmacother. 2012;13:2511–31.
75. Girela JL, Gil D, Johnsson M, Gomez-Torres MJ, De JJ. Semen parameters can be predicted from environmental factors and lifestyle using artificial intelligence methods. Biol Reprod. 2013;88(4):99.
76. Ainsworth C, Nixon B, Jansen RP, Aitken RJ. First recorded pregnancy and normal birth after ICSI using electrophoretically isolated spermatozoa. Hum Reprod. 2007;22:197–200.
77. Grunewald S, Reinhardt M, Blumenauer V, Said TM, Agarwal A, Abu HF, Glander HJ, Paasch U. Increased sperm chromatin decondensation in selected non-apoptotic spermatozoa of patients with male infertility. Fertil Steril. 2009;92:572–7.
78. Dirican EK, Ozgun OD, Akarsu S, Akin KO, Ercan O, Ugurlu M, Camsari C, Kanyilmaz O, Kaya A, Unsal A. Clinical outcome of magnetic activated cell sorting of non-apoptotic spermatozoa before density gradient centrifugation for assisted reproduction. J Assist Reprod Genet. 2008;25: 375–81.

Index

A
Abamectin, 185–186
Acrosin, 21
Adipocytokines, 32, 38
Adipose tissue
    adipocytokines, 32
    aromatase cytochrome p450, 41
    suprapubic region, 42
    THC, 94
ADMA. *See* Asymmetric dimethylarginine (ADMA)
Age
    alcohol consumption, 84
    comorbidities (*see* Age-related comorbidities)
    cryptorchidism and hypospadias, 199–200
    diapers, 114, 115
    glucocorticoids, 232
    paternal, 250–251
    population-based studies, 249–250
    prostate cancer, 203
    reproductive hormones, 248
    semen parameters, 247–248
    strengths and limitations, 252
    testosterone and sexual function, 248–249
Age-related comorbidities
    BPH and prostate cancer, 251
    hypertension and atherosclerosis, 251
    mental diseases, 252
    overweight and diabetes, 251–252
ALA. *See* Alpha-lipoic acid (ALA)
Alcohol consumption
    adults, 84
    chronic diseases, 83
    description, 83
    ethanol-induced oxidative stress, 85
    GST M1 genotype, 88–89
    male reproduction, 87–89
    prenatal exposure, 85
    semen parameters and spermatozoa, 85–87
    and smoking, 83
    testicular lipid peroxidation, 85
    vitamin A, 85
    world population, 84
    xanthine dehydrogenase, 85
    Zn and Mg, 89
Alexithymia, 143

Alkylphenols, 197
Alpha-lipoic acid (ALA), 74–76
5-Aminosalicylic acid (5-ASA), 236
Anabolic steroids
    marijuana, 100, 101
    resistance training, 49
    supraphysiological doses, 100
    testosterone, 100
Androgenic-anabolic steroids (AAS)
    definition, 99
    oral administration, 99
    resistance training, 50
Anejaculation, 145, 147, 239
Antibiotics
    adverse effects, 237
    antitumor, 234
    epididymitis, 132
    erythromycin and gentamicin, 237
    tetracycline and nitrofurantoin, 237
    U. urealyticum, 133
Antihypertensives
    beta-blockers, 240
    classes, 239
    diuretics, 240
Antioxidants
    DNA damage, 164
    endogenous and exogenous, 62
    glutathione, 69
    and histone kinase, 171
    human semen, 22
    indirect/direct activity, 64
    and L-arginine, 66
    properties, 62
    psychological stress, 153
    RCTs, 72
    and ROS, 26, 32, 217
    SOD, 150
    spermatozoa, 25–26
    superoxide anion and peroxide (H_2O_2), 153
    and supplementation, 75–76
    testicular, 168
    vitamin A, 75
Antipsychotics, 230–231, 240
Antisperm antibodies (ASA), 127, 130, 131
5-α reductase inhibitors, 238–239

S.S. du Plessis et al. (eds.), *Male Infertility: A Complete Guide to Lifestyle and Environmental Factors*,
DOI 10.1007/978-1-4939-1040-3, © Springer Science+Business Media New York 2014

Index

Aromatase
    cytochrome p450, 34
    inhibitors, 41–42, 50
    LH, 194
ART. *See* Assisted reproductive technique (ART)
ASA. *See* Antisperm antibodies (ASA)
5-ASA. *See* 5-Aminosalicylic acid (5-ASA)
Ascorbic acid, 22, 89
Assessing testicular temperature
    accuracy and reproducibility, 109
    continuous measurements, 112
    methods, 109–111
    single/discontinuous measurements, 109, 112
Assisted reproductive technique (ART)
    diet and obesity, 63
    glutathione, 69
    IVF and ICSI, 220
    pentoxifylline, 71
    smoking, 27
Asymmetric dimethylarginine (ADMA), 38

B

Bakers, 117
Benign prostatic hyperplasia (BPH), 238, 239, 251
Biocides, 199
Bisphenol-A (BPA), 195, 198
Blood-testis barrier (BTB), 162, 163
Body mass index (BMI)
    classification, 31–32
    leptin levels, 37
    reproductive system, 35–36
    ROS and semen quality, 32
    semen quality, 63
    sperm parameters, 32–35
    and WHO, 31
BPA. *See* Bisphenol-A (BPA)
BPH. *See* Benign prostatic hyperplasia (BPH)
BTB. *See* Blood-testis barrier (BTB)

C

Calcium channel blockers, 237–238
Cannabidiol (CBD), 94, 95
Cannabinol (CBN), 6, 94, 95
Carbaryl, 183
Carcinogens, 6, 20
Catecholamines, 23, 95, 152
CBD. *See* Cannabidiol (CBD)
CBN. *See* Cannabinol (CBN)
Cell phones
    description, 161
    male reproduction (*see* Male reproductive system)
    radiation, intracellular effects, 165, 166
    SAR, 164–165
    sound waves, 164
Cellular stress, 163–164
Ceramic oven operators, 117
Chewing (smokeless) tobacco, 23–24
Chlamydia trachomatis, 132–133

Chlordane, 183
Chlorpyrifos, 184
Cigarette smoking
    ART, 27
    carcinogens, 20
    chromosomal damage, 23
    description, 19
    DNA fragmentation, 24
    gaseous and particulate phases, 19–20
    main stream and sidestream, 20
    male reproductive system, 20, 21
    prenatal tobacco exposure, 24
    RNS and OS, 22–23
    ROS (*see* Reactive oxygen species (ROS))
    semen parameters, 20
    seminal plasma and sex glands, 21–22
    spermatozoa, 20–21
    toxic compound and hormone mechanisms, 26–27
    varicoceles, 23
Cimetidine, 233
Clothing, 112, 114
Clusterin, 40, 42, 194, 251
Cobalamin (vitamin B12), 67–68
Cocaine
    coca plant, 98
    human spermatozoa, 98
    hydrochloride, 98
    lifestyle factors, 202
    testicular function, 100
Co-enzyme Q10 (CoQ10), 68
Colchicine, 237
Cryptorchidism
    and hypospadias, 199–200
    Sertoli and Leydig cells, 109
    supra-scrotal position, 109
    testicular hyperthermia, 108
    TGCT, 203
    UDT, 200–201
CuZn-SODs, 26
Cyclosporine, 233

D

DBCP. *See* 1,2-Dibromo-3-chloropropane (DBCP)
DDT. *See* Dichlorodiphenyltrichloroethane (DDT)
Delayed ejaculation, 146–147
Delta-9-tetrahydrocannabinol (THC)
    CB1 receptor, 96
    endo-cannabinoids, 95
    lipid soluble compound, 94
    marijuana, 233
DETP. *See* Diethylthiophosphate (DETP)
Diapers, 114–115
1,2-Dibromo-3-chloropropane (DBCP), 183–184
Dichlorodiphenyltrichloroethane (DDT)
    alkylphenols, 197
    BPA, 198
    exposure and semen parameters, 182–183
    NP, 197–198
    POPs, 197

Index

Diet
- and exercise, 40
- lifestyle, 196
- low-fat, 56
- and obesity, 63–64
- plant and animal origin, 99
- radionuclides, 215

Diethylthiophosphate (DETP), 184

Difference gel electrophoresis (DIGE) technique, 40

Dimethylphosphate (DMP), 184

DMP. *See* Dimethylphosphate (DMP)

DNA fragmentation
- blood pressure, 251
- fertility evaluations, 247–248
- oxidative stress, 248, 253
- paroxetine, 252
- phosphatidylserine, 248

Drug abuse
- cocaine, 98
- creatine and steroids, 99–100
- male infertility (*see* Male infertility)
- marijuana, 94–96
- methamphetamine and MDMA, 97–98
- opioids, 96–97

E

EBV. *See* Epstein-Barr virus (EBV)

Ecstasy, 94, 97

ED. *See* Erectile dysfunction (ED)

EDCs. *See* Endocrine disrupting chemicals (EDCs)

Ejaculatory dysfunctions
- anejaculation, 147
- delayed ejaculation, 146–147
- description, 145–146
- premature ejaculation (PE), 146
- retrograde ejaculation, 146

Electromagnetic waves (EMWs)
- absorption process, 162
- BTB, 163
- calcium ions and PKC, 162–163
- cell phone effects (*see* Cell phones)
- cellular stress, 163–164
- computational analysis, 171–172
- description, 161
- DNA damage, 164
- oxidative stress, 164
- thermal effects, 162

Electroporation, 162

Emotional behavior
- alexithymia, 143
- depression, anxiety and sleep disturbance, 142
- donor insemination, 142
- grief, 142
- self-esteem, 142–143
- sexual adequacy, 143
- stigma, 143

EMWs. *See* Electromagnetic waves (EMWs)

Endocrine disrupting chemicals (EDCs)
- definition, 193
- dose responses, 195
- exposure, 196–197
- HPG axis, 194–195
- humans and wildlife, 195–196
- mechanisms and mode of action, 193–194
- metals and metalloids, 199
- MRH, 199–204
- vulnerable periods, 195

Endurance and ultra-endurance exercise
- hormonal effects, 51–53, 56
- oxidative stress biomarkers and DNA damage, 54–57
- seminological effects
  - athletes, 53, 54
  - ED, 54
  - ironman triathletes, 54
  - runners, 53
  - semen parameters, 56
  - sperm morphology, cycling, 53–54
  - training modalities, 54

Environmental factors
- clothing, 114
- diapers, 114–115
- nuclides, 216
- posture, 112
- radionuclides, 214, 216
- sitting, 112–114
- tight underwear, boxers and Jockey shorts, 114
- uranium, 214, 216

Epidemiology
- anti-endocrine disruptor theory, 2
- cryptorchidism and hypospadias, 1
- estrogen-like activity, 4
- fertile and subfertile men, 7
- GU, 9–10
- human sperm production
  - cigarette smoking, 6
  - factors, 6
  - marijuana, 6
  - semen quality, 5
- male reproduction system, 7–9
- meta-analysis, 4
- semen analysis, 6
- seminal parameters, 2–3
- sperm count, 4, 5
- WHO guidelines, 7

Epididymal epithelium, 26

Epididymitis, 131, 132

Epididymo-orchitis, 131

Eppin protein complex (EPC) proteins, 40, 42

Epstein-Barr virus (EBV), 134

Erectile dysfunction (ED)
- adipocytokines, 38
- cycling, 54
- obesity-induced pathways, 38–39
- physical barriers, 39
- psychological stress, 145
- psychosexual disorders, 144
- reflex and psychogenic erection, 145
- renin-angiotensin system, 38
- sexual activity, 38

Erectile dysfunction (ED) (*cont.*)
    subconscious memory, 145
    and testicular temperature, 42
Estrogen
    anti-androgenic activity, 197
    BPA, 198
    cytochrome p450 aromatase enzyme, 34
    environmental, 8–9
    LH secretion, 34
    pesticides, 181–182
    and spermatogenesis, 41, 42
    and testosterone (*see* Testosterone)
Ethylparathion (EP), 184
Exposures
    EMWs (*See* Electromagnetic waves (EMWs))
    heat (*see* Scrotal heat stress)
    heavy metals (*see* Heavy metals)
    lifestyle, 196–197
    non-occupation, 196
    occupation, male reproduction, 7–9, 196
    prenatal tobacco, 24
    travel and recreation, 196

F
Factors affecting testicular temperature, 118–121
Febrile episodes, 108
Folic acid (vitamin B9), 68–69, 75, 76
Follicle-stimulating hormone (FSH)
    cadmium, 186
    environmental estrogens, 9
    gonadal steroidogenesis, 231
    and inhibin B levels, 185, 248
    and LH (*see* Luteinizing hormone (LH))
    nonsmokers, 27
    pituitary hormone, 218–219
    and testosterone production, 37
FSH. *See* Follicle-stimulating hormone (FSH)

G
Genitourinary (GU)
    Chlamydia trachomatis, 132–133
    cryopreservation, 1
    epididymo-orchitis, 132
    genetic factors, 1
    genital ureaplasmas and mycoplasmas, 133
    inflammation and infections, 127
    leukocytes, 130
    Mollicutes, 133–134
    Neisseria gonorrhoeae, 132
    neoplasms, 9
    sperm counts, 10
    testicular cancer, 9
Ghrelin, 37
Glucocorticoids
    athletes, 52–53
    cortisol, 151
    testosterone levels, 232
    TSH, 152

Glutathione
    class and mechanism, 69
    data supporting use, 69
    GPX, 26, 62, 72, 107, 168
    GST M1 genotype, 88–89
    intramuscular administration, 69
    and polyenoic fatty acids, 85
Glutathione peroxidases (GPX), 26
Glutathione *S*-transferase (GST) M1 genotype, 88–89
GnRH. *See* Gonadotropin-releasing hormone (GnRH)
Golgi-phase spermatids, 23
Gonadotoxic
    BTB, 163
    chemotherapeutic medications, 234–235
    methotrexate, 236
    sulfasalazine, 236
Gonadotropin-releasing hormone (GnRH)
    anterior pituitary, 218
    antiandrogens, 229, 241
    antipsychotics, 240
    beta-endorphins, 152
    CRH, 152
    and exogenous dopamine, 51
    exogenous hormones, 229, 241
    gonadal steroidogenesis, 231
    hypothalamus, 34, 41, 49, 218
    marijuana, 95
    MDMA, 97
    pituitary gonadotrophs, 34
    serum testosterone, 51
    sperm parameters, 41
GPX. *See* Glutathione peroxidases (GPX)
GU. *See* Genitourinary (GU)

H
HAART. *See* Highly active antiretroviral therapy (HAART)
Heat shock proteins (HSP), 107, 116
Heavy metals
    arsenic, 188
    cadmium, 186–187
    creatine kinase (CK) enzyme, 186
    human population, 186
    lead, 187
    manganese, 188
    mercury, 187–188
    molybdenum, 188
Herpes simplex virus (HSV), 130, 134–135
Highly active antiretroviral therapy (HAART), 134, 135
HIV. *See* Human immunodeficiency virus (HIV)
Homeostatic effects
    cellular/molecular changes, 153
    description, 148–149
    hormonal changes, 150–152
    L-arginine–NO pathway, 149–150
    neurotransmitters, 152–153
Hormones
    acute and chronic effects, 56
    androgens, 56

Index

aromatase, 34
CNS, 150–151
CRH, 152
depression, 150
FSH and inhibin B, 248, 249
FT/TT, 51
ghrelin, 37
GnRH, 34
gonadotrophin and prolactin, 152
HPA and HPT axes, 151
HPG axis, 34
inhibin B levels, 37–38
leptin, 34, 36–37
LH, 34
mechanisms and toxic compound, 26–27
obesity, 249
PRL and LH, 51
qualitatively and quantitatively, spermatogenesis, 51
reproductive hormones and semen quality, 51
resistance exercise, 50
resistin, 38
SHBG, 56
testosterone and estrogen, 34, 37, 152
ultra-endurance exercise, 52–53, 56
Hot baths, 116
HPG axis. *See* Hypothalamic–pituitary–gonadal
(HPG) axis
HPV. *See* Human papillomaviruses (HPV)
Human immunodeficiency virus (HIV), 134
Human papillomaviruses (HPV), 135
Hypogonadism
glucocorticoids, 232
hypogonadotropic, 42, 50, 94, 241
Leydig cell injury, 242
overweight and diabetes, 252
prevalence, opioids, 231, 232
prolactin, 231
testosterone, 229, 249
Hypopituitarism, 242–243
Hypothalamic–pituitary–gonadal (HPG) axis
AAS, 50
epilepsy, 229
estrogen, 41
glucocorticoids, 232
hormonal feedback relationships, 194
methamphetamine and MDMA, 97
prolactin, 194–195
Sertoli cells, 194
sex determination, 194
SSRIs, 231
testosterone, 49

I

IBD. *See* Inflammatory bowel disease (IBD)
ICSI. *See* Intracytoplasmic sperm injection (ICSI)
iGH. *See* Immunoreactive growth hormone (iGH)
Immunoreactive growth hormone (iGH), 55–56
Infertility. *See* Male infertility
Inflammatory bowel disease (IBD)

antibiotics, 237
calcium channel blockers, 237–238
colchicine, 237
description, 235–236
infliximab, 236–237
sulfasalazine and methotrexate, 236
Infliximab, 236–237
Intracytoplasmic sperm injection (ICSI), 63, 67, 220, 250
Ionizing radiation (IR)
artificial sources
diagnosis and therapy, 213–214
diet, 215–216
environmental factors, 216
occupational exposure, 215
definition, 212
dose and duration, 220
hypothalamic-anterior pituitary-testicular axis,
218–219
molecular injury, 218
natural sources
cosmic rays, 212–214
description, 212, 213
environmental factors, 214
OS, 216–217
spermatogenesis, 217–218
treatment, 219–220
UMI prevalence, 211
IR. *See* Ionizing radiation (IR)

K

Ketoconazole, 232
Kisspeptin, 34, 37, 194

L

LAC. *See* L-Acetyl carnitine (LAC)
L-Acetyl carnitine (LAC), 66–67
Laptop computers
nonthermal effects, 170
portable computers, 169
thermal effects, 169–170
L-Arginine, 66, 76
L-Arginine–NO pathway, 149–150
L-Ascorbic acid, 72–73
LC. *See* L-Carnitine (LC)
L-Carnitine (LC), 66–67, 76
Leptin
and adiponectin, 32
BBB, 34, 36
BTB, 34
description, 34
and insulin, 40, 42
kisspeptin, 37, 194
Leydig cells, 34
NPY, 37
OS, 32
receptors, 34
and testosterone, 37
LH. *See* Luteinizing hormone (LH)

Lifestyle factors
  cycling, 116
  diagnosis and therapy, 213–214
  diet, 215–216
  environmental factors, 216
  hot baths, 116
  industrial development, 211
  laptop usage, 116
  obesity, 115
  occupational exposure, 215
  sauna, 115–116
Lipid peroxidation
  alcohol abuse, 88
  and ATP depletion, 150
  membrane injury and gonadal dysfunction, 85
  ROS, 25, 61
Lower urinary tract symptoms (LUTS)
  alpha-blockers, 239
  5-α reductase inhibitors, 238–239
Luteinizing hormone (LH)
  cocaine, 98
  and FSH, 34, 49, 50, 87
  interstitial cell stimulating hormone, 218
  Leydig cells, 53, 194
  marijuana, 231
  opiates, 234
  opioids, 96
  pituitary gland, 51
  and PRL, 51
  and prolactin, 27, 34
  spermatogenesis, 219
  testosterone and estrogen, 34, 219
LUTS. *See* Lower urinary tract symptoms (LUTS)

M
Male accessory gland infection (MAGI), 131–132
Male fertility
  aging, 247–253
  epidemiology and evidence, 1–11
  nutrition, 63–74
  physical exercise, 47–57
Male infertility
  alcohol consumption, 83–90
  BMI, 31–43
  and cell phones, 164–169
  drug abuse
    hormone replacement therapy, 101
    pre and common testicular, 94
    reproductive damage, 100
    sperm transport, 100
    substance abuse, 94, 95
  EMWs (*see* Electromagnetic waves (EMWs))
  laptop computers, 169–170
  microwaves, 170–171
  obesity, 31–43
  and psychological stress (*see* Psychological stress)
  smoking, 19–28
Male reproductive health (MRH)
  DNA damage, 202

hypospadias, 199–200
male infertility, 201
prostate cancer, 203
sperm count, 201–202
sperm morphology, 202
sperm motility, 202
systemic diseases and ejaculatory dysfunction, 204
TDS, 203
testicular cancer, 201
UDT, 200–201
Male reproductive system
  adipocytokines, 32
  apoptosis, 168
  chronic alcohol consumption, 154
  EMW, 162
  environmental pollution and factors, 9
  estrogen hypothesis, 9
  germ-cell differentiation, 8
  histopathological changes, 168–169
  IR, 217–221
  Leydig cells, 169
  OS (*see* oxidative stress (OS))
  pituitary gland, 169
  potential effects, 172
  radiation-induced oxidative stress, 216–217
  semen quality (*see* Semen quality)
  spermatogenesis, 7
  spermatozoa, 22
  sperm DNA damage, 167, 168
  steroidogenesis and testosterone secretion, 37
  TDS, 8
  xenobiotics, 8
Malnutrition, 9, 64
Marijuana
  cannabinoids, 96
  cannabis plant, 94
  CBN and CBD, 95
  GnRH, 95
  hypo-androgenism, 233
  recreational drug, 95
  seminal fluid leukocytes, 6
  testes and germ cells, 96
  testosterone, 233
  THC, 94, 233
MBP. *See* Monobutyl phthalate (MBP)
MDMA. *See* 3, 4-Methylenedioxymethamphetamine
    (MDMA)
Mechanism of heat stress, 106–108
Medications
  drug classes, 227–229
  post-testicular, 238–241
  pre-testicular, 229–233
  testicular, 234–238
Mental diseases, 252
Methamidophos, 184
Methamphetamine, 97–98
Methotrexate, 236
3, 4-Methylenedioxymethamphetamine (MDMA), 97–98
Microwaves
  antioxidant enzymes and histone kinase, 171

cell cycle regulatory enzymes, 164
description, 161, 172
Leydig cells, 171
SAR levels, 171
thermal and nonthermal effects, 170
Mild scrotal heating, 118
Modulating factors, psychological stress, 153–154
Mollicutes, 133–134
Monobutyl phthalate (MBP), 185, 198, 202
Morphology
alcohol consumption, 86
altered semen characteristics, 131
cell phone radiation exposure, 167
cigarette smoke, 20
fasalazine's gonadotoxic effects, 236
glutathione, 69
high temperature exposure, 108
laptop Wi-Fi exposure, 170
LC and LAC, 66
NAC, 70
newborns, 54
OS, 63
selenium and Vitamin E, 72, 73
sperm axonemes, 21
sperm characteristics, 32
SSRIs, 231
TCAs, 231
urinary MBP levels and MBzP levels, 202
vitamin A supplementation, 88
vitamin C and E, 73
Motility
BMI, 33
cell phone radiation exposure, 167
cobalamin (vitamin B12), 67
CoQ10, 68
DDT, 183
glutathione, 69
HPV, 135
L-arginine, 66
LC and LAC, 66–67
lifestyle, 115
MDMA, 97
mitochondrial energy, 133
NAC, 70
NO, 149, 150
pentoxifylline, 71
percentage, 6
PKC, 163
selenium, 72
sperm DNA integrity, 32
SSRI, 231
vitamin C and E, 73–74
MRH. *See* Male reproductive health (MRH)

N
N-Acetyl cysteine (NAC), 70, 76
National Toxicology Program (NTP), 195
Neisseria gonorrhoeae (NG), 132
Neuropeptide Y (NPY), 37

Neurotransmitters, 152–153
Nicotine
cigarettes and produce free radicals, 6
receptors, 20
and tar, 19–20
Non-monotonic dose response curves (NMDRCs), 195
Nonylphenol (NP), 197–198
NTP. *See* National Toxicology Program (NTP)
Nutrition
ALA, 75
antioxidant efficacy, 75–76
cobalamin (vitamin B12), 67–68
CoQ10, 68
deficiencies, 64
diet and obesity, 63–64
folic acid (vitamin B9), 68–69
glutathione, 69
LAC, 66–67
L-arginine, 66
LC, 66–67
lycopene, 69–70
malnutrition, 64
NAC, 70
pentoxifylline, 70–71
PUFAs, 71
RCTs, 64, 75
selenium, 72
spermatozoa, 21
supplementation, 64–66
vitamin A and D, 75
vitamin C, 72–73
vitamin E, 73–74
zinc, 74

O
Obesity
adipocytokines, 32
adipose tissue, 32
definition, 31
and diet, 63–64
fertility outcomes, 62
hormonal abnormalities (*see* Hormones)
lifestyle modifications
aromatase inhibitors, 41–42
bariatric surgery, 41
environmental factors, 40
gastric bypass, 41
natural/surgical weight loss, 40–41
scrotal lipectomy, 41
sperm parameters, 41
low testosterone level, 154
physical effects
erectile dysfunction, 38–39
heat stress, 39–40
scrotal temperature, 39
testicular temperature, 39
and proteomics, 40
ROS, 32
scrotal hyperthermia, 115

Obesity (*cont.*)
scrotal lipomatosis, 115
  sperm parameters and reproductive potential
    BMI, 33–36
    characteristics, 32–33
    hip and waist circumference, 33
    overweight and obese men, 33
  testicular temperatures, 115
Occupational exposure
  bakers, 117
  BPA, 198
  IR, 215
  lead, 187
  male reproduction system, 7–9
Occupational risk factors
  ambient temperature and seasonality, 117–118
  bakers, 117
  ceramic oven operators, 117
  professional drivers, 117
  submariners, 117
  welders, 116
Oligospermia
  and azoospermia, 20
  cimetidine, 233
  colchicine, 237
  lycopene, 70
  marijuana, 233
  NAC, 70
  opiates, 232
  and teratospermia, 148
Opiates, 231–232
Opioids
  intrathecal, oral and transdermal, 231
  LH, 96
  poppy plant, 96
  spermatozoa, 97
  testosterone, 231
Organochlorine pesticides, 182–184
Organophosphate pesticides, 184
OS. *See* Oxidative stress (OS)
Oxidative stress (OS)
  antioxidants and ROS species, 217
  biomarkers and DNA damage, 54–57
  cellular components, 216–217
  cigarette smoking, 22–23
  CoQ10, 68
  and DNA fragmentation, 164, 168
  8-hydroxy-2′-deoxyguanasine (8-OH-2G), 167
  mitochondrial membrane potential (MMP), 164
  ROS and antioxidant defense mechanisms, 32
  spermatozoa, 164
  vitamins C and E, 167–168

P
PAE. *See* Paternal age effect (PAE)
PAHs. *See* Polycyclic aromatic hydrocarbons (PAHs)
Paraquat, 184
Paternal age effect (PAE)
  disorders, 250, 252, 253
  telomere hypothesis, 250–251

PCBs. *See* Polychlorinated biphenyls (PCBs)
Penile erection, 145
Pentoxifylline, 70–71, 76
Persistent organic pollutants (POPs), 197
Pesticides
  abamectin, 185–186
  antiandrogenic/estrogenic properties, 181–182
  non-persistent, 199
  organochlorine, 182–184
  organophosphate, 184, 199
  phthalates, 184–185
  TDS hypothesis, 182
  types, 181, 182
  uses, 198–199
Phthalates
  DEHP and DBP, 185
  dust particles, vinyl tiles, 196
  metabolites, 198
  monobutyl, dose–response relationships, 185
  and PCBs, 185
  solvents, additives and plasticizers, 198
  urinary concentrations, 185
Physical exercise
  catabolic and oxidation events, 48
  description, 47
  endurance (*see* Endurance and ultra-endurance
    exercise)
  GnRH, 49
  HPG axis, 49
  LH and FSH, 49
  muscle contraction, 48
  negative effects, 49
  parameters, 48–49
  positive effects, 55
  resistance (*see* Resistance exercise)
  strength training, 48
  training density and intensity, 49
  training load, 48
PKC. *See* Protein kinase C (PKC)
Polychlorinated biphenyls (PCBs)
  congeners and cadmium, 203
  and MBP, 185
  PCB-153 concentration, 183
  sealants and insulating agents, 197
  semen parameters, 183
  UDT, 200
Polycyclic aromatic hydrocarbons (PAHs), 26–27
Polyunsaturated fatty acids (PUFAs), 71, 218
POPs. *See* Persistent organic pollutants (POPs)
Post-testicular
  antidepressant-related sexual dysfunction, 240–241
  antihypertensives, 239–240
  antipsychotics, 240
  exogenous hormones, antiandrogens and GnRH
    agonists, 241
  LUTS, 238–239
  mechanisms, 228
Pregnancy
  ART, 63
  CoQ10, 68
  IVF, 133

L-arginine, 66
LC and LAC, 66
methotrexate, 236
NAC, 70
prolactin, 194
rates, 75
vitamin E, 73
Premature ejaculation (PE), 86, 146, 231
Pre-testicular
antiepileptics, 229
exogenous hormones, antiandrogens and GnRH
agonists, 229, 230
glucocorticoids, 232
miscellaneous drugs, endocrine disturbances,
232–233
opiates, 231–232
psychotherapeutic agents, 229–231
Professional drivers, 117
Protein kinase C (PKC), 163, 166
Proteomics, 40
Psychological stress
counseling and behavioral therapy, 155
description, 141–142
emotional behavior, 142–143
homeostatic effects, 148–153
manifestations, 142
modulating factors, 153–154
reproductive function, 143–148
treatment, 154–155
PUFAs. *See* Polyunsaturated fatty acids (PUFAs)

R
Radiation
cell phones (*see* Cell phones)
chemotherapy, 241
EMWs (*see* Electromagnetic waves (EMWs))
germinal epithelium, 241–242
hypopituitarism, 242–243
IR (*see* Ionizing radiation (IR))
Leydig cells, 242
microwaves, 170–171
nonionizing, 169
Reactive nitrogen species (RNS), 22–23
Reactive oxygen species (ROS)
cigarette smoking, 22–23
CuZn-SODs, 26
dietary supplementation, 62
and DNA, 26
endogenous and exogenous antioxidants, 62
epididymal epithelium, 26
GPX, 26
interleukins (IL-6 and IL-8), 26
leukocytes, 130
obesity and BMI, 32
OS gene families, 26
production, 61
and RCTs, 62–63
scavengers, 26
seminal plasma and spermatozoa, 61–62
spermatozoa, 25–26

and sperm motility, NO level, 149, 150
vitamins, minerals and fatty acids, 62
Reproductive function
anejaculation, 147
ejaculatory dysfunctions, 145–147
erectile dysfunctions, 145
loss of libido, 145
male sexual cycle, phases, 143–144
oligospermia and teratospermia, 148
psychosexual disorders, 144
sperm parameters, 147–148
Resistance exercise
hormonal effects, 50
iGH, 55–56
muscle adaptation, 55
seminological effects, 50
steroids, 49
testosterone, 55
TT and FT, 55
Resistance training, 50, 55
Retrograde ejaculation, 145, 146
RNS. *See* Reactive nitrogen species (RNS)
ROS. *See* Reactive oxygen species (ROS)

S
SA. *See* Semen analysis (SA)
Saunas, 115–116
Scrotal cooling, 118, 119
Scrotal heat stress
lifestyle, 115–116
measurement, methods, 109–112
mechanisms, germ cell apoptosis, 106–108
risk factors, 112–115
scrotal cooling, 118
semen parameters, 108
testicular thermoregulation, 105–106
varicocele, 109
Scrotal lipectomy, 41, 42
Selective serotonin reuptake inhibitors (SSRIs)
5-hydroxytryptamine (5-HT), 155
prolactin levels, 231
sexual dysfunctions, 154–155, 240–241
Selenium, 72–75
Semen
alcohol consumption, 86
BMI, 34
cell phone exposure, 168
cryopreservation, 243
DNA damage, 168
EBV, 134
folic acid, 68
hormonal serum levels, 87
leukocyte concentration, 6
lycopene, 70
pregnant women, 85
SE, 56
seasonal fluctuation, 6
seminiferous tubules, 86
sexual dysfunction, 86
spermatogenesis and sperm output, 53

Semen (*cont.*)
  sperm count, 2
  testicular dysgenesis syndrome, 8
  toxic effects and hormonal disruption, 2
  zinc, 74
Semen analysis (SA)
  cobalamin (vitamin B12), 67
  L-arginine, 66
  lycopene, 69–70
  selenium, 72
  sperm parameters, 108
  U. urealyticum, 133
Semenogelin-1, 40, 42
Semen quality. *See also* Semen
  cell phone radiation
    animal, 167
    human, 165–166
  diet and obesity, 63
  HIV infection, 134
Semen quality decline, 181, 187
Seminal plasma
  cadmium, 186
  CoQ10, 68
  infertile men, 96
  NO, 150
  proteins, 40
  and sex glands, 21–22
  and spermatozoa, 61, 149
Sex glands, 21–22
Sex-hormone-binding globulin (SHBG), 38, 40–42,
    56, 229
Sexually transmitted infections (STIs)
  ASA, 127, 128
  EBV, 134
  epididymitis and epididymo-orchitis, 131
  genitourinary, 132–134
  HIV, 134
  HPV, 135
  HSV, 134–135
  leukocytes, 130
  MAGI, 131–132
  male factor infertility, 127
  mechanisms, 127
  pathologic organisms, 128, 129
  spermatogenesis, 130
  spermatozoa, 128
  urethritis, 130–131
SHBG. *See* Sex-hormone-binding globulin (SHBG)
Sidestream smoke, 20
Sitting position
  chair types, 113
  insulating effect, 113
  poor ventilation, groin area, 112
  surfaces, 114
  wheelchairs, paraplegic men, 113
Smoking. *See* Cigarette smoking
SOD. *See* Superoxide dismutase (SOD)
Sperm
  apoptosis, 248
  count, 53

cryopreservation, 251
DNA fragmentation (*see* DNA fragmentation)
levels, diabetes, 251–252
morphology and weekly training volume, 53
motility, 54, 56
and non-sperm cell elements, 53
PAE, 250
parameters, 50
quality, 50, 53
Spermatogenesis
  AAS, 50
  alcohol consumption, 86–88, 90
  chromosomal abnormalities, 218
  data collection, 218, 220
  heat stress (*see* Scrotal heat stress)
  hypothalamus, 218
  IR doses, 220
  medical therapy (*see* Medications)
  meiosis, 218
  PAHs, 26–27
  ROS (*see* Reactive oxygen species (ROS))
  Sertoli cells, 219
Spermatozoa
  alcohol-induced alteration, 88
  chronic smokers, 20
  CK isoenzymes, 100
  cocaine, 98
  creatine and steroids, 100
  DNA-damage, 23, 47
  DNA fragmentation, 33
  dose-dependent effects, 86
  germinal epithelium, 8
  HIV, 134
  marijuana, 96
  MDMA, 97–98
  nicotine receptors, 20
  nonsmokers, 20
  nutrition and protection, 21
  OS, 22, 164
  ROS-induced damage, 25, 26
  and semen parameters, 85–87
  and seminal plasma, 61–62
  smokers, 21–22
  sophisticated biological process, 1
  sperm parameters, 147
  structure and proteins, 20–21
Sperm count
  adult EDC, 201
  AGD, 201
  bilateral cryptorchidism, 200
  BMI measurements, 33
  cervical penetration, 67
  cyclosporine, 233
  epididymal, 171
  estrogen hypothesis, 9
  hormonal effects, 233
  HSV, 135
  hypothalamic pituitary axis, 8
  meta-analysis, 4
  motility, 118

PCB concentration, 183
reproductive toxicity, 201–202
seeking infertility, 3
seminal parameter modi?cations, 6
seminal plasma, 68
sperm concentration, 3
testicular cancer, 10
Sperm DNA fragmentation
antioxidants, 168
clastogenic effects, 164, 168
histone kinase, 168
and oxidative stress, 164
ROS levels, 167
Sperm quality
chromosomal damage, 23
creatine kinase, 171
obesity, 42
and testicular heat stress (*see* Scrotal heat stress)
Spironolactone, 232, 239, 251
SSRIs. *See* Selective serotonin reuptake
inhibitors (SSRIs)
Steroids
AAS, 50
and creatine, 99–100
exogenous hormones, 229, 241
receptor pathways, 199
resistance exercise, 49
StAR, 37
STIs. *See* Sexually transmitted infections (STIs)
Submariners, 117
Sulfasalazine, 236
Superoxide dismutase (SOD)
and catalase, 153
copper-zinc, 26
CoQ10, 68
PUFAs, 71
and ROS, 22, 25
Suppressor of cytokine signaling 3 (SOCS-3)
pathway, 38, 42

T
TAC. *See* Total antioxidant capacity (TAC)
Tar, 19–20
TCAs. *See* Tricyclic antidepressants (TCAs)
Telomere, 250–251
Teratospermia, 132, 148, 232
Testes
AAS, 50
bone marrow transplantation and malignant
cells, 220
cannabinoids, 96
chronic ethanol administration, 85, 88
creatine and steroids, 100
germ cells, 220
lycopene, 69
methamphetamine and MDMA, 97
opioids, 96–97
PAE, 250
recovery period, spermatogenesis, 220

Sertoli cells, 9
UDT, 200–201
Testicular
antibiotics, 237
atrophy, 84, 85
calcium channel blockers, 237–238
chemotherapy, 234–235
colchicine, 237
IBD, 235–237
lipid peroxidation, 85, 88
mean testicular weight, 87
membranes, 85
polyenoic fatty acids and GSH, 88
spermatogenesis, 87
and testosterone, 90
toxin and chronic, 88
Testicular dysgenesis syndrome (TDS)
foetal development, 203
hypospadias, 200
TGCT, 203
Testicular germ cell tumors (TGCT), 183, 201, 203
Testicular thermoregulation
cremasteric and dartos muscles, 106
febrile episodes, 108
germ cell apoptosis, 106–107
homeothermic birds and mammals, 105
scrotum, 105–106
semen parameters, 108
spermatic cord, 106
varicocele and cryptorchidism, 109
Testosterone
cimetidine, 233
cyclosporine, 233
DHT, 100, 194
and estrogen, 34
and FSH, 37
FT/TT, 51, 55
ghrelin receptors, 37
gonadotropin, 232
ketoconazole, 232
and leptin, 37
LH secretion, 34
opioids, 96
protein synthesis and muscle growth, 50
resistance training, 50
and sexual function, 248–249
and SHBG, 40
spironolactone, 232
and steroidogenesis, 37
steroids, 99
TGCT. *See* Testicular germ cell tumors (TGCT)
THC. *See* Delta-9-tetrahydrocannabinol (THC)
TNF-α. *See* Tumor necrosis factor alpha (TNF-α)
Tobacco
chewing (smokeless), 23–24
prenatal tobacco exposure, 24
smoking, 20
Total antioxidant capacity (TAC), 64, 68, 70
Toxicity
alcohol-associated testicular, 85, 88

Toxicity (*cont.*)
  heavy metals (*see* Heavy metals)
  mitochondrial, 134
  thermal, 169–170
Training intensity, 49
Training load, 48, 51, 54
Training volume, 49–51, 53, 54
Treatment
  cancer, 220
  counseling, 154
  NG, 132
  opioids, 97
  psychological and behavioral therapy, 154
  radiation (*see* Radiation)
  SSRI medicines, 154–155
  vitamins C and E, 167–168
Tricyclic antidepressants (TCAs), 229, 231, 240
Tumor necrosis factor alpha (TNF-α)
  and IL-6, 32
  infliximab, 236

U
UDT. *See* Undescended testes (UDT)
UMI. *See* Unexplained male infertility (UMI)

Undescended testes (UDT), 10, 200–201
Unexplained male infertility (UMI), 161, 173, 211
Ureaplasma, 130, 133
Urethral stricture disease (USD), 131, 132
Urethritis, 130–131
USD. *See* Urethral stricture disease (USD)

V
Varicoceles
  cigarette smoking, 23
  scrotal temperature, 109
Vitamins
  cobalamin, 67–68
  vitamin A, 75
  vitamin C, 72–73
  vitamin D, 75
  vitamin E, 73–74

W
Waist-to-hip ratio (WHR), 32
Welders, 16

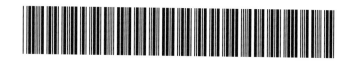